T0258425

Science on Stage

WRITING SCIENCE

EDITORS Timothy Lenoir and Hans Ulrich Gumbrecht

Science on Stage

EXPERT ADVICE AS
PUBLIC DRAMA

Stephen Hilgartner

STANFORD UNIVERSITY PRESS
STANFORD, CALIFORNIA

Stanford University Press
Stanford, California

© 2000 by the Board of Trustees of the
Leland Stanford Junior University

Assistance for the publication of this book
has been provided by the Hull Memorial
publication fund of Cornell University

Library of Congress Cataloging-in-Publication Data

Hilgartner, Stephen.
   Science on stage : expert advice as public drama /
   Stephen Hilgartner.
      p.   cm. — (Writing science)
   Includes blibliographical references and index.
   ISBN 0-8047-3645-6 (alk. paper) —
   ISBN 0-8047-3646-4 (pbk. : alk. paper)
   1. National Academy of Sciences (U.S.) 2. Science
   consultants — United States.   3. Science and
   state — United States.   I. Title.   II. Series.

Q127.U5 H55 2000
338.973'06—dc21   00-055706

To my mother

ACKNOWLEDGMENTS

All authorship has a collective dimension, and this book is no exception. Many people in many places have helped me in many ways, and without their assistance, I would have been unable to complete this work. Thanking them here is a pleasure and a privilege. It goes without saying — and yet must be said anyway — that none of them bears any responsibility for the remaining shortcomings of this book. I am deeply indebted to the scientists, Academy officials and staff, trade association executives, consumer advocates, and other participants in the debates examined in this book who talked with me, provided documents, and helped in many other ways. In particular, I thank the National Academy of Sciences, Dorothy Kamin, and Dr. Frank Press for granting me permission to quote and reprint material. The Hull Memorial publication fund of Cornell University awarded subvention funds to help offset the costs of producing this book, and I am pleased to acknowledge its contribution. Early versions of this work were presented in talks or seminars at Cornell University, the University of Illinois, Virginia Polytechnic Institute, and the Society for Social Studies of Science. These forums, among others, provided occasions for provocative questions and invaluable criticism, and I particularly thank Dick Bell, Geoffrey Bowker, Richard Burian, John Carson, Eileen Crist, Michael Dennis, Gary Downey, David Guston, Bruce Lewenstein, Michael Meyer, Andy Pickering, Trevor Pinch, and Leigh Star for helpful comments and interesting discussions.

I am especially grateful to my colleagues and friends who read and commented on various incarnations of the manuscript or parts of it. Their efforts made this a better book, and even when I did not follow their advice, I found their suggestions helpful and challenging. In this regard, I thank Fred Buttel, Peter Dear, Thomas F. Gieryn, Patrick Hamlett, Jim Hilgartner, and Michael Reich. I am particularly indebted to Michael Lynch and Judith Reppy, whose critical comments near the end of the project immeasurably improved this work. Timothy Lenoir, editor of the Writing Science series, was also an enormous help and I greatly appreciate his advice and enthusiasm. I want to spotlight the exceptional contributions of three people, who not only read and provided invaluable comments on the work presented in this book but have played significant roles in my broader scholarly development. Charles Bosk's ethnographic example inspired my sociological imagination, and he also helped me develop my interest in dramaturgy. Sheila Jasanoff profoundly influenced my scholarly sensibilities, and I thank her for her intellectual vision, demanding standards, and many forms of guidance. Dorothy Nelkin deserves special credit for helping me launch a career in science studies; she introduced me to STS, encouraged me to pursue my path, and helped me along the road in ways too varied and numerous to mention.

I am also grateful to my former colleagues at the Center for the Study of Society and Medicine at Columbia University—especially David J. Rothman, for seeing the possibilities. I also thank Sherry Brandt-Rauf, Stephanie Kiceluk, Nancy Lundebjerg, and Sheila Rothman for their encouragement and support. Martin Rivlin was a dedicated research assistant. My colleagues at the Department of Science and Technology Studies at Cornell deserve special thanks, not only for their advice and helpfulness, but also for creating the stimulating environment that has become my intellectual home. Debbie Van Galder, our administrative manager, has earned my heartfelt thanks in so many ways, and I greatly appreciate the assistance of the department's dedicated staff. At Stanford University Press, I thank Nathan MacBrien, my editor, for his expert guidance; Peter Dreyer, who copyedited the manuscript, for doing a splendid job; and Helen Tartar for her contributions earlier in the process. Sheila Jasanoff, Nathan MacBrien, and Peter Dear all played roles in the ongoing game of anagrams that ultimately produced the book's title.

My family also has earned my gratitude. I thank my mother and my father for their love and support. My mother, a connoisseur and writer of children's books, cultivated my appreciation of the wonders of the written text. My father's enthusiasm for science rubbed off on me at an early age. My brothers and sisters have celebrated and commiserated with me as needed. I am also grateful to Mel Schlank for all his endearing Mel-ness, and especially for the grandfatherly attentions he lovingly bestows on my children. Mrs. O. is sorely missed and her memory remains an inspiration to me.

I owe thanks of a special kind to Nathan and Kevin, whose magical imaginations bring me unparalleled joy, and to Erin, who, as this book took final form, began her human adventures by smiling benignly through engaging eyes.

Finally, I owe a special debt to Kate, who has shared in every stage of this work's evolution. Throughout, she provided valuable comments and steadfast support, exhibited patience and good humor, and remained tolerant of an often inhuman work schedule. I am grateful to her for all that and, now that this project is completed, for her unflagging enthusiasm for the new book that I am writing. Most of all, however, I thank her for the depth of her love and for the richness of our life together.

CONTENTS

TABLES AND FIGURES

Tables

Figures

Science on Stage

CHAPTER I

Introduction

Behind the headlines of our time stands an unobtrusive army of science advisors. Panels of scientific, medical, and engineering experts evaluate the safety of the food we eat, the drugs we take, and the cars we drive. Science advisors estimate the scope of global warming and investigate industrial accidents. They inspect weapons sites in far-off lands and analyze outbreaks of *E. coli*. They weigh the risks of mammograms and examine threats to computer security. They predict the course of the economy and set standards for highway design. They compare strategies for exploring Mars and assess the future of genetic engineering. In sum, they advise the government on nearly every area of policy, playing an indispensable role in the modern state. For this reason, it is important to understand how science advisors work to achieve credibility and defend themselves against critics who challenge their objectivity, expertise, or integrity.

This book examines struggles over the credibility of science advice, using a theoretical framework grounded in the metaphor of performance. The empirical focus of the study is the National Academy of Sciences (NAS), an influential advisor to the U.S. state. The NAS is an appropriate advisory body to examine, both as an example of a producer of authoritative advice and as an important institution, worthy of scholarly attention in its own right. Its prestige is unmatched by other advisory bodies in the United States today, and although the NAS is not a government agency, in many areas its recommendations carry a quasi-regulatory force. To explore how the credibility of NAS advice is produced, contested, and maintained, I concentrate on the debates surrounding three controversial NAS reports on diet and health. This research method permits a detailed comparative analysis, sensitive to nuances of meaning and the complexity of events. The three reports, and the NAS, are introduced below. First, however, it is necessary to elaborate the theoretical framework of the study and to pose its central questions.

Science advice is a ubiquitous source of authority in contemporary Western societies. In the United States, a variety of advisory bodies—including the expert committees established by federal agencies, the consensus conferences held by the National Institutes of Health (NIH), and the panels appointed by the NAS—channel advice into countless government decisions. Government officials rely on these sources of scientific and engineering knowledge to help make and justify a wide range of regulatory decisions.[1] Even more significantly, science advice shores up the legitimacy of state institutions by removing some issues from the domain of politics. Many contemporary public problems are complex "hybrids" of the scientific and the political. Science advice plays an important role in "purifying" these hybrid issues, separating them into "scientific" and "political" components, and thereby defusing some of their destabilizing tendencies.[2]

Yet even if mountains of evidence show that science advice enjoys enormous influence, equally strong data demonstrate that it no longer commands automatic respect. As Dorothy Nelkin has documented, the new social movements of the 1960s initiated unprecedented challenges to the "technical" decisions of experts.[3] Environmental and consumer activists today often demand extensive public participation in decisions about science and technology. Advocates of patients' rights challenge the scope of physician authority. Feminists argue that scientific institutions and knowledge display a masculine orientation. Religious groups object to developments in genetic engineering and reproductive technology. AIDS and breast cancer activists train "lay experts" of their own. These movements undercut the authority of expertise on many fronts, calling for greater citizen involvement in expert deliberations, questioning the objectivity of technical analyses, and, in a variety of policy disputes, charging that a veneer of scientific rationality masks the political nature of important societal decisions.[4]

Science advice, in this social context, is often developed on contested terrain. As Sheila Jasanoff has shown, the U.S. regulatory process—with its open, adversarial style of decision making—subjects science advice to relentless deconstruction.[5] For example, in debates over the environment, the combatants often highlight the contingent elements in opposing technical analyses, bringing into full view limitations in data, simplifying assumptions, and other sources of uncertainty. Policymakers thus find themselves facing a double bind: in a political culture that demands openness, they need to draw legitimacy from allowing technical arguments to unfold visibly, yet they must do so in situations where critics can easily take these arguments apart.[6]

Problems with the legitimacy of science advice are embedded in cultural trends that extend well beyond the regulatory arena. In the United States today, the claim that technical experts offer a value-laden vision has become a familiar idea—a cliché that stands in uneasy opposition to the even more commonplace notion that science-based expertise is universal and objective. To some extent, the spectacle of a steady stream of scientific controversies may have undermined confidence in the objectivity of science (at least in policymaking contexts)—as suggested by the courtroom image of scientific experts as "hired guns," or the by now tired joke that "for every expert there is an equal and opposite expert." But the deeper issues lie beyond a glib cynicism. More important are nagging questions about the nature of knowledge, about the politics of technology, and about the viability of democracy in a world where decisions with vast consequences involve the esoteric knowledge of technical elites.[7] Is scientific knowledge really neutral? Do technologies have politics built into their very design? When analyzing public policy, can matters of fact be convincingly separated from matters of value? If science does not simply reveal the facts of nature but is socially conditioned, then the very procedures for creating knowledge acquire political significance. The historians of science Steven Shapin and Simon Schaffer do not exaggerate when they write: "To entertain these doubts about our science is to question the constitution of our society."[8]

SCIENCE ADVICE AS PUBLIC DRAMA

In a polity that is familiar not only with the concept of objective science but also with the notion that expertise has a politics, the credibility of science advice will often be problematic. The ability to offer authoritative advice is obviously not an entitlement, automatically bestowed on any group that seeks it, but something that advisors must actively assert, cultivate, and guard—sometimes in the face of intense opposition.[9] How do advisory bodies lay claim to the cultural authority of science?[10] How do they cast themselves as trustworthy advisors? And how do they create credible voices for themselves?

The existing literature on science advice—which concentrates on the quantity and quality of advice, on the political dimensions of expertise, and on the interactions between advisors and agencies—pays scant attention to these questions.[11] Many observers argue that effective science advice stems from sound science and judicious expert deliberation.[12] Some analysts suggest that the successful advisor must strike a viable balance (given the particular institutional context) between neutrality and partisanship.[13] Others stress the importance of building strong relations between advisor and advisee, giving advisory bodies a clear mandate, providing adequate resources, and appointing effective committee chairs.[14] But pointing to these factors (no matter how significant they may be) does little to explain *in operational terms* precisely how advisory bodies achieve and defend their credibility. To a surprising degree, the social machinery used to produce, present, and defend science advice remains an unexamined "black box."[15]

The theoretical framework employed in this book—which treats expert advice as performance—provides a way to open the black box of advising, permitting a sociological investigation of the apparatus through which advisory bodies produce credibility. Through the metaphor of the theater, I analyze science advice as a form of drama, examining how it is produced, performed, and subjected to critique. From this viewpoint, an advisory body's reports and recommendations are performances; advisors are performers who display their work before audiences. Science advisors use a variety of dramatic techniques to create—or better, to *enact*—the basis of their authority as experts. Critics of advice are also performers who use theatrical techniques to challenge advice. Debates about advisory reports are theatrical contests. An advisory body's recommendations are artfully presented and intended to persuade. Likewise, public comments on science advice are stylized productions.

This analytic framework concentrates on how advisory bodies and their critics strategically present themselves in ways intended to foster favorable impressions in their audiences. These performers do not simply appear before audiences; they construct the personae they display, managing information and appearances in complex ways. Nor do events arrive ready-made on the public stage: the protagonists give them narrative structure, fitting them into stories and defining the identities of the characters. As they struggle to frame the "same" events, competing performers respond to, and even preempt, opposing stories. At the beginning of the show, the identities of the characters, their interests, and the meaning of the action are not firmly established, although these entities tend to solidify as the plot thickens. Collective judgments about who should be considered credible emerge through interactive "theater," as performers act and audiences react, sometimes quite unpredictably.

This perspective offers distinct advantages over the more traditional frameworks found in previous studies of science advice, most of which analyze interest-group bargaining and bureaucratic politics in fairly conventional ways.[16] The theatrical metaphor highlights a number of issues that receive only peripheral attention in the existing literature and provides a framework for systematically examining the "apparatus" that advisors use to underwrite their authority. In particular, with its focus on how science advisors present themselves to audiences, the theatrical perspective offers a means to examine how credibility is produced in social action, rather than treating it as a preexisting property of an advisory body. It also fits neatly with a world in which debates about expert advice are often played out in the mass media, and is well suited to analyzing debates in which the identities of the actors are among the central issues at stake. Finally, and most important, this viewpoint illuminates the significant role that stage management—that is, techniques for controlling what is publicly displayed and what is concealed—plays in constituting expert authority.

The Metaphor of Performance

The dramaturgical perspective on society, especially as expressed in the work of Erving Goffman, provides theoretical inspiration for my approach.[17] Goffman uses the metaphor of the theater to examine how individuals present themselves in everyday interaction and how audiences appreciate them. Marshaling a variety of ethnographic materials, he analyzes individuals as *performers* who engage in selective self-revelation and concealment to project a *character* (typically one with admirable traits) by fostering the desired appearances. Performers manage the impressions they create, tailoring their performances to particular situations and presenting different "selves" depending on the circumstances. He explores the many techniques of "information control" (that is, means for managing what audiences are capable of perceiving) that people deploy to create and sustain favorable impressions, casting themselves in particular roles and defining the nature of the occasion.[18] Goffman's point is not simply that the sociologist who observes an interaction can analyze it as if it were a drama; his point is rather that the participants in social interactions experience an active, theatrical self-consciousness.[19] They are well aware that their actions create impressions, and—like actors onstage—use a range of dramatic devices to create and maintain appearances.

But while performers may intend to control the perceptions of audiences, they can only do so imperfectly. The performances of everyday life, like Broadway plays, can fall flat. The observers of a person's act may conclude that he or she is merely going through the motions or playing a part. Indeed, all performances are in principle susceptible to being discredited, and circumstances that the performer would rather conceal often leak out and compromise the show. An unsteady gaze may suggest that a person is carefully editing what is being said rather than speaking freely. A jittery voice may reveal a performer to be less poised than he or she would have others believe. Ultimately, the audience builds impressions using not only what performers intentionally display but also what they unintentionally communicate.[20]

The notion of performance offers an apt metaphor for analyzing the production of science advice. To win the confidence of their audiences, advisory bodies actively display their competence and credibility. They present themselves as knowledgeable and trustworthy. They comport themselves in ways that exhibit their integrity and good judgment. The science advisor thus does not merely offer recommendations but also conveys an impression of the advisory body's *character*—in both the literary and moral senses of that term. An expert committee, for example, not only provides advice but also explains, in direct and indirect ways, who it is and why it should be believed. Self-presentation is central to the science advisor's work.

Theatrical metaphors also help address the reception of advice. After an advisory body publishes recommendations, audiences react to them—sometimes quite vigorously. But in a sense, interactions between advisors and their audiences begin long before publication. Advisors, like all performers, envision the audience their work will eventually encounter and, at least to some extent, tailor their presentations accordingly. Because advisors "respond" in advance to imagined audiences, the production and reception of science advice cannot be completely disentangled.

When advisors present recommendations, much of the audience remains in the role of observer, keeping any reaction to the show private. Often, however, some members of the audience, especially those with a professional connection to the issue at hand, publicly evaluate reports. The goals of these commentators—as critics, interpreters, or supporters of advice—may differ greatly, but they all work to package their ideas for public display, sometimes in sophisticated and self-conscious ways. Indeed, because Washington, D.C., is densely populated with public relations operatives, media consultants, and political professionals, the actors who comment on science advice are often skilled manipulators of the theatrical dimensions of politics. As in some participatory forms of theater, these vocal members of the audience stop being mere spectators and become another set of performers, who (like advisors) also face the challenges of assuming creditable characters and presenting credible messages. Public debates over science advice are therefore theatrical contests in which the protagonists perform opposing dramas before audiences that include (but are not limited to) one another.

My analysis explores how the protagonists in these theatrical contests work to create persuasive performances, exploring the art and artifice they employ to foster impressions and shape the experience of their audiences. Scientists, as we know from numerous contemporary and historical studies of laboratory practices, employ a wide variety of tools and techniques to produce knowledge.[21] But the tools that science advisors use to produce authoritative advice have been much less thoroughly studied. The analysis developed below examines the techniques, props, and procedures that advisors deploy to build credibility, paying special attention to self-presentation and "information control."

Persuasive Rhetoric

Among the most important means that advisors use to persuade audiences of their credibility are rhetorical and narrative techniques. A variety of studies of scientific writing and speech have explored how scientific texts function as rhetorical devices aimed at persuading audiences to reach particular conclusions.[22] Like all persuasive texts, scientific ones apply many familiar rhetorical techniques, such as anticipating the reader's objections and trying to demolish them in advance.[23] The framing of problems, the presentation of evidence, and the basic structure of the text are intended to direct the reader down specific logical channels, while blocking off others.[24] In particular, Bruno Latour argues, the persuasive force of scientific texts lies in the extensive network of "allies" that scientists recruit from such places as the technical literature (through citations) and from "inscriptions" (e.g., data, charts, graphs) produced in laboratories.[25] By mobilizing and disciplining these allies, an author can tie his or her paper to many sources of support, which collectively serve to bolster its claims.

The advisory report, as a genre of scientific literature, is no exception. Advisors use a variety of rhetorical devices to mobilize support from the literature and package advice persuasively. This study builds on existing work on scientific rhetoric to analyze the literary structure of the advisor's performances, examining how reports are narrated, the rhetorical devices that they use, and the narrative techniques that they employ to define the story, present the characters, and control the plot.

In the advising context, one particularly important form of rhetorical struggle concerns efforts to define the "contested boundary" that separates "science" from "policy."[26] These boundary-drawing struggles—examples of what Thomas F. Gieryn terms "boundary work"—are consequential, because whether a question is classified as "scientific" or "political" shapes judgments about who should resolve it.[27] The authority of science advisors stems from their status as representatives of science, yet many of their activities can easily be interpreted as policymaking. To be effective, as Jasanoff has shown, advisory bodies must engage in successful boundary work, securing their legitimacy and resisting efforts to portray them as having overstepped their proper authority. In other words, the legitimacy of advisory bodies depends on persuading their audiences, not only to accept their knowledge claims and recommendations, but also to accept the rhetoric they use to define the boundary that separates science from policy.[28]

Just as scientific writing uses rhetorical techniques, a variety of scientific procedures have performative dimensions. In their study of the emergence of a culture of experiment in seventeenth-century England, Shapin and Schaffer contend that Robert Boyle's procedures for practicing experimental science served performative ends. Boyle's techniques for conducting experiments and making the laboratory into a "public space" were not simply methods for investigating nature; they were also a means of policing the production of knowledge, of making experiment into a collective act, and of assuring the community that the experiments had been properly performed.[29] Similarly, statistical analysis—a routine procedure in many areas of science—often serves important rhetorical functions. Theodore M. Porter argues that quantitative analysis does not simply reflect the technical requirements for investigating complex subjects; it also provides a means of fortifying claims against charges of subjectivity. Because quantification imposes rigid, algorithmic rules that everyone must follow, it creates a form of "mechanical objectivity": not necessarily by ensuring a perfect match between nature and numbers, but by reducing individual discretion and holding researchers to a consistent and observable standard. Indeed, Porter contends, it is precisely in controversial areas with many actors and high stakes that mechanical objectivity, grounded in the impartiality of rigid procedures, becomes an especially useful means of underwriting knowledge.[30] Quantitative methods are "technologies of trust"—mechanisms that help to secure the assent of skeptics and bind communities together.[31]

These observations suggest that the procedures advisory bodies use to produce advice may serve rhetorical functions. Preparing science advice is a complex enterprise, entailing such activities as constituting panels of experts, reviewing literatures, developing recommendations, and subjecting drafts to review. How do advisory bodies describe the procedures that they use to develop advice? Does a rhetoric of procedures play a significant role in building the credibility of advice?

Stage Management

We have every reason to expect that many forms of rhetoric and narrative are central to the means advisors use to assert their credibility. But the metaphor of the text, which lies at the core of rhetorical analysis, carries implications that differ from those implied by the metaphor of the stage, which stands at the heart of dramaturgy. Indeed, the theatrical metaphor casts a spotlight on a number of questions that rhetorical analysis often leaves waiting in the wings. In particular, a dramaturgical perspective calls attention to the dialectic of self-revelation and concealment through which advisors present themselves. Put otherwise, it focuses attention not only on the rhetoric and narrative of the performance itself but also on the way performance expresses — and is embedded in — modes of information control.

Consider Goffman's provocative concept of "region behavior."[32] In the theater, performers work hard to maintain a division between the "backstage" (which is carefully concealed from the audience) and the "front stage" (which is deliberately displayed). Indeed, the typical play uses a variety of machinery—scaffolding, sets, lighting, costumes—to create and sustain this separation. Controlling what the audience sees is fundamental to successful drama. The most profound tragedy becomes a farce if the audience grows too aware of the world behind the curtain. (In one ill-fated performance of Shakespeare's most famous tragedy, the lights are said to have accidentally come on, revealing the ghost of Hamlet's father to be roller-skating about the stage.)[33] Analogous staging techniques, Goffman argues, are ubiquitous in everyday life. For example, restaurants and hotels, like other establishments where a staff presents a performance to a clientele, divide physical space into regions: a "front stage" where the performance takes place and a "backstage" where the performers prepare the show. Typically, the audience is not allowed to observe the backstage; restaurants—especially posh ones—seldom encourage their customers to inspect the kitchen. A white-linen, black-tie performance might be spoiled if patrons watched the staff clean their fish or learned how the waiters refer to them behind the double doors.

Just as social establishments partition physical space into regions, the participants in interpersonal encounters attempt to separate their activities into front- and backstage. Through the strategic use of words, gestures, facial expressions, clothing, posture, and countless other devices, people attempt to highlight their creditable attributes, while artfully drawing attention away from stigmatizing characteristics. But these elaborate techniques of information control do not always operate according to plan. Performers may attempt to manage the stage tightly, but audiences often observe much that the performer might not have meant to communicate, and discrediting impressions often escape from the backstage.[34]

These distinctively dramaturgical observations help bring into focus the techniques of stage management that science advisors use to display and mask various aspects of the process of preparing advice. What do science advisors publicly present and what do they relegate to the backstage? How do they create divisions between backstage and front stage, and how do these divisions contribute to creating credibility? How well does stage management function, and what happens when it breaks down?

Another useful concept is Goffman's notion of "dramaturgical cooperation"—collective work to stage a performance. In many contexts, social actors collaborate to create impressions, forming what Goffman calls a "team." On Broadway, a team consists of an assortment of actors, set designers, directors, stagehands, and others who work to help the audience suspend disbelief. Similarly, at a memorial service, the gathering mourners may constitute a team, supported by the funeral home staff and the clergy, that silently conspires to overlook any awkward facts about the deceased. At a school play, the gathered parents—ostensibly the audience—become a team of performers when they wink, applaud, and enthusiastically forgive glaring flaws in the production. For Goffman, teams are social groups whose members are defined, not with respect to formal organizational structures, but by virtue of their engagement in mutual cooperation to manage impressions.[35]

Extending this concept to science advice, we can see that the teams that produce advisory reports include a number of actors, such as the staff members and the individuals who serve on expert panels. Thus, it is important to consider the kinds of dramaturgical cooperation in which team members engage and to examine how advisory bodies orchestrate it. How, for example, are novice team members introduced to the characters that they are supposed to play? Moreover, because perfect cooperation is unattainable, it is important to explore what happens when conflicts develop. When dramaturgical cooperation is compromised, what effect does this have on the performance? What happens to science advice when dramaturgical cooperation breaks down?

Identity and Interests

In preparing advice, an advisory body does more than simply review scientific evidence and develop recommendations; it also presents—even creates—itself as a character. It must form some sort of collective understanding of itself, define its role and perspective, and constitute its public persona. Because its credibility hinges on convincing audiences that it is trustworthy and knowledgeable, a team has every incentive to enact an identity that possesses these characteristics. Dramaturgical analysis can tease apart the techniques through which teams strategically present the character of the advisor. Similarly, examining performance can show us precisely how critics seek to discredit that character.

This emphasis on strategies for shaping appearances does not rest on the assumption that science advisors (or their critics) are fundamentally cynical performers who—like con men or impostors—knowingly seek to project false identities. For Goffman, individuals do not possess a single true self, but exhibit multiple identities that emerge in different situations; the self is not a psychological state but a social phenomenon created through interaction.[36] In a short space of time, a man may find himself playing the roles of husband, father, salesman, sports fan, and customer at a convenience store. He may present himself as macho at one moment and sensitive at the next. But such variation need not be understood as a contrast between the "real person" and the "mask." Instead, such conflicting images of the self reflect the ways in which people have a multiplicity of identities, expressed in ongoing practices of speech and comportment. People enact their identities, actively creating the "selves" that they display.[37] Although we may judge some of these performances to be honest and others to be false, from a dramaturgical perspective the key point is not this difference but their similarity. As Goffman puts it:

> Whether an honest performer wishes to convey the truth or whether a dishonest performer wishes to convey a falsehood, both must take care to enliven their performances with appropriate expressions, exclude from their performances expressions that might discredit the impression being fostered, and take care lest the audience impute unintended meanings.[38]

Performers typically seek to display themselves in ways that make them appear to conform to the "identity norms" befitting a person of their status given the nature of the occasion.[39] Sometimes these self-presentations are frankly deceptive, and sometimes they are wholly honest. At times, people feel fully justified in misrepresenting themselves, and at other times, they are unwilling to project an identity that sharply contradicts their own sense of self. Indeed, performers often experience a profound need to *be* a certain kind of character, such as a good scientist or a public servant, and to act in keeping with this role even when no one else is watching. But the poles of sincerity and cynicism are not the only possibilities; performers vary in the extent to which they are, as Goffman puts it, "taken in by their own act."[40] In a reciprocal way, audiences express a range of responses to the possibility of being "taken in"—sometimes tactfully suspending disbelief in the identity the performer projects and sometimes warily searching for signs that they are being intentionally or unintentionally misled.

In the world of science advice, one of the central identity norms concerns the objectivity (in the sense of disinterestedness) with which advisory bodies approach their charge. Thus, as we shall see in detail below, advisors work hard to enact objectivity, sharply separating themselves from "vested interests" that might seek to influence their advice. Critics of advice, for their part, often attribute interests to the advisor, charging that the impression of objectivity is merely a mask. Much of the drama surrounding science advice consists of efforts to expose, disclaim, or disavow putative interests, as competing performers present conflicting assessments of the character of the advisor. Judgments about the credibility of advice thus cannot be separated from moral judgments about the people and institutions that produce it.[41] When controversies flare, claims of expertise, integrity, and disinterestedness battle against accusations of incompetence, dishonesty, and bias, in a war of dramatic narratives, as competing performers fit events into stylized plots that allocate blame and suggest ways to restore social order.

A dramaturgical framework is well equipped to examine the structure, operation, and consequences of the morality plays that surround science advice.[42] But, as the above discussion suggests, the analyst need not attempt to settle questions about the identities and motives of the actors permanently. Most of the time, inherent ambiguities require us to leave these questions open. On some occasions, however, it is useful (following Brian Wynne) to make the "first order approximation" that actors possess identifiable interests that one can treat as stable for a defined period of time.[43] In this spirit, I shall make the crucial assumption that established advisory bodies have a broad interest in maintaining their credibility and influence, and that this represents an important institutional goal. In addition, at a few points in the argument, I shall introduce assumptions about the goals of some critics of advisory reports.

Information Control and Written Documents

Goffman's theoretical framework was designed for (and has largely been applied to) the analysis of interactions among individuals during face-to-face encounters—a context that may seem far removed from the written reports that are the centerpieces of much science advice. Accordingly, it is necessary to elaborate more fully on how a dramaturgical perspective can be employed in the analysis of scientific advisory reports and other written documents.

Goffman has had relatively little influence in social studies of science, but his perspective is clearly applicable to situations, such as courtrooms or congressional hearings, in which individual scientific or technical experts perform in face-to-face encounters.[44] In court, the expert witness becomes a performer attempting to inspire the jury's confidence. The words he speaks and facial expressions he displays, the explanations he gives of laboratory techniques, the visual displays he uses to train the jury to see things "through" his professionally informed eyes—these form the core of his performance, a show that the opposing attorney (also a performer) attempts to disrupt through the ritualized interrogation of courtroom Q and A.[45] In such settings, expertise is quite literally *embodied* in the person of the expert witness, so Goffman's analysis of interpersonal encounters is well suited to examining how these performers and their audiences interact.[46] But it may be less obvious how dramaturgy is relevant to advice produced by committees, rather than individuals, and presented mainly in written reports, not face-to-face interaction. For this reason, developing a dramaturgical analysis of science advice involves adjusting Goffman's perspective to make it suitable for analyzing written documents and the collective modes of information control that permeate and surround them.

The first step in bringing a dramaturgical approach to the analysis of scientific writing is to recognize that Goffman's most general observations about performances also apply to written documents such as the advisory reports that concern us here. Face-to-face interactions, in which performers rely mainly on speech and the idiom of bodily appearances and gestures to present themselves, differ from written texts in many ways, but they share fundamental structural features that arise in all performance.[47] Viewed dramaturgically, the written document becomes a device for self-presentation that the performer uses to project his or her "voice" and create the desired impression on the audience: the production, editing, and presentation of written texts become means of impression management; the strategic control of information becomes a central feature of the activity of writing; and the written document, like the verbal and bodily displays that constitute interpersonal encounters, becomes a potentially discreditable performance.

But if written documents and face-to-face interactions can both be regarded as performance, they must also be understood as performances of different kinds. The technology of writing offers performers and audiences alike a different mix of opportunities and constraints than is available in interpersonal encounters. For one thing, the linguistic and material form of written documents creates performative possibilities different from those afforded by talk and bodily display. Moreover, because writers and readers rarely occupy the same physical and temporal location, their "encounters" have a virtual character that lacks the immediacy and directness of interpersonal interaction. Thus, in written performance the performer cannot monitor the audience's response during the show, making real-time adjustments as things unfold. Nor can the audience draw on many of the cues, such as facial expressions or faltering speech, that are crucial sources of information in interpersonal settings. Audiences may deem the writer to be insincere, stupid, or hostile, but they cannot base such judgments on shifty eyes, a bovine stare, or a surly tone of voice.

These differences suggest that the task of preparing and displaying written performances involves a particular set of practices and problems. For example, the physical separation of writer and reader allows the performer the luxury of deliberately and repeatedly revising a written performance in ways that are impossible during face-to-face encounters, which can be prepared for and even rehearsed in advance, but must be delivered in real time. Similarly, the relative permanence of written performances (when compared to verbal ones) creates its own problems of information control.[48] Written texts, like other performances, are intended for certain audiences, and all manner of trouble may ensue if they fall into the wrong hands. The author of a passionate love letter (usually) prepares it for a single, special person, and the exclusive nature of the audience is typically a central theme of the genre. This theme is expressed, not only in the text of the letter, but also in how access to it is handled: the authors and recipients of extremely personal letters tend to restrict their distribution, blocking the vision of unwanted readers with opaque envelopes and other technologies of privacy.[49] Even so, the material form of the letter leaves open the potential for embarrassing revelations — owing, say, to a breach in security or a conflict between the couple.

As this example suggests, a dramaturgical perspective on written documents entails examining the complex manner in which they internally encode — and the same time are embedded in — collective modes of information control. Documents may be implicated in efforts to control impressions on several intertwined levels: performers actively reveal some information to their intended audience by displaying it in written text; they actively conceal other information from the intended audience by omitting it from the text; and they create nonaudiences by restricting access to the document, preventing unwanted persons from reading it at all. Thus, the text of a love letter might strategically manage information by employing language that presents a self that is passionately "in love" with the recipient, while simultaneously avoiding topics (such as the past recipients of similarly phrased letters) that might weaken the performance. At the same time, one might expect the couple to employ various information-control practices to protect the letter — possibly imperfectly — from leaks or snooping.

The misadventures of intimate communications have inspired countless novelists and playwrights, and the declaration of passion that reaches the wrong person is a well-worn feature of the bedroom farce. But problems of information control are by no means confined to the context of the couple; they are also important to the life of much larger, more formal organizations, which often develop extensive procedures for managing what documents reveal and conceal and to whom they are (and are not) made available. Indeed, forms of "region behavior" are inscribed directly into the written texts that organizations produce and the practices that govern their disposition. Bureaucracies—well known for their elaborate external and internal boundaries—typically segregate audiences and separate information into multiple regions, carefully controlling access to written materials. Some documents form the centerpieces of public performances and are dramatically unveiled at news conferences. Others are prepared with the understanding that they will remain backstage, and they are contained through informal practices or formal rules of confidentiality.[50] Some documents are filed; some are shredded; and some especially sensitive things are never written down.[51]

Like rhetoric and narrative, the practices that selectively grant access to an organization's filing cabinets, computerized records, and official pronouncements play an important role in impression management. But the official regimes of information control that organizations attempt to establish function only imperfectly; public relations operatives and information officers may seek to manage the messages and impressions that emanate from their organizations, but accidental and intentional "leakage" of information is ubiquitous. As the recent history of the U.S. presidency demonstrates with a particular vengeance, the participants in the struggles that surround and permeate organizations may strategically leak confidential documents, bringing fragments of information from the "backstage" to the "front stage"—often with great dramatic effect.[52] The division between backstage and front stage, thus, is not a firmly fixed feature of organizational life but a contestable and flexible boundary that is continually being (re)constructed as competing performers actively work to "backstage" some bits of information, while "front-staging" others.

As the above discussion suggests, a dramaturgical perspective on written documents entails examining the ways in which they express collective modes of information control. In this context, the concept of information control refers both to what is contained in the text and to what is absent from it. The concept also includes the performer's efforts to control who gets access to the document. Viewed in this light, written texts become not only carriers of meaning but also means of social organization implicated in effecting divisions between performers and audiences and structuring the relations among them. In short, written texts emerge as devices that performers—whether individuals or organizations—incorporate into their ongoing efforts to manage the stage and to shape what audiences perceive.

By highlighting stagecraft and information management, the dramaturgical approach advocated here provides a fresh look at scientific writing. From this perspective, scientific texts emerge, not just as semiotic assemblages, rhetorical constructions, or forms of discourse, but also as crucial parts of systems for organizing and controlling the enclosure and disclosure of information. The differences between formal scientific texts and the activities required to produce them are well known in science studies: scientists tinker in the privacy of the laboratory until they are ready to "go public" with neatly packaged results; their published work systematically elides the contingencies of actual research; and at times, they even stage spectacular public demonstrations, displaying results dramatically and visually in a carefully arranged "theater of proof."[53] Scientific texts conceal the history of their own production, but they do so neither automatically nor in a single, uniform way. The dramaturgical perspective calls attention to systems of stage management and the role of various modes of information control in creating authorized voices, authoritative knowledge, and credible science advice.

Experts perform in many different contexts, and many local features of particular situations shape the enclosure and disclosure of information. For example, documents produced in the context of committee investigations are, generally speaking, more susceptible to leakage than are those prepared by individuals or small, homogeneous groups.[54] Similarly, an oral briefing offers an audience opportunities for engaging with expertise that little resemble those afforded by a written report, which arrives on the desk neatly typeset and bound, or by a televised hearing, which—through its audiovisual richness—provides observers with an illusory sense of having experienced the action in an unmediated way.[55] The variety of performative contexts cannot be captured in a simple typology, but it is clear that countless local details structure the extent to which performers can guide the perceptions of audiences down prefigured pathways, enforce dramaturgical cooperation, and control what appears onstage. Local details also shape opportunities for dissident team members to subvert the official show, and influence the possibilities for audience participation.

The dramaturgical perspective offers a framework for empirically investigating struggles over the enclosure and disclosure of information. The terms *information enclosure* and *disclosure*, so central to this approach, resonate linguistically with one of the most important concepts in contemporary science and technology studies: *closure*, a word used to refer to the stabilization of knowledge claims or technological artifacts.[56] The connection among these terms, however, is not merely a matter of shared linguistic roots; struggles to control access to information are an integral part of struggles over the creation of knowledge. In contemporary science and technology, especially in areas of political and economic importance, maneuvering that shapes the social, temporal, and spatial availability of information plays a central role in reaching closure and reopening issues. Systems of stage management are key technologies for making credible knowledge, and the dramaturgical perspective is well suited to examining how these systems operate, what they achieve, and under what circumstances they break down. These phenomena will be explored through the analysis of the National Academy of Sciences and its controversial reports on diet and health.

THE ACADEMY COMPLEX

Owing to its prestige and prominence, the National Academy of Sciences offers an excellent focus for a study of the authority of expert advice. Several interlocking organizations make up what is known as the Academy complex: the National Academy of Sciences, the National Academy of Engineering, the National Research Council (the operating arm of the two Academies), and the Institute of Medicine. The organization that evolved into the present Academy complex—a sizable operation with about 1,200 staff members—was founded in 1863. Created by an act of Congress, the National Academy of Sciences is a private, nonprofit honorary society of members elected by their peers. Each year, individuals who have made outstanding contributions to science are honored with Academy membership, one of highest forms of recognition bestowed on American scientists.[57] Over the years, the NAS has expanded, growing into the four organizations that now comprise the Academy complex. The National Research Council (NRC) was founded in 1916 as the operating arm of the NAS. The Academy's charter was modified in 1964 to create a parallel National Academy of Engineering, which honors outstanding engineers. The Institute of Medicine, an honorary society for eminent members of the health professions, was established in 1970. At present, the NAS and NAE each have about 1,800 members, while the IOM has about 600. These scientists, engineers, and health professionals constitute the "honorary apex" of American science.[58] Following common practice, I shall use the terms *the Academy* or *the NAS* more or less interchangeably to refer to the entire Academy complex, unless otherwise noted. (In keeping with this practice, the references use "National Academy of Sciences" as the author of all Academy complex reports, brochures, and other publications.)

The Academy occupies a curious position on the boundary that separates public from private institutions. It is not a federal agency but a private organization, so it therefore is not subject to federal oversight and does not receive direct appropriations from the public purse. Most of its revenues come from government grants and contracts awarded to fund specific projects (see Table 1). Yet, during the half-century since World War II, especially since the 1960s, the Academy has served as an important actor in the U.S. state, and it is generally considered a "quasi-official organization." Its congressional charter explicitly directs it to provide advice on scientific matters to the U.S. government. (It also advises state and local governments.) To this end, the Academy's expert committees currently produce some 300 reports per year, channeling valuable expertise into virtually every conceivable area of policy. Its reports address a stunning diversity of topics, covering everything from arms control to genetic testing, immigration, beach erosion, sexually transmitted disease, computer privacy, and the radiation risks of interplanetary travel. Most Academy reports are received without incident, often making notable yet quiet contributions to policy and sometimes being politely ignored. But on occasion—as in the case of diet and health—NAS reports become the subject of bitter debates that expand into conflicts about the credibility of the Academy itself.

How Academy advice fits into governmental decision making varies with the substantive area, but it enjoys considerable influence. Public policy benefits enormously from its advice on important matters concerning international security, transportation, space, health, and the environment. Its

TABLE I
Academy Reports by Topic Area, January 1993–June 1997

Report topic area	Number of reports issued	% of total reports issued
International affairs	45	3.4%
Education	52	3.9
Defense and space	79	5.9
Natural resources/environment	116	8.7
Industry, commerce, technology	127	9.5
Scientific enterprise	154	11.6
Health and safety	234	17.6
Transportation	524	39.4
TOTAL	1,331	100.0%

SOURCE: U.S. General Accounting Office, 1998, p. 4.

NOTE: During this period, the Academy's annual budget averaged about $150 million. Work for the federal government provided about 87% of this revenue and the Academy complex produced an average of about 300 reports per year.

most successful reports play a major role in framing policy problems and building consensus behind new initiatives. Even in the midst of controversies, where science advice might be expected to have little impact, the Academy often makes its presence felt. In fact, many of its standing committees and boards perform what very nearly amount to regulatory functions. The Food and Nutrition Board (FNB), a standing NAS committee that presided over two of the reports examined below, is a case in point. Since 1941, the board has set nutritional standards, such as the Recommended Dietary Allowances (RDAs), exerting a powerful influence on the U.S. food system. The RDAs, originally intended for planning wartime food production, later achieved many other uses. They now appear on food labels, and government agencies use them to shape food-assistance programs and plan diets for institutionalized populations. Nonprofit organizations also deploy the RDAs to guide nutrition research and education, and food manufacturers use them to develop and market new products.[59]

Academy reports vary widely in size and scope, ranging, as one NAS publication explains, "from a brief document on a narrowly defined, highly technical problem to a comprehensive review of an important public-policy issue."[60] Government agencies and private foundations commission the vast majority of the Academy's reports, although at times it chooses to fund studies using its own endowment. The "consensus report"—which surveys scientific knowledge about a subject and offers recommendations—is the most common type of Academy study. Each consensus report is prepared by an expert panel, expressly convened for that purpose. These expert committees do not perform new research, but review the literature, hold workshops and symposia, and consult with relevant specialists. The Academy instructs its committees to strive to reach unanimous agreement on their findings and recommendations.[61]

A Reputation for Excellence

The Academy enjoys a long-standing reputation for expertise and objectivity. Its standing compares favorably with other centralized sources of expert advice, including the White House Office of Science and Technology Policy, private think tanks such as the RAND Corporation, and the Office of Technology Assessment (OTA)—a congressional research agency that the Republicans summarily eliminated after winning control of the legislative branch in 1994.[62] Even in today's climate of mistrust in government and declining confidence in U.S. institutions, the Academy is highly regarded. It remains a trusted institution in distrustful times.

The Academy's science advice gains considerable prestige from its association with the elected memberships of the NAS, NAE, and IOM. However, members of the honorary societies play a limited role in preparing Academy advice. Some members occupy posts on the bodies that establish the Academy's overall policies and oversee its advising operations, such as its governing board, commissions, and divisions. Members also often participate on the committees that prepare reports, but there they are greatly outnumbered: the vast majority of the experts who serve on Academy panels come from the scientific community at large. (In fiscal year 1990, about 6 percent of the members of Academy committees were members of one of the honorary societies.)[63] In addition, Academy staff typically play a major (and sometimes central) role in preparing NRC reports. In essence, the Academy bureaucracy and the committees it appoints—not the members of the honorary societies—produce its science advice.

The Academy has developed extensive procedures for maintaining the quality and integrity of its advice and safeguarding its reputation for independence. These procedures (examined further in Chapter 2) are intended to guard against conflict of interest, to prevent the sponsors of studies from influencing conclusions, and to assure that qualified experts review all Academy reports prior to publication. Academy procedures also require confidentiality: committees are instructed to keep their deliberations, draft reports, and internal documents private. The Academy sees insulation from public scrutiny as a prerequisite for candid discussion among panel members and as a means of preventing government, industry, and private groups from pressuring committees to reach particular conclusions.[64]

Despite its reputation, the Academy has not been immune from criticism. In recent decades (especially during the 1970s), a number of observers have argued that the Academy too seldom produced reports of the highest quality, too rarely took the lead on important social problems, and too often succumbed to the influence of powerful interests in government and industry.[65] Not surprisingly, given the distrust with which experts are often viewed in American political culture, the Academy was also criticized for elitism, for failing to seek enough public input, and for lack of public accountability.[66]

The most detailed critique of the Academy appeared in *The Brain Bank of America*, a 1975 book by the science writer Phillip M. Boffey, commissioned by Ralph Nader's Center for Responsive Law.[67] Boffey's study scrutinized the Academy through the ideological lens of the consumer movement, focusing on public accountability. Arguing that the Academy had all too often fallen short of serving the public interest, he blamed its failings on its structural relationships with government agencies and industrial interests. Dependence on funding from such clients as the Department of Defense, for example, limited its ability to offer truly independent advice. Patterns of committee appointments only made matters worse. The Academy, Boffey argued, rarely named "activist boat-rockers" to advisory committees, and its expert panels underrepresented women, minorities, and the young.[68] The problem, according to Boffey, was not that committee members were swayed by direct, financial conflict of interest so much as that they were "influenced by the viewpoints of the institutions and professional worlds within which they routinely operate."[69] Similarly, Boffey contended, the Academy's commitment to the narrow interests of the scientific community tempered its dedication to the wider public. Boffey also faulted the Academy for lack of openness, arguing that its internal deliberations should be subject to public scrutiny.[70]

Boffey and other critics had a limited impact on the Academy's influence and activities, however, although the NAS did implement some significant reforms during the 1970s and 1980s. For example, it established an institutionwide oversight committee in 1970 to guide the review of all draft reports. Later that decade, Academy President Philip Handler introduced new procedures requiring committee members to disclose potential conflicts of interest. These measures represented minor adjustments, however, not the wholesale overhaul that the Academy's critics sought. Academy officials managed to defuse the potentially explosive charge that its advice systematically favored powerful interests, and the NAS retained its reputation for being an independent voice. The Academy also defeated efforts to open its decision-making process to public view. When critics sued for public access, the Academy successfully argued that a policy of openness would inhibit committees from conducting frank discussions and would subject them to outside pressures, thus compromising their objectivity. Until recently, the courts consistently supported the Academy's confidentiality procedures, holding that the Federal Advisory Committee Act (FACA) and the Freedom of Information Act did not apply to the NAS.[71]

New Uncertainties

Although the Academy's prominent position has proven resilient, recent developments have also shown that this status cannot be taken for granted. In January 1997, the U.S. Court of Appeals held that Academy committees that advise the federal government must comply with the Federal Advisory Committee Act. This dramatic decision threw the future of Academy procedures for preparing reports into doubt, for FACA requires advisory committees to open their meetings and documents to the public. In addition, federal officials would have to "sign off" on meeting agendas and even on the composition of committees, ending the Academy's ability to select its expert panels as it sees fit. Arguing that FACA strictures would fundamentally compromise the independence of its advice, the Academy appealed, but the U.S. Supreme Court allowed the circuit court ruling to stand. To the great relief of Academy officials, however, Congress passed a law in December 1997 that exempts the NAS from FACA. The new law allows confidentiality to continue and keeps committee composition squarely under Academy control, but it also calls for more transparency in institutional procedures than before.[72]

The Academy's legislative victory ended the immediate threat posed by the court decisions, but the broader meaning of the FACA episode remains unclear. Arguably, the Academy's success in Congress gave it an opportunity to consolidate its strength. But one might well wonder whether the court decisions are harbingers of an emerging uncertainty about the correct place of this institution, with its unique quasi-public status, in the policy process. A mood of uneasiness about the role of the Academy is also reflected in perceptions that the organization needs reform. A number of critics—connected both with the Academy and with federal agencies—contend that the NRC bureaucracy has grown bloated, and that its process for producing reports is often too slow and too expensive to serve a shrinking government.[73] Some are even asking whether the Academy in its current configuration remains capable of adequately representing a changing American society. Writing in *Science* in 1997, Andrew Lawler reported that some Academy observers believe that the status quo puts the NRC

> at risk of becoming an increasingly irrelevant think tank attached to a
> prestigious society made up primarily of elderly, white, and male scientists
> and engineers. "There was a time when that demographic group could speak
> with authority on anything," says one agency manager who deals with the
> [National Research] council. "But that is no longer the case." The challenge
> for NRC officials is finding a new voice to speak to a changing world.[74]

Such contentions surely overstate the risk of irrelevance, but they vividly capture a new sense of disquiet about the role of the Academy that has recently taken hold. At the close of the 1990s, the future of the Academy in the U.S. state seems less secure and more open to renegotiation than before, making this venerable institution a particularly ripe topic for analysis.[75]

For all of the reasons discussed above, the Academy offers an appropriate body for a study of the credibility of science advice. Its prestige and influence make understanding it especially important. Nevertheless, one must recognize that science advice varies greatly across nations and historical periods, and the Academy, as presently constituted, has unique institutional features and distinctly American qualities. As Jasanoff points out, U.S. policy culture is "open, adversarial, formal and legalistic," and American science advice reflects this fact; in contrast, for example, British advisory mechanisms, part of a much less open political culture, are "closed, cooperative, informal and consensual."[76] Even within the United States, science advice takes diverse institutional forms. The Academy differs greatly from such devices as the presidential commission, the advisory committees that serve federal agencies, the consensus conferences held by the National Institutes of Health, the variously structured panels and commissions that provide bioethical advice, private think tanks, and the late Office of Technology Assessment.[77] But despite the Academy's unique character, examining this institution can yield insights that are relevant to other advisory systems.

THE REPORTS ON DIET AND HEALTH

To analyze how the Academy works to construct credibility, this study focuses on three reports: *Toward Healthful Diets* (1980), *Diet, Nutrition, and Cancer* (1982), and the unpublished 1985 Draft of the Tenth Edition of the Recommended Dietary Allowances.[78] Each provoked strong reactions, both positive and negative, from scientific experts on nutrition and health.[79] Consider, for example, what several scientists had to say about *Diet, Nutrition, and Cancer*, a 478-page consensus report that reviewed the literature on the role of diet in causing cancer and presented a set of "interim dietary guidelines" for cancer prevention.[80]

> Bandaru S. Reddy of the American Health Foundation, a nonprofit organization dedicated to preventive medicine, called *Diet, Nutrition, and Cancer* "a comprehensive assessment and detailed appraisal of the current knowledge."[81]
>
> Robert E. Olson, one of the authors of *Toward Healthful Diets*, called *Diet, Nutrition, and Cancer* "a somewhat superficial and uncritical review of the scientific literature . . . followed by a series of [dietary] recommendations which, in fact, do not follow logically from a critical review."[82]
>
> Albert I. Mendeloff of the Johns Hopkins School of Medicine described the report as "a remarkably well written and clear summary of the epidemiologic, laboratory, and clinical evidence," although he did not endorse all of the committee's recommendations.[83]
>
> Milton L. Scott, Jacob Gould Schurman Professor Emeritus of Nutrition at Cornell University, said the report was a "lengthy, verbose and often contradictory tome," calling it "one of the most unscientific reports I have ever read."[84]

These conflicting assessments of the same document provide a succinct introduction to the challenge of constructing authoritative science advice about diet and health in the early 1980s. All three reports, as noted above, generated significant public controversies. In the case of the 1985 Draft of the Tenth Edition of the RDAs, debate within the Academy led its president, Frank Press, to take the extreme measure of halting publication, a move that amplified an already bitter dispute. Although *Toward Healthful Diets* and *Diet, Nutrition, and Cancer* were both successfully completed, each encountered hostile critics and generated unusually intense debate. Advocacy groups released rebuttals at news conferences. Congress held hearings. Federal agencies prepared official responses. Four U.S. senators and seven members of the House of Representatives asked the General Accounting Office to conduct an investigation. The protagonists in these debates charged each other with scientific incompetence, bias, and conflicts of interest. In all three cases, the disputes expanded beyond the reports themselves to encompass questions about the adequacy and integrity of NAS procedures for preparing reports, and, ultimately, to questions about the Academy's ability to provide objective, credible science advice.

As a methodological strategy, focusing on three reports has the advantage of permitting a detailed interpretive analysis. The debates surrounding these reports provide unusually good material for comparative analysis: they share subject matter and characters; they were all written within a five-year period; and they all met different fates—permitting systematic investigation of diverse outcomes. Moreover, the extensive controversies over these reports provide a rich source of data on how the credibility of expert advice is contested. Finally, because only a tiny minority of Academy reports (less than 1 percent) engender such extensive debate, these episodes cast problems of credibility into especially stark relief.[85]

Even so, this research strategy has limitations. I do not undertake a comprehensive survey of the Academy's advisory activities and make no pretense to statistical validity. In addition, the highly controversial nature of these reports might tempt some observers to dismiss my findings. How, they might ask, can such abnormal situations tell us anything about the routine operation of the Academy? If you want to understand the credibility of science advice, why concentrate on episodes in which its authority was relentlessly challenged? Why examine controversial reports rather than ordinary ones? These are reasonable questions. A long tradition of social research demonstrates, however, that studies of extreme situations are often deeply revealing about mundane events, because examining incidents that stretch or tear the social fabric exposes how it is woven together. In research on face-to-face interactions, looking at awkward moments illuminates smoother interpersonal encounters. Similarly, in science and technology studies, analyzing scientific controversies sheds light on the mechanisms that produce scientific agreement, and studying accidents displays with striking clarity the sociotechnical networks that underlie the everyday operation of technology.[86] From the perspective of this methodological tradition, the episodes surrounding the Academy's nutrition reports are excellent cases; not because they were typical but because they subjected the institution to extreme situations. Analyzing them offers an unusually good opportunity for examining how cultural authority is constructed and contested.

Nutrition Reform

Like most contemporary issues, the question of what people should eat in order to maintain good health cannot be neatly split into matters of "fact" and matters of "values." To ask, for example, whether the public should be told to eat low-fat foods inevitably brings up many additional questions. How strong is the evidence that fat is risky? According to whom? Do scientists agree about this issue, and, if not, which ones should be believed? More generally, how much evidence should be required before a knowledge claim can be considered a fact? When making health recommendations, how important are economic impacts and the pleasure of the palate? Should decision making in this area be managed by private nonprofit organizations and the market, or is government intervention required? These questions do not fit into the tidy dichotomy of facts versus values.[87] The question "What are the facts?" is entangled in questions about the criteria for determining facts, which in turn are connected to questions about who can be believed, which institutions are credible, what scientific methods are reliable, and how much evidence is needed to justify altering the status quo.

Controversy about nutrition promises to continue for the foreseeable future. To understand the disputes over the three Academy reports, however, one must consider the specific context of the diet and health debate in the 1970s and early 1980s. At that time, much more than today, people argued about the very idea of using dietary change to prevent chronic diseases, such as heart disease, hypertension, cancer, and diabetes. Claims about specific diet-disease relationships—such as the link between cholesterol and heart disease, or the cancer-preventing properties of fruits and vegetables—were more controversial than they are now. The debate included many questions.

How strong was the technical evidence? Which research methods were adequate? By what criteria should scientists weigh the sufficiency of evidence that virtually all observers agreed was incomplete, uncertain, and contested?[88] The most acrimonious disagreements surrounded dietary advice for the general public. Some researchers and health professionals actively promoted a "prudent diet" — low in fat, cholesterol, and sodium and high in fiber, fruits, and vegetables. Others contended that beyond admonishing people to avoid gaining too much weight, the scientific evidence was too weak to justify dietary recommendations. This perspective offered another brand of prudence: caution about the medical advice given to the public.[89]

Prior to the 1970s, government nutrition policy focused on eliminating dietary deficiencies. It aimed to prevent conditions such as scurvy, rickets, and pellagra, not cancer, heart disease, and strokes. The U.S. Department of Agriculture (USDA), the lead agency in nutrition, worked to ensure that people obtained adequate supplies of protein, vitamins, and minerals. USDA advice emphasized what were then known as the "Basic Four Food Groups" — meat, dairy, vegetables and fruits, and grains.[90] The recommended dietary allowances (RDAs), set by the NAS Food and Nutrition Board, were also aimed at dietary deficiencies.

Debate over diet and health heated up considerably in the 1970s when a group of nutrition reformers mounted a concerted attack on "the American diet." They mobilized a variety of resources, data, and rhetoric in an effort to define the American diet as a major public health problem. They attacked the long-standing premises of federal nutrition policy, contending that the emphasis on dietary deficiencies was outdated and that the problem that plagued Americans in the late twentieth century was not malnutrition but overnutrition. They sought to redirect nutrition policy toward the chronic diseases that kill most Americans. Senator George McGovern, the South Dakota Democrat, perhaps best expressed their sense of urgency:

> We have reached the point where nutrition . . . may be the Nation's number one public health problem. The threat is not beriberi, pellagra, or scurvy. Rather we face the more subtle, but also more deadly, reality of millions of Americans loading their stomachs with food which is likely to make them obese, to give them high blood pressure, to induce heart disease, diabetes, and cancer — in short, to kill them over the long term.[91]

McGovern, who chaired the Senate Select Committee on Nutrition and Human Needs, held a series of congressional hearings during 1974–77 that spotlighted advocates of dietary change: scientific experts on diet and chronic disease; public health specialists; advocates of preventive medicine; consumer groups; dietitians; and representatives of the American Heart Association (AHA), which had begun issuing warnings about dietary cholesterol and fats in 1960s.[92] At these hearings, nutrition reformers advocated nothing less than a wholesale transformation of American eating habits in favor of a diet low in fat, cholesterol, and sodium, and high in whole grains, fruits and vegetables, and dietary fiber. They pushed for nutrition education programs that would alter people's food choices. They proposed regulatory changes designed to reform food marketing. And they argued that nutrition policy should be controlled by the Department of Health, Education, and Welfare (DHEW)—and later its successor, the Department of Health and Human Services (DHHS)—rather than the USDA, which they believed was too strongly committed to agricultural interests to implement the necessary changes.

The nutrition-reform agenda, however, encountered serious criticism from some scientists. One axis of controversy concerned putative links between diet and disease, as researchers debated whether dietary cholesterol causes coronary artery disease, whether sodium increases the risk of hypertension, and whether high-fiber foods protect against colon cancer. A second axis of debate concerned the relative credibility of the different methods scientists use to address such questions. The proper role of epidemiology was particularly controversial. Some researchers argued that in the area of nutrition, epidemiology should be regarded primarily as a source of hypotheses rather than a means of testing them.[93] In their view, experimental studies in laboratory animals—or, better yet, clinical trials in humans—were needed to resolve the scientific issues. Other researchers placed much more confidence in epidemiology, arguing that its critics displayed an unscientific bias against a valid research method.[94] Still another axis of debate concerned the standards of proof that should apply when incomplete evidence bears on public health. In particular, the question of whether public health agencies should aim dietary recommendations intended to reduce chronic disease at the general public was controversial, with some health professionals arguing that physicians should assess risks and offer advice on an individual basis.[95] Disputes also broke out about what types of nutrition information should appear on food labels, and about whether fast food restaurants should be required to disclose the nutritional content of their burgers, shakes, and fries.[96]

The agenda of the nutrition reformers brought them into direct conflict with some of the most powerful actors in the food system, especially meat, dairy, and egg producers and manufacturers of foods high in fat and sodium, who saw the new diet advice as a profound threat, with ominous implications for the size and structure of markets. To lower fat intake to 30 percent of calories, for example, most Americans would need to reduce their consumption of meat and dairy products; shift to lean meats, skim milk, and low-fat cheeses; cut down on eggs, butter, margarine, oils, and salad dressing; and eat more fruits, vegetables, legumes, and cereal products. Observers expected these changes, if widely adopted, to have major economic effects on agriculture and the food industry, and perhaps to lower the value of land in states dependent on animal agriculture.[97]

The New Diet Advice

The three Academy reports on diet and health emerged in the context of this complex, multifaceted debate. Each of these reports was a separate Academy project, written by a different committee. To understand how these reports fit into the evolving controversy, one must position them alongside other nutrition reports published during this period. In the late 1970s and early 1980s, the debate about dietary recommendations was sufficiently polarized that observers often classified reports as "pro" or "con" dietary change. Table 2 summarizes the major recommendations on nutrition and health issued to the U.S. public by expert panels between 1977 and 1989. In keeping with the prevailing perceptions of participants in the debate over nutrition advice at the time, reports are designated as "pro" or "con" dietary change. During the period, support grew for reducing intakes of fat, cholesterol, and salt; for increasing consumption of whole grains, fruits, vegetables, and high-fiber foods; and for replacing simple sugars with complex carbohydrates. Many of the reports offer complex recommendations that cannot be described fully here. As indicated, some expert groups offered quantitative guidance on issues such as maximum levels of fat, cholesterol, and salt consumption, or desirable intake of fiber. Most expert panels also explicitly advised people to maintain a desirable body weight by balancing intake of calories with energy expenditure (not shown); many also called for limiting alcohol consumption. Viewed through this simple pro/con frame, the general trend over the 1970s and 1980s was clearly in the direction of increasing support for the new nutrition advice.

In 1977, under McGovern's leadership, the Senate Select Committee on

Nutrition and Human Needs published the federal government's first dietary recommendations aimed at chronic disease. *Dietary Goals for the United States* was merely a report by a congressional committee, however; it constituted neither a resolution of Congress nor a policy of the executive branch. Yet despite its weak official standing, the report became both controversial and influential. The meat and dairy industry, joined by some nutrition professionals, attacked the report, leading the committee to issue a revised, and slightly toned-down, edition. Even so, many observers saw the very existence of *Dietary Goals* as an indictment of the USDA and DHEW for failing to address a serious public health problem. These agencies were quite critical of the report and felt that they had to respond, which further increased government attention to diet and health.[98]

Between 1977 and 1980, the proponents of dietary change made more progress toward reforming nutrition policy. In the late 1970s, McGovern pressured the National Cancer Institute (NCI) to devote more attention to the role of diet in cancer, and the NCI's director, Arthur Upton, presented the agency's first dietary recommendations (a set of "prudent interim principles") before the senator's committee in 1979.[99] More important, the Carter administration appointed supporters of dietary change to important positions in the USDA. In February 1980, the USDA and DHHS jointly issued *Dietary Guidelines for Americans*, a report widely seen as a watershed in federal nutrition policy; for the first time, two executive branch agencies advised the American public that dietary change could lower the risk of chronic disease.[100]

When *Toward Healthful Diets*, the first of the three Academy reports examined below, was released in May 1980, most observers perceived it as an attack on the new diet advice, such as the American Heart Association's recommendations, *Dietary Goals*, and *Dietary Guidelines for Americans*. The NAS Food and Nutrition Board prepared *Toward Healthful Diets*—a short report only 24 pages long—using its own funds, rather than under a contract with an external sponsor, taking this unusual step with the aim of reducing public "confusion" about diet and health. As the introduction explained:

> The Food and Nutrition Board is concerned about the flood of dietary recommendations currently being made to the American public in the hope that a variety of chronic degenerative diseases may be prevented in some persons. These recommendations, which have come from various agencies in

TABLE 2
Trends in Dietary Advice, 1977–1989

Report	"Pro" or "Con"	Focus	Reduce Total Fat (% total calories)	Reduce Saturated Fat (% total calories)	Reduce Cholesterol (mg/day)	Reduce Simple Sugars	Increase Complex Carbohydrates	Increase Fiber (g/day)	Decrease salt (g/day)	Other (selected)
U.S. Senate, "Dietary Goals," 1st ed. (1977)	pro	overall health	Yes (30%)	Yes	Yes (300)	Yes	Yes	Yes	Yes (3)	Eat less meat, more poultry, and fish. Eat fewer eggs, less butterfat. Eat more fruits, vegetables, and whole grains.
U.S. Senate, "Dietary Goals," 2d ed. (1977)	pro	overall health	Yes (27–33%)	Yes	Yes (250–350)	Yes	Yes	Yes	Yes (4–6)	Choose meats, poultry, and fish that will lower intake of animal fat. Eat fewer eggs, less butterfat, more fruits, vegetables, and whole grains.
American Heart Association (1978)	pro	heart	Yes (30–35%)	Yes	Yes (300)	NC	Yes	No	Yes	Limit alcohol.
Surgeon General (1979)	pro	overall health	Yes	Yes	Yes	Yes	Yes	NC	Yes	Increase fish, poultry, legumes; less red meat. Limit alcohol.
National Cancer Institute (1979)	pro	cancer	Yes	NC	NC	NC	NC	Yes	NC	Well-balanced diet. Ample fresh fruits and vegetables. Limit alcohol.

Organization	Position	Focus								Recommendation
American Medical Association (1979)	con	overall health	No	No	No	Yes	NC	NC	Yes (12)	Moderation in diet. MDs should give high-risk patients individualized diet advice.
USDA–DHHS, "Dietary Guidelines" (1980)	pro	overall health	Yes	Yes	Yes	Yes	Yes	Yes	Yes	Variety of foods. Choose low-fat meats, dairy products. Eat fruits, vegetables, whole grains. Limit alcohol.
Toward Healthful Diets (1980)	con	overall health	No	No	No	No[a]	No[a]	No	Yes (3–8)	Variety and moderation in diet. If overweight, decrease intake of fats, sugars, and alcohol.
American Heart Association (1982)	pro	heart	Yes (30%)	Yes	Yes (300)	Yes	Yes (55%)	NC	Yes	Public education about heart disease risks.
Diet, Nutrition, and Cancer (1982)	pro	cancer	Yes[b] (30%)	Yes	NC	NC	Yes	NC	NC	Eat fruits, vegetables, and whole grains.[c] Minimize intake of smoked and salt-cured foods. Limit alcohol.
American Cancer Society (1984)	pro	cancer	Yes (30%)	Yes	NC	NC	Yes	Yes	NC	Eat high-fiber foods, such as whole grains. Eat foods rich in vitamins A and C and cabbage-family vegetables. Limit salt-cured and smoked foods. Limit alcohol.
National Cancer Institute (1984)	pro	cancer	Yes	Yes (30%)	NC	NC	Yes	Yes (25–35)	NC	Eat high-fiber foods, such as whole grains. Eat foods rich in vitamins A and C and cabbage-family vegetables. Choose barbecued, grilled, smoked foods less often. Limit alcohol.

(continued)

TABLE 2 (continued)

				Recommendations						
Report	"Pro" or "Con"	Focus	Reduce Total Fat (% total calories)	Reduce Saturated Fat (% total calories)	Reduce Cholesterol (mg/day)	Reduce Simple Sugars	Increase Complex Carbohydrates	Increase Fiber (g/day)	Decrease salt (g/day)	Other (selected)
NIH Consensus Conference (1985)	pro	heart	Yes (30%)	Yes (10%)	Yes (250–300)	Yes[d]	Yes[d]	NC	Yes	Food industry should intensify effort to market products that help individuals meet dietary goals. Doctors should treat patients with high blood cholesterol.
USDA–DHHS, "Dietary Guidelines," 2d ed. (1985)	pro	overall health	Yes	Yes	Yes	Yes	Yes	Yes	Yes	Variety of foods. Limit alcohol.
The 1985 Draft (canceled Oct. 1985)	con	avoiding nutrient deficiency			not published					Critics argued that the draft report was inconsistent with recent anticancer advice.
National Cancer Institute (1987)	pro	cancer	Yes (30%)	Yes	NC	NC	Yes	Yes (20–35)	NC	Eat high-fiber foods, such as whole grains. Eat foods rich in vitamins A and C and cabbage-family vegetables. Choose barbecued, grilled, smoked foods less often. Limit alcohol.

Surgeon General (1988)	pro	overall health	Yes	Yes	Yes	Yes	Yes	Yes	Yes	Yes	Limit alcohol. Adolescent girls and women should increase calcium intake to help avoid osteoporosis.
National Academy of Sciences, "Diet and Health" (1989)	pro	overall health	Yes (30%)	Yes (10%)	Yes	Yes	Yes	Yes	Yes	Yes	Daily intake of 5 servings of fruits and vegetables and 6 servings of cereals, breads, and legumes. Population mean for saturated fat should be 7–8%. Avoid dietary supplements. Limit protein intake to moderate levels. Limit alcohol.

SOURCES: American Cancer Society 1984; American Heart Association 1978, 1982; American Medical Association, Council on Scientific Affairs 1979; National Academy of Sciences 1980, 1982, and 1989a; U.S. Department of Health and Human Services 1980 and 1985; U.S. Department of Health, Education, and Welfare 1979; U.S. National Cancer Institute 1979b, 1984b, and 1987; U.S. National Institutes of Health 1985; U.S. Senate Select Committee on Nutrition and Human Needs 1977b, pp. 12–13 and 1977 f., pp. xxvi, 4–5; and U.S. Surgeon General 1988. See also tables summarizing nutrition advice and McNutt 1980, Palmer and Bakshi 1983, Pariza 1986, and National Academy of Sciences 1989a, ch. 28.

NOTE: The three Academy reports that provide the empirical focus of this book are indicated in boldface. NC: no comment; not discussed.

[a] The report recommended that persons at high risk for diabetes reduce sugar and increase complex carbohydrates.

[b] The committee chose 30% as a practical target, but stated that the data might justify even lower intakes.

[c] The committee stated that the data especially point to vegetables and fruits high in vitamins A and C and in the cabbage family.

[d] The conference endorsed the dietary approach of the American Heart Association.

government, voluntary health groups, consumer advocates, and health-food interests, often lack a sound scientific foundation, and some are contradictory to one another. In an effort to reduce the confusion in the mind of the public that has resulted from these many conflicting recommendations, the Board has prepared the following statement. . . .[101]

Toward Healthful Diets contended that it was "scientifically unsound to make single, all-inclusive recommendations to the public regarding intakes of energy [i.e., total calories], protein, fat, cholesterol, carbohydrate, fiber, and sodium."[102] In general, *Toward Healthful Diets* argued that putative links between diet and chronic disease were too weak to support broad recommendations to the public at large (as opposed to advice that doctors tailor individually to particular patients based on their specific medical problems).[103] The report said that there was insufficient evidence to advise the American population to reduce cholesterol intake. It also contended that there was "no basis" for recommending changes in consumption of macronutrients such as fat, carbohydrates, and protein to prevent cancer.[104] As discussed below, proponents of nutrition reform attacked *Toward Healthful Diets*, calling it unscientific and charging that its authors included food industry consultants. The president of the NAS, Philip Handler, appeared before Congress to defend the Academy and the Food and Nutrition Board against charges of bias.

The second Academy report, *Diet, Nutrition, and Cancer*, was widely perceived as supporting significant change in the American diet, although its recommendations were cautiously worded. In 1980, the NCI asked the Academy to conduct a comprehensive survey of the literature on nutrition and cancer and prepare dietary recommendations where warranted. The Academy formed an expert panel, which released a 478-page report, *Diet, Nutrition, and Cancer*, in 1982. This offered a set of "interim dietary guidelines" that it said might reduce cancer risks, although it cautioned that the evidence was not conclusive. These guidelines included lowering intake of fat to 30 percent of calories (from the 40 percent then consumed); including vegetables, citrus fruits, and whole grains in the daily diet; and reducing consumption of smoked and salt-cured foods.[105] Critics of the new dietary advice, including several authors of *Toward Healthful Diets* and meat and dairy groups, attacked the report. Producers of smoked meats, such as ham and hot dogs, were particularly vocal. Although controversial, *Diet, Nutrition, and Cancer* was influential; it focused scientific attention on the subject and helped consolidate interest in diet as a cancer-prevention strategy.[106]

TABLE 3

Members of the Committees That Prepared the Three Academy Nutrition
Reports, 1980–1985

"Toward Healthful Diets" (1980)	"Diet, Nutrition, and Cancer" (1982)	The 1985 RDA Draft
Alfred E. Harper, chairman	Clifford Grobstein, chairman	**Henry Kamin,** chairman
Henry Kamin, vice chairman	John Cairns, vice chairman	James Olson, vice chairman
Roslyn B. Alfin-Slater	Robert J. Berliner	Philip Farrell
Sol H. Chafkin	Selwyn A. Broitman	Helen Guthrie
George K. Davis	T. Colin Campbell	**Victor Herbert**
Richard L. Hall	Joan Dye Gussow	Robert Hodges
Gail G. Harrison	Laurence N. Kolonel	Max Horwitt
Victor Herbert	**David Kritchevsky**	Orville Levander
Ogden C. Johnson	Walter Mertz	Peter Pellet
David Kritchevsky	Anthony Bernard Miller	
Robert A. Neal	Michael J. Prival	
Robert E. Olson	Thomas Joseph Slaga	
George M. Owen	Lee W. Wattenberg	
Willard B. Robinson	Takashi Sugimura, advisor	
Irwin H. Rosenberg		

NOTE: Those who served on more than one panel are indicated in boldface.

Although the third report, the 1985 Draft of the Tenth Edition of the Recommended Dietary Allowances (hereafter referred to as the 1985 Draft), was never published, most observers believed it to be incompatible with the agenda of the nutrition reformers. Since 1941, the Food and Nutrition Board has periodically updated the RDAs, and its Committee on Dietary Allowances began work on the Tenth Edition in 1980. As the draft report approached publication, it became entangled in bitter debate. As we shall see, the disputing parties disagreed about the causes of the conflict, but a key issue was whether the RDAs should remain focused on avoiding nutrient deficiencies or begin to address prevention of cancer and other chronic disease. The Committee on Dietary Allowances objected to expanding the scope of the RDAs to encompass chronic disease; critics charged that the draft was inconsistent with the recent guidelines of *Diet, Nutrition, and Cancer* and the NCI. For the opponents of the new advice, NAS President Frank Press's decision in the fall of 1985 not to publish the 1985 Draft was a major setback.[107]

Table 3 shows the members of the panels that prepared each of the three reports. During the period 1980–85, the membership of the Food and Nutrition Board, which rotated, completely turned over. In 1980, when it issued *Toward Healthful Diets*, the board was dominated by scientists skeptical of the new nutrition advice. These skeptics also controlled the board when the Committee on Dietary Allowances, which wrote the 1985 Draft, was appointed later that year. But by the time Frank Press canceled that report in 1985, these skeptics had been replaced. The new board members, who were far more sympathetic to nutrition reform, opposed publishing the 1985 Draft. As this discussion suggests, the Academy's outlook on diet and health changed significantly during the first half of the 1980s.

Over the same period, the new diet advice also gained increasing support beyond the Academy. Debate about nutrition did not stop, but a relatively robust core of recommendations took shape, with a cascade of reports recommending broadly similar changes (Table 2). Scientific critics of this advice found their views increasingly marginalized. The core advice became the conventional wisdom, and growing numbers of health professionals advised patients to make dietary changes. As the 1980s progressed, agricultural interests and food manufacturers also changed their perspective on the new diet advice. Rather than attacking nutrition guidelines, they increasingly developed and promoted new "healthy" products, seeking to transform a threat into a market segment.[108] This general trend in the debate over dietary advice is important to keep in mind as we analyze struggles over the credibility of the Academy nutrition reports.

THE CHAPTERS AHEAD

The bulk of this book applies the dramaturgical framework to the Academy reports on diet and health, examining the relationship between stage management and credibility and analyzing the particular modes of information control that surround Academy advice. Chapter 2 focuses on the production of reports, examining the Academy's system of stage management and its role in creating a credible persona that can speak authoritatively. After considering *Diet, Nutrition, and Cancer*, a report that was successfully produced, the chapter turns to the 1985 Draft, which provides an example of a breakdown in stage management. Chapter 3 addresses the reception of reports, comparing how critics attacked *Toward Healthful Diets* and *Diet, Nutrition, and Cancer*, analyzing the critics' performative techniques, assessing the results of their attacks, and explaining the different outcomes.

Amid charges of bias and institutional problems, the debates over all three reports expanded to encompass questions about the credibility and integrity of the Academy. Chapter 4 examines struggles to define the institution's character, using the cancellation of the 1985 Draft as a case in point. I develop a detailed account of how the main protagonists in this debate emplotted the story into conflicting dramas about the maintenance of social order. The final chapter briefly summarizes my findings.

The analysis draws on a wide range of publicly available documents, including Academy reports, brochures, and memoranda; articles and letters in scientific journals; government reports; congressional hearings; media accounts; news releases; and the publications of consumer groups and trade associations. Additional information—some of which provides a peek backstage—was obtained from unpublished correspondence and interviews with Academy employees and other participants in these debates. Most sources are clearly indicated by full citations. In a very few cases, however, documents cannot be quoted or individuals who provided information must remain anonymous.

CHAPTER 2

Staging Authoritative Reports

What is a National Academy of Sciences report? Who writes these reports and how? What underwrites their authority? This chapter explores these questions by examining how the Academy, the nation's premier producer of science advice, brings its reports to the public stage. Academy reports use a number of rhetorical and discursive devices to present compelling narratives of scientific authority, and I analyze these techniques below. But to understand how Academy reports dramatize their own authority entails looking, not only at the literary structure of its reports, but also at the modes of information control in which they are embedded. Like other performers, the Academy employs a variety of techniques to control what its audiences can perceive; for example, by dividing the work of producing its reports into two parts—a "front stage" performance, which is actively displayed to the audience, and a "backstage," which is carefully concealed. As we shall see below, these stage-management practices, along with the rhetorical devices that reports employ, function in an integrated manner and together form a system for preparing reports that enact compelling dramas of scientific authority.

To understand the operation of this system, this chapter undertakes a comparative analysis of two reports—one that was successfully produced and one that was not. In the case of *Diet, Nutrition, and Cancer*, the Academy's practices for producing reports functioned normally, and the report was published in 1982.[1] In contrast, these practices broke down in the case of the 1985 Draft of the RDAs, which the NRC president canceled prior to publication. Comparing these two reports, thus, provides an excellent opportunity for investigating the narrative structure of Academy reports, its system of stage management, and what happens when its techniques of information control fail.

We begin with *Diet, Nutrition, and Cancer*, focusing on what this report brings to the front stage. After analyzing the visible features of Academy reports, the chapter turns to the techniques that the Academy uses to shape how audiences perceive the backstage. This entails, first, considering the confidentiality procedures through which the Academy creates a backstage region that its audiences cannot directly observe, and second, examining how the Academy describes the backstage to outsiders. Next, the chapter analyzes the case of the 1985 Draft, an instance in which the usual means of staging reports failed in two ways: not only did the official, authorized performance end up being canceled, but confidentiality was breached, internal documents were leaked, and unauthorized accounts of the backstage were widely circulated. The conclusion discusses the lessons learned from the comparison, exploring the role of stage management in creating unified performances that present credible advice in an authoritative voice.

FRONT STAGE: "DIET, NUTRITION, AND CANCER"

To begin our analysis of the Academy's stage-management techniques, let us consider one of its public performances, *Diet, Nutrition, and Cancer*. Imagine someone handed you a copy. You would find yourself holding a fat green book, 478 pages long. What sort of book? The title would tell you something, but not very much. After all, a book of that title could be a guide to natural foods, a theoretical treatise by a self-proclaimed expert, or perhaps even a novel. Much more informative than the title itself are the other words that appear on the title page:

> Committee on Diet, Nutrition, and Cancer
> Assembly of Life Sciences
> National Research Council
> National Academy Press
> Washington, D.C. 1982

These few lines tell the reader much. They signal that this book belongs to a specialized genre — the science advisory report — and was produced by a distinguished organization: the National Academy of Sciences' operative branch, the National Research Council.

What is this "National Academy of Sciences"? From a dramaturgical perspective, the key issue is not the true nature of the Academy but what we might call its "public identity": the stylized image by which an actor is broadly identified. Public identities provide maps of the dramatis personae of social life; they offer guides to who's who and how particular actors can be expected to behave. In the theatricalized world of contemporary policy discourse, an actor's public identity can be thought of as consisting of two main things: the assignment of the individual or organization to a relevant "type" and the attribution to the actor of the kinds of characteristics associated with that type in collective understandings. In the case of an individual person, for example, the most important aspects of public identity are often the sort of shared understandings that are invoked by the stylized shorthand of an official title, a curriculum vitae, a business card, or (more to the point in the public arenas we are examining) an identifying phrase in a newspaper article. These means of signaling do not so much identify the person as an individual as position him or her in cultural space. A "scientist" is understood to be a different sort of person from a "government official," a "trade association executive," or a "drug kingpin." A similar set of signals indicate the cultural position of organizations. Thus, a "university" is considered to be a different kind of entity from a "corporation" or a "government agency."

What are the main features of the public identity of the National Academy of Sciences? We must approach the question with some caution owing to the multiple, intertwined ambiguities of public identity.[2] Because public identities, along with the cultural categories that define "types" of actors, are constantly being both contested and reshaped, the identity of the "National Academy of Sciences" cannot be taken as a unitary, well-defined thing, frozen into a stable social structure and immune to change.[3] But neither can it be considered totally amorphous or infinitely malleable, at least in the short term. That the National Academy of Sciences stands at the pinnacle of American science is a well-established social fact. Thus, we can safely assume that although people who encounter references to "the Academy" may regard it somewhat differently, they are quite likely to view it as a prestigious scientific organization. For this reason, we may conclude that the mere fact that *Diet, Nutrition, and Cancer* is a product of the Academy positions the report in cultural space and informs readers that it represents authoritative fact, not fiction or imaginative writing.[4] The connection to the Academy thus establishes a (potentially rebuttable) case for treating the report as the product of serious scientific inquiry.

The public identity of the Academy, then, is a crucial resource that helps to construct the credibility of the report. When presenting itself, the Academy carefully emphasizes its specialness. The Academy, as one of its own brochures puts it, is "a unique national resource."[5] No other U.S. institution has the same mix of characteristics: unquestionable scientific and technological expertise; an official congressional charter to provide scientific advice to the federal government; and independence from the political chain of command. NRC reports draw a great deal of credibility from these aspects of the Academy's identity. But public identities cannot simply be used; they must also be cultivated and maintained. To foster and protect its identity as an authoritative source of science advice, the Academy works hard. Building credibility is a goal that influences the narratives of its reports, the process by which they are produced, and the practices that selectively reveal and conceal aspects of this process.

The Narrative of the Report

The public identity of the Academy clearly provides some grounds for expecting its reports to be authoritative documents, but the NAS does not rest its case there. For one thing, if reputation alone were the only tool for making Academy reports persuasive, then in the short run each report would be easy to challenge, and in the long run confidence in the institution would be hard to preserve. We thus need to take a closer look at the techniques the teams that produced the reports on diet and health used to make them persuasive. In particular, what literary techniques did these teams use to create a strong case for the reports' cultural authority? To address these questions, I shall examine the text of *Diet, Nutrition, and Cancer*, drawing on recent studies of scientific rhetoric, especially the work of Bruno Latour, that provide useful tools for examining how the authors of scientific texts try to make them persuasive. As Latour and others have shown, scientific texts are rhetorical devices aimed at persuading audiences to reach particular conclusions.[6] Advisory reports are no exception. But what rhetorical features and narrative structures are employed in the peculiar genre of the science advisory report? Let us examine this question, using *Diet, Nutrition, and Cancer* as a concrete example.

Diet, Nutrition, and Cancer is a large text and refers to many thousands of semiotic entities, ranging from "epidemiologists" to "mucosal cells," from "broiled beef" to "alcoholics admitted to mental hospitals in Massachusetts," from "Marshall *et al.*" to "2-aminofluorene." Rather than examining *Diet, Nutrition, and Cancer* in all of its complexity to uncover the secrets of its persuasive force, however, let's look at the apparently simple story that the team that produced it tells of its history in the front matter, where it is presented as conforming to the institutionalized definition of what constitutes an advisory report, a definition from which it draws much credibility.[7]

Like the "materials and methods" section of a scientific paper, the front matter of *Diet, Nutrition, and Cancer* is in fact an intense polemic.[8] As Latour has shown, the rhetorical structure of a scientific text can be revealed starkly by envisioning a confrontation between the text and an imaginary skeptic predisposed to doubt its conclusions.[9] Let us imagine a dialogue between this skeptic, who stubbornly raises questions, and answers from *Diet, Nutrition, and Cancer* itself (with verbatim quotations from the report):[10]

SKEPTIC: Who performed this study? Some fly-by-night food-fad group?

REPORT: "In June 1980, the NCI commissioned the National Research Council (NRC) to conduct a comprehensive study of the scientific information" on diet, nutrition, and cancer.[11]

SKEPTIC: Well, the NRC certainly is a prestigious scientific organization, but it's also a complex one. How can we be sure that this represents the Academy's considered judgment, not merely the opinions of a fringe group within the institution?

REPORT: "The project that is the subject of this report was approved by the Governing Board of the National Research Council, whose members are drawn from the Councils of the National Academy of Sciences, the National Academy of Engineering, and the Institute of Medicine."[12]

SKEPTIC: Yeah, sure! I might have guessed you'd say something like that. But who actually conducted the study?

REPORT: "The NRC Governing Board assigned administrative responsibility for this project to the Executive Office of the Assembly of Life Sciences (ALS). Subsequently, a 13-member committee and one advisor were appointed to conduct the study.[13]

"The members of the committee responsible for the report were chosen for their special competences and with regard for appropriate balance."[14]

SKEPTIC: You claim they were competent, but why should I believe you?

REPORT: "Institutional affiliations and major research interests of the committee members and the staff are presented in Appendix A."[15]

SKEPTIC [*looking over the list*]: Hmmm . . . John Cairns—I've *heard* of him. And Harvard, Columbia, Cornell, and the Wistar Institute are all top-rank places. And these people seem to be well established, too. They all seem to be director of this or full professor of that. Look, here's the head of the cancer research center at Tokyo University! And the dean of the Yale School of Medicine! On paper, it surely looks like a distinguished panel. But still—

REPORT: "The diverse expertise represented on the committee includes such disciplines as biochemistry, microbiology, embryology, epidemiology, experimental oncology, internal medicine, microbial genetics, molecular biology, molecular genetics, nutrition, nutrition education, public health, and toxicology. . . . . This multidisciplinary composition has served to ensure comprehensive coverage of the scientific literature and to provide a broad perspective to the committee's conclusions."[16]

SKEPTIC: Even if they are top-of-the-line experts, how could a mere thirteen people—no matter how prominent—possibly keep track of all the literature in all these fields?

REPORT: "The work of the committee has been aided by extensive consultation with scientific colleagues, by specially arranged technical conferences on specific subjects, and by a public meeting to receive such additional information and advice as scientists and others wished to provide.[17]

"The committee particularly wishes to commend the able and devoted assistance of an NRC staff headed by Dr. Sushma Palmer, and consisting of [seven additional people].[18]

"The committee is also greatly indebted to [six scientists—names and affiliations are given], who served as consultants and in this capacity wrote manuscripts for the consideration and use of the committee, and extends thanks to those who gave testimony at the public meeting or, upon request, presented data and engaged in discussions during committee meetings, conferences, or workshops. Many others, especially [six more names], also provided valuable advice to the committee. . . . "[19]

SKEPTIC: Perhaps. But the *real* question is whether the committee was objective, isn't it?

REPORT: "The committee has attempted to present the evidence as objectively as possible and to indicate the range of scientifically acceptable interpretation. It hopes that the results will be useful to all interested parties."[20]

SKEPTIC: You say, "as objectively as possible." That sounds perfect in principle, but what does it really mean in practice? This is an extremely controversial area.

REPORT: "The committee is aware that several aspects of its charge are matters of controversy, either within the scientific and medical community or among the general population. Controversies are inevitable when data are neither clear-cut nor complete. Interpretations then depend on the criteria selected for evaluation and are influenced by individual or collective judgment."[21]

SKEPTIC: That's my point! How can we be sure that the committee used appropriate criteria?

REPORT [*flipping ahead to the 21-page chapter on "Methodology"*]: This chapter "explains the approach adopted by the committee in evaluating the epidemiological and experimental evidence."[22]

SKEPTIC: Okay. Let's see this "approach" spelled out.

REPORT: "Because no studies of this difficult subject are without limitations, the committee did not wish to place too much emphasis on the results, especially the precise quantitative data (e.g., relative risks in epidemiological studies or tumor incidence in animal experiments), from any single study. Rather, it reviewed all the data and based its conclusions on the overall strength of all the evidence combined."[23]

SKEPTIC: This sounds laudable, but it's rather vague. Give me details!

REPORT: "Although the committee considered the evidence from all types of epidemiological studies, it had the most confidence in data derived from case-control studies and from the few cohort studies that have been reported. Instead of relying on aggregate correlation data, these studies are based on the collection and analysis of data on individuals, and investigators can control for confounding variables. Therefore, the committee concluded that the evidence on diet and cancer provided by these two types of studies is more definitive and indicative of meaningful associations. . . . "[24]

SKEPTIC: And what about laboratory studies? How were those factored in?

REPORT: "In evaluating laboratory evidence, the committee placed more confidence in data derived from studies on more than one animal species or test system, on results that have been reproduced in different laboratories, and on the few data that indicate a gradient in response.

"The preponderance of the data and the degree of concordance between the epidemiological and laboratory evidence determined the strength of the conclusions in the report."[25]

SKEPTIC: Well, was the report carefully peer-reviewed?

REPORT: "This report has been reviewed by a group other than the authors according to procedures approved by a Report Review Committee consisting of members of the National Academy of Sciences, the National Academy of Engineering, and the Institute of Medicine."[26]

Let us now interrupt this imaginary dialogue and consider what the team that constructed the report has accomplished. Obviously, the skeptic is free to remain unconvinced, so the questioning could in principle continue.[27] But who and what must the skeptic challenge in order to persist? The committee, for one. Who make up this committee? The report leaves no doubt: it is a group of highly qualified experts, chosen according to Academy procedures for their "special competences" and for "appropriate balance." According to the logic of the report, the members of the committee should not be thought of simply as individual scientists—they are *representatives* of domains of expertise.[28] These individuals, it is important to note, do not speak for particular organizations or constituencies; they represent the viewpoints of their specific areas of knowledge.[29] The committee's "multidisciplinary composition" makes it more than the sum of its parts; the mix of expertise (in some thirteen disciplines) ensures "comprehensive coverage of the scientific literature" and provides "a broad perspective to the committee's conclusions."[30]

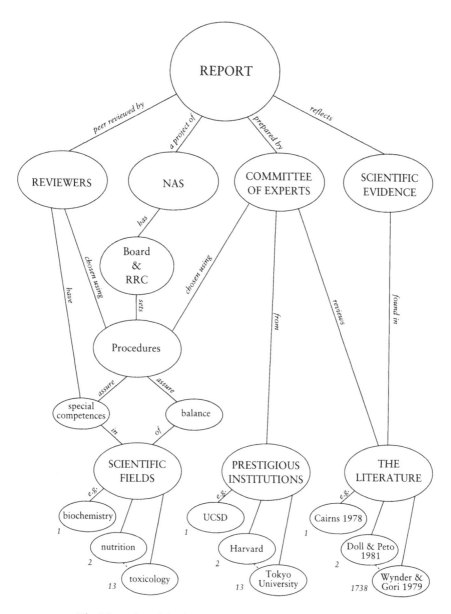

FIGURE 1. The Narrative of Authoritative Science Advice. The "concept map"
above presents the arguments that *Diet, Nutrition, and Cancer* makes to warrant
its authority. Reading through the nodes and links of the map produces statements
that summarize aspects of the narrative. The conceptual structure of the narrative
is thus displayed. (On concept maps, see Novak and Gowin 1984.)

The persona of the committee is also established through many chains of associations that link it, via its members, to outstanding research institutions, where these scientists occupy high posts. In effect, the report implicates each of these institutions—via its public identity as a pinnacle of scientific excellence—in a network of what Steven Shapin calls *vouching* for the credibility of the people associated with the report.[31] By appointing Robert J. Berliner as dean of its School of Medicine, Yale University vouches for his scientific competence and integrity. In turn, by allowing his name to appear on *Diet, Nutrition, and Cancer*, Berliner vouches for the credibility of the claims contained therein. To be sure, no representative of Yale reviewed the report on the university's behalf, but the report has constructed a chain of associations through which the reputational resources of Yale are gathered into the report. The same arguments apply to Harvard, Columbia, Cornell, the University of California at San Diego, and every other institution that supplied an expert to the committee.[32] Challenging the credentials of the committee, thus, entails questioning judgments about scientific competence made by the National Academy of Sciences and some of the world's leading research universities. The skeptic is welcome to *make* the argument that these institutions have erred in appointing a given committee member as a professor or dean, but most skeptics (especially those lacking conspicuous scientific credentials) may find it hard to persuade audiences to agree.

As the example of the persona of the committee suggests, the text sets up some rather formidable defenses against challenges by constructing a web of associations with entities that carry the cultural authority of science. The report draws a bit of scientific credibility from each link with an authoritative expert or a well-known university, and of course it draws much prestige from its connection to the membership of the National Academy of Sciences itself, the honorary elite of American science. The team that produced the report also uses many other "props" to bolster its authority. The most important are "the literature" and "the evidence," formally invoked by 1,738 citations (Fig. 1).[33] These references have a complex character: not only do they tie the report to established knowledge, but they simultaneously link it to prestigious institutions, such as well-known journals, and to reliable procedures, such as peer review. Facts, reputations, and procedures are all deployed to attest to the credibility of the report. The team's overall narrative about the authority of the report is thus grounded in a widely distributed, mutually reinforcing network of assurances about the credibility of the elements of its story.[34]

Beyond knitting together a wide range of characters all linked to the cultural authority of science, advisory reports use discursive devices that frequently appear in scientific writing and help render it authoritative. Like other formal scientific texts, advisory reports are written mainly in what Nigel Gilbert and Michael Mulkay call the "empiricist repertoire"—a linguistic register that conveys the impression of simply allowing evidence to speak for itself.[35] This form of discourse helps separate the report's conclusions from possible sources of contingency, such as the capricious decisions of opinionated individuals. On occasion, especially when dealing with conclusions that are classified as interpretive judgments rather than matters of fact, advisory reports also use what we might call the rhetoric of "expert judgment." Although this rhetoric does not simply give a voice to the evidence, it presents conclusions as the rational and carefully considered opinions of qualified experts who have carefully reviewed the evidence. Reports are expected, as one NAS publication puts it, to strike an impartial tone and to treat "sensitive policy issues . . . with appropriate care."[36] Advisory reports thus weave together rhetorics that enhance their authority in one of two ways: either by letting scientific evidence simply speak for itself or by displaying interpretive conclusions reached by qualified experts through judicious, rational deliberation.[37]

The rhetorical force of the report is also intensified by the fact that *Diet, Nutrition, and Cancer* appears to speak with a single voice; it is in this respect a monologue, not a dialogue or a multilogue. To increase the impact of its reports, the Academy instructs its committees to make a mighty effort to reach consensus, and the great majority of reports succeed in creating a public display of unanimity. In rare cases, however, "reaching consensus either is not possible or would substantially skew what otherwise would be the considered report of the majority."[38] Thus, Academy reports occasionally present "majority and minority views—fully explaining the rationale for each." At times, they also describe "the pros and cons of alternative policies—without indicating the extent to which committee members subscribe to one view or another." Finally, as "a measure of final recourse," reports may include a signed dissent by the member(s) of the committee who disagree with the rest of the group.[39] But *Diet, Nutrition, and Cancer* is not one of these rare cases: it presents no majority and minority reports, no split decisions, no dissents, no competing claims. The report often describes conflicting studies, but it provides a unified assessment of their meaning; members of the audience are not asked to evaluate opposing views. In short, the report speaks with a unified voice whose authority is grounded in the scientific evidence, thirteen disciplines, a committee of experts, and the Academy.[40] The fact that many diverse authorities apparently agreed about what the text should say reinforces the notion that the report represents, or at least approaches, a universal form of knowledge.

Backstaging Negotiation, Front-Staging Unity

Much of the dramatic force of *Diet, Nutrition, and Cancer* stems from its public display of unity. The report presents a drama of agreement: a single, unified voice is performatively forged out many, diverse ones. But how did it come to pass that the report speaks with one voice? Clearly, the report was created by no single individual; it was collectively constructed. Not even "the committee" can be considered the sole creator of the report. To be sure, the report designates the committee as its author (e.g., by putting its name on the title page and making it the official "author of record"), but clearly the committee did not act alone. According to the report, many other actors played important roles—"the National Cancer Institute" (which commissioned the report), "the National Research Council" (which agreed to perform the study), "the NRC staff" (which aided the committee), "scientists and members of the public" (who provided advice, drafted manuscripts, made presentations, attended meetings), and a "group other than the authors" (which reviewed the report). It would be a great oversimplification to say that the report was created by the committee, especially since one of the critical steps in preparing the report consisted of *creating the committee itself*—a task that entailed selecting its members, and prior to that, defining its formal charge.

We have every reason to believe that producing *Diet, Nutrition, and Cancer* required extensive negotiations. Scientists at the frontiers of research often interpret evidence differently, and scientific texts, as many studies have shown, emerge through complex and continuing negotiations.[41] Moreover, anyone who has ever served on a committee of any kind—whether formed to plan picnics or frame foreign policy—might imagine that achieving a unanimous consensus on such a report would pose challenges. Not only would it be surprising if Academy committees reached agreement automatically, but in its general accounts of how its committees operate, the Academy itself describes "the consensus-building process" as "difficult, frustrating, yet rewarding."[42] For these reasons (not to mention the extensive debate surrounding diet and cancer), it seems extremely likely that the large team that prepared *Diet, Nutrition, and Cancer* engaged in protracted negotiations. But the report tells us little about the dynamics of this process, the entry and exit of different actors, the efforts to define their roles, the bargaining among them, the conflicts, the deals. The report tells us only in the most general terms how the NCI came to commission the report, and it says nothing about why the agency chose the NRC to perform the study or whether it considered and discarded other options.[43] Nor does it show us the negotiations that took place between the NCI and the NRC regarding the goals, scope, timing, and cost of the study. It does not provide any detail about how the committee members were selected; it contains no discussion of who else was considered, no lists of possibilities, no picture of the alternative configurations that the committee might have assumed. A Congressional Research Service report on *Diet, Nutrition, and Cancer* states that 500 names were considered before the 13-member committee was established.[44] Since there are some 17,000,000,000,000,000,000,000,000,000 ways to choose a committee of 13 from a list of 500 names, only the most unreasonable person would expect the Academy to provide an exhaustive list of alternative configurations. The point, however, is that the issue is systematically unaddressed. We cannot see the committee's internal dynamics; all we are told about its organizational structure is that it had a chairman, a vice-chairman, eleven members, and an advisor. The report does not tell us what was required to make the committee—once constituted—into something more than a collection of individuals, something capable of acting as a whole. Nor does it show us the discussions that took place as the report evolved through successive drafts. We cannot see the discarded wordings or the arguments over proposed changes in the text. We cannot tell, simply from reading the text, which claims were controversial and which were uncontested, which sentences were readily agreed to and which were hammered out in debate. Nor can we identify the points in the report (if any) where changes were made in response to the reviewers. In short, we cannot see the series of negotiations that drew together the members of the team who collectively prepared the report, defined their goals, and managed their differences. Nor can we see how these negotiations created manuscripts, edited them into successive drafts, and stabilized them to form the final text.

These omissions, of course, are not random; they are an integral *part* of the report. Indeed, as a matter of policy, the Academy specifically instructs its committees and staff to omit discussions of their deliberations from reports.[45] Doing so is one way the Academy "backstages" details that almost certainly would complicate, call into question, or otherwise muddy its clean narrative of credibility. Exposing the debates within the committee would undermine the sense of unity that is a central theme of this narrative. Describing the revisions made to the report would project a sense of contingency. Discussing the many possible structures of alternative committees would highlight the roads not taken. By omitting such information, the report conceals contingency from its audiences and reinforces the impression of objectivity, unity, and credibility that the performance is designed to foster.

BACKSTAGE: THE NRC PROCESS

As the above analysis shows, the text of *Diet, Nutrition, and Cancer* places a powerful narrative of credibility center stage. But the dramatic force of this narrative lies not only in what is presented in—and omitted from—the text itself, but also in the ongoing modes of information control associated with its production, and in which it continues to be embedded even after publication. The Academy reinforces the visible features of its performances by regulating access to information. In particular, the Academy prevents audiences from examining the process through which its reports are produced by preparing them in a private space and denying outsiders access to committee records. Thus, to understand how Academy advice achieves credibility, we must analyze not only the narratives that reports actively display but also the means that the Academy uses to create an enclosed "backstage," inaccessible to audiences, where the work of preparing reports takes place. This backstage—needless to say, a metaphoric space rather than a physical location—is constructed through the Academy's ongoing practices of information control. Let us examine how these practices produce a backstage and its role in constructing credible advice.

An Enclosed Space

The Academy considers it essential to create a private space in which the teams that prepare reports can operate. The institution regards the confidentiality of its deliberations as essential to its independence and indispensable to its ability to offer sound science advice. Concealing the negotiations that produce reports enables Academy insiders to engage in frank discussion and informal bargaining without fearing that every word or deed, no matter how tentative or exploratory, may be subjected to searing public scrutiny.

Procedures that create a closed environment, the Academy maintains, protect committees "from outside pressures and thereby safeguard the credibility and integrity of their work."[46] As Bruce Alberts, president of the NAS and chairman of the NRC, put it in a 1997 statement:

> We believe that keeping the committee deliberations and our review process closed and confidential is fundamental for ensuring the independence of our studies and the scientific quality of our reports, enabling our recommendations and findings to be based on science rather than politics. A frank, confidential discussion of the merits of a committee draft during review is our most effective quality assurance mechanism.[47]

Because it considers confidentiality essential to its operation, the Academy has developed formal practices intended to regulate who may have access to what information and when. The Academy's confidentiality procedures specify which forums outsiders may observe:

> "Many of the institution's meetings are open to interested individuals and the media."[48]

And which are off limits:

> "Meetings are always closed . . . when the committee is developing findings, conclusions, and recommendations."[49]

They state which documents are confidential:

> "All files associated with a project are privileged and not open to sponsors or others, with certain exceptions decided on a case-by-case basis."[50]

And which are not:

> "Material available to the public prior to completion of the project includes a copy of the statement of task, committee membership, and signed contract."[51]

They stipulate restrictions on who may obtain information:

> "Sponsors . . . may not be informed of the committee's findings and recommendations until review of the report has been successfully completed."[52]

And name gatekeepers authorized to release it:

> "The Report Review Committee and . . . the major unit responsible for the study" must "sign off" before a report is released.[53]

In short, these procedures aim to designate the spatial, social, and temporal boundaries of a "backstage" in which information about privileged deliberations is contained.

In its effort to seal this space, the Academy strives to establish a tight regime of information control—inscribed in a system of rules governing who can see and say what—that extends over observers, documents, and talk. Thus, in addition to banning outsiders from closed meetings, the Academy instructs committees, reviewers, and other participants who are granted access to privileged committee materials about their responsibilities vis-à-vis confidentiality. Committee members, for example, are "expected to reject any requests for early briefings or interviews on the committee's findings, and to treat committee deliberations and draft products as confidential."[54] The Academy also asks committee members to limit their public comments (written or spoken) to three areas until the report is officially released: the scope of the project and charge of the committee; the name of the sponsor and estimated cost; and the makeup of the committee, including names and affiliations.[55] Leaks and premature briefings are seen as particularly threatening, as one might expect in the context of Washington, D.C.:

> Conclusions and recommendations can change up to the final sign-off; premature briefings for sponsors or others outside the institution may lock committees into a position not fully supported by the evidence. Early briefings also damage the final report by subjecting the committee to the accusation that it permitted the sponsor to preview and approve the conclusions and recommendations—a serious charge that undermines the independence and integrity of both the committee and the institution. In such cases, the hard work of the committee can be discredited, diminishing the report's value to the sponsor and to the nation.[56]

After the final sign-off authorizes publication of a report, the Academy orchestrates its release. Its Office of News and Public Information "works closely with committee members and staff to plan dissemination activities" that maximize the impact of NRC reports.[57] Committee members, of course, are cautioned to avoid premature disclosures to the media:

> Many . . . reports are newsworthy, and the news media serve as an important channel for disseminating report contents. It is critical, however, to observe carefully the rules of confidentiality until the report is ready for release to the public. The report first must have successfully completed review and been thoroughly edited.[58]

Publication transforms a draft into a report, bringing it to the public stage. But when the curtain rises, the backstage remains a restricted space. For one thing, as we saw in the case of *Diet, Nutrition, and Cancer*, the

Academy builds the closure of this space right into the texts of its reports, which systematically omit discussion of negotiations. For another, the Academy continues to limit access to backstage information and documents associated with its reports long after publication. Closed files remain confidential: reviewers are "asked to return or destroy copies" of draft manuscripts, and committee members, reviewers, and staff "are asked to refrain from disclosing any contents" of drafts or review comments.[59] In fact, the Academy routinely denies outsiders access to these internal documents, which it retains in a closed part of its archives for at least the first 25 years after a report's publication. This is a long-standing policy, evenhandedly applied to outsiders of all kinds, be they critics of specific Academy reports, science writers, government agencies, or academics. For example, when the General Accounting Office (GAO) conducted an investigation of NAS procedures regarding *Diet, Nutrition, and Cancer* and *Toward Healthful Diets*, the Academy declined to permit GAO personnel to examine such internal documents as reviewer comments on the reports or statements on committee members' potential conflicts of interest. NAS officials also declined to provide confidential documents concerning the diet and health reports that I requested for this study, although they were generally quite helpful, meeting with me on several occasions and providing documents on general Academy procedures.[60]

The Academy's confidentiality practices constitute a system aimed at strictly regulating the entry of observers and exit of information from the privileged space in which reports are prepared. We can now summarize the principles of the system as follows: Only authorized observers are permitted to enter this metaphoric space, and information only can leave with authorization. The public and the press are barred; confidential documents may not be removed; reports can leave (after receiving clearance) but they must omit discussions of backstage deliberations. Personnel must police their remarks: committee members, Academy staff, and others who have observed the privileged discussions or texts are asked not to reveal what they have learned. Through this ongoing, collective work, the Academy seeks to constitute a protected space where the teams that produce reports can operate independently: discussing issues openly without fearing that their words will be freely circulated, working to forge agreement, while concealing the negotiations required to do so. In this backstage space, the Academy assembles the dramatic displays of univocality that it later presents fully formed and neatly packaged. In this way, its stage-management techniques are intended to limit what its audiences can observe and know, closing off certain lines of perception in order to create a more effective performance. At the same time, these techniques are also designed to constrain the ability of members of the audience to communicate by closing off potential lines of influence. Shutting in information is also a way of shutting out pressure groups and publics, preventing them from commenting on draft recommendations and incomplete reports. Thus, the Academy's system of closure aims not only to furnish committees with a protected environment where they can operate independently but also to deprive vested interests of a space for influence peddling.

As one might expect, given the distrust of closed processes characteristic of American political culture, critics of the Academy have sometimes charged that the confidentiality of its deliberations does not guarantee objectivity, but rather creates a space where vested interests can operate unobserved. In his 1975 book on the Academy, *The Brain Bank of America: An Inquiry into the Politics of Science*, Phillip M. Boffey argued that it should open its advisory proceedings and committee records to public inspection. Academy policies for controlling information, he wrote, make it

> extraordinarily difficult to monitor the performance of an Academy committee. Even experts find it hard to evaluate a committee's judgment without access to the original data on which that judgment is based. And the public has no way to judge whether special interests have influenced the committee's deliberations. The excuse generally given for this secrecy is that the committee members can speak more frankly, and with less fear of outside pressure, if the public is barred. But if the process were opened up more—if all meetings and records were made public—then the committees might benefit from unexpected insights volunteered by the interested public, and the public could assure itself that the project was being well handled.[61]

Such contentions have not only appeared in books; Academy critics have also sued for access, and the NAS has repeatedly defended its confidentiality procedures in court—until recently, with considerable success. In the 1975 case *Lombardo v. Handler*, the federal courts held that the NAS was an "ally of the government," not an "agency," and therefore was exempt from the provisions of the Freedom of Information Act (FOIA) and Federal Advisory Committee Act (FACA).[62] The limits of the Academy's entitlement to confidentiality were also explored in litigation surrounding *Diet, Nutrition, and Cancer*. Following publication of the report, several food-supplement manufacturers, including the General Nutrition Corporation (GNC), began marketing tablets said to have anticancer properties. Their advertising materials used the Academy's name, suggesting that *Diet, Nutrition, and Cancer* recommended consuming such tablets (which was clearly untrue). When the Academy brought legal action before the Federal Trade Commission (FTC), charging false advertising, GNC lawyers sought access to "backstage" records. They subpoenaed all documents in the Academy's possession pertaining to the production of the report, including all drafts of the report, "all memoranda, notes, minutes of meetings, correspondence, and other documents by, between, and among . . . any and all persons who participated in the review and preparation" of the report, and "all studies, tests, reports, memoranda, correspondence and other documents submitted to and/or considered by the Committee."[63] The Academy moved to limit discovery, arguing that the confidentiality of these documents was essential to its functioning. For the NAS, a fundamental principle was at stake. The FTC administrative law judge agreed, ruling that GNC's interest in obtaining the documents was unclear and "must yield to the demonstrated needs of the Academy":[64]

> Were it not for the shielding of its deliberative and review process, participants in the Academy's studies would be inhibited in the candid exchange of views concerning often controversial scientific subjects. Such disclosures would have a chilling effect upon the conduct of vigorous internal debate and seriously impair the Academy's ability to produce reports of the best possible quality for the Government. Moreover, the revealing of unfinished or working drafts could result in the dissemination of incomplete or even misleading information.[65]

In 1997, however, the deference that the courts had previously displayed toward the Academy's confidentiality procedures came to an abrupt end. In *Animal Legal Defense Fund v. Shalala*, a federal court held that FACA applied to NRC committees that provided advice to federal agencies.[66] The Academy's appeal failed; the U.S. Supreme Court refused to intervene. The Academy was stunned by these developments, which it perceived as a fundamental assault on its independence and integrity; its executive officer, for example, described the situation as "a true crisis for the Academy, probably the most serious one we have ever faced."[67] Conforming with the provisions of FACA would require extensive modifications to the NRC process. Under FACA, the government agency that requested a study would have to certify the composition of committee, approve all meetings and agendas, and send a government official to chair or attend each meeting. In addition, the law would require all committee meetings—including those where recommendations were debated and discussed—to be open to the public. The Academy perceived these requirements as completely unacceptable and mounted an extensive legal and legislative effort to resist the decision.[68] Ultimately, in a major legislative victory, the Academy persuaded Congress to amend FACA to exempt its committees from some of the act's requirements and specify precisely what NRC committees were required to do.[69] The resulting changes in NRC procedures increased openness in some ways (see the accompanying text box); for example, the names of those who have reviewed a report are now made public upon its release. (The Academy is using the World Wide Web to provide the required public information on open meetings, committee memberships, and so forth.)[70] The Academy's president, Bruce Alberts, told Congress in 1998 that the new law has "had a positive effect by making our deliberations and processes more accessible and transparent to the interested public."[71] Nevertheless, the constraints on access that remain are more significant than the increases in openness introduced: the FACA amendments retain the essence of the Academy's previous practices, permitting it to produce a closed "backstage" where it can assemble reports in private.

The NRC Process: A Drama of Procedures

The Academy considers it essential to create a backstage and carefully defend its boundaries. But although the Academy conceals backstage action from its audiences, it finds it unavoidable—and even advantageous—to produce public descriptions of the *kinds* of activities that go on backstage. In other words, the Academy's system of closure does not simply hide the NRC process but strategically presents it through a dialectic of revelation and concealment. Outsiders are not allowed to see the action itself, but the Academy presents official accounts of its general form in many places and publications. Official descriptions of how reports are prepared appear in documents such as booklets and memoranda for committee members and other participants in report preparation, which the Academy provides to outsiders on request. They also appear in congressional testimony, material distributed to journalists, and on the NAS website. By describing the NRC process to many opinion leaders, these accounts help the Academy bolster its public

New Openness Requirements under the Federal Advisory Committee Act (FACA)

Under the 1997 FACA amendments, federal agencies that contract with the National Academy of Sciences to prepare advice cannot use it unless the following procedures have been followed:

1. The Academy shall provide public notice of the names of all individuals that it appoints or intends to appoint to serve on the committee. The Academy shall provide a reasonable opportunity for public comment on appointments.

2. The Academy shall allow public access to meetings of the committee intended to gather data. The Academy can close meetings at which committees deliberate. The public must be notified in advance of open meetings.

3. The Academy shall provide the public with a brief summary of all closed meetings. The summary shall identify the individuals present, the topics discussed, and other matters that the Academy determines should be included.

4. The Academy shall provide public access to written materials that are provided to the committee by persons who are not connected to the Academy.

5. After publication of a committee report, the Academy shall make public the names of the main reviewers (from outside the Academy) who examined the report in draft form.

As amended in 1997, FACA exempts the Academy from most of the Act's provisions, such as opening all meetings to the public. However, the amendments state that Academy committees that prepare advice for federal agencies must meet several provisions, including the openness requirements summarized above.

SOURCE: Federal Advisory Committee Act Amendments of 1997, Public Law 105-153, H.R. 2977, An Act to Amend the Federal Advisory Committee Act to Clarify Public Disclosure Requirements That Are Applicable to the National Academy of Sciences and the National Academy of Public Administration, Approved Dec. 17, 1997, §15.

identity as an authoritative advisory body, defend itself against criticism, and respond to legal challenges, such as the 1997 Supreme Court decision.

The Academy's official descriptions of the NRC process provide few details. They consist of schematic summaries of the general process of report preparation and never describe the negotiations surrounding specific reports. They are written in a narrative voice that presumes its own authority, making assertions with little effort to mobilize support from additional evidence or arguments. Their central theme—that a well-designed system of procedures ensures the objectivity and quality of Academy reports—is dramatized in many Academy documents. As one brochure puts it:

> The value of the institution's work is based on its ability to provide *independent* [emphasis in original] expert advice. The National Academy of Sciences, National Academy of Engineering, Institute of Medicine, and National Research Council have special procedures and practices to safeguard the credibility and integrity of projects.[72]

And elsewhere in the same document:

> Every project is given scrupulous attention. Study and oversight committees deliberate in an environment independent of government, sponsors, and special interest groups. Continuous oversight and formal, anonymous review of the final product assure objectivity and quality. It is this process that undergirds the institution's credibility and accounts for its important role in influencing public policy on scientific and technological issues.[73]

In accounts of how reports get prepared, Academy documents and officials typically describe the stages of report preparation, stressing the procedures that safeguard the process at each step, from project formulation, to committee selection, to committee work, to report review, to report dissemination (see Fig. 2). Thus, the Academy explains, before a study is initiated, a prospectus is developed describing the task to be undertaken by the committee and providing a preliminary study plan, a picture of the kinds of expertise required, a tentative budget, an outline of anticipated meetings and workshops, a discussion of means of deliberation, and an assessment of what may be required to achieve consensus. The prospectus is then vetted at multiple levels within the organization, including review by an executive committee that must sign off before the project can proceed.

Similarly, once a project is funded, the selection of the committee is governed by "specific procedures . . . to achieve appropriate balance . . . and to

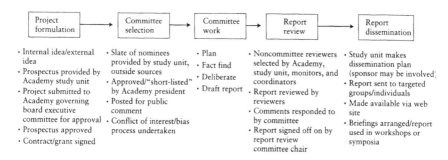

FIGURE 2. Academy Report Preparation Procedures, 1998. Note that this diagram depicts the procedures as described in official Academy statements. Adapted from U.S. General Accounting Office 1998, p. 8.

avoid conflicts of interest."[74] In this context, the term *balance* entails obtaining adequate representation from all areas of relevant expertise and from diverse "perspectives" on the issue under consideration. The Academy collects suggestions for committee appointments from a number of sources, including the members of the Academy's honorary societies, the NRC's standing committees and staff, and the study sponsor. "Actual selection of committee members, however, is the sole responsibility of the institution, and final approval rests with the Research Council chair."[75] Avoiding conflicts of interest is a special concern (Fig. 3):

> At the time of appointment, each committee member is required to list all
> professional, consulting, and financial connections, as well as to describe
> pertinent intellectual positions and public statements by filling out a confi-
> dential form, "Potential Sources of Bias and Conflict of Interest." As part
> of the process of becoming acquainted with each other . . . , committee
> members discuss this information in executive session at the beginning
> of their first meeting and annually thereafter. The information also is
> reviewed by officials of the institution, and if a potential conflict becomes
> apparent—which is rare—the committee member may be asked to resign.
> When a question of balance arises, the usual procedure is to add members
> to the committee to achieve the appropriate balance.[76]

The Academy's accounts of the NRC process emphasize how its procedures protect committees from outside pressures. An Academy booklet for prospective sponsors notes the role that they play in developing ideas for Academy projects—from initial, informal discussions through the negotiations that produce a "statement of task" that "clearly defines the scope of

On Potential Sources of Bias

Reports of appointed committees and other bodies of the National Academy of Sciences/National Academy of Engineering/Institute of Medicine/ National Research Council which consider technical matters directly relevant to issues of public interest or policy frequently contain conclusions and recommendations that necessarily rest upon professional value judgments as well as upon findings arguable on purely scientific or technical grounds.

When this is the case, some instances will arise in which it is inappropriate to appoint to membership an individual who has a substantial professional or financial interest that would be affected by the outcome of the deliberations. In other instances it may be necessary, in order to ensure that the committee is highly competent, to appoint members in such a way as to represent a balance of potentially biasing backgrounds or interests

It is for these reasons that you are requested to complete the form on the reverse hereof, showing: (1) remunerative affiliations over the last five years, as an employee, director, officer, or consultant; (2) sources of research support in excess of $10,000 over the last five years; (3) any company in which you or your spouse or minor children hold a financial interest in an amount exceeding $10,000 in market value, which also represents more than 10% of your or their current holdings.

More subtle is the question of other potential sources of bias. These might be, for example, prejudgments implicit in views to which you are publicly committed, or conclusions given as an expert witness in administrative or legislative proceedings. You are asked on the reverse hereof to indicate any such factors that in your opinion might reasonably be construed as _potentially_ compromising your independence of judgment in matters within the assigned task of the group to which you have been appointed.

If, during your term of service, any of these conditions should change, a letter explaining the circumstances should be provided for the file.

Each of our committees and similar bodies is asked to discuss the matter of potential sources of bias at its first meeting and once annually thereafter. On these occasions the chairman will share with the other members such excerpts from these statements as appear relevant. A record of the discussion will be made, for use at the discretion of the Chairman of the National Research Council in defense of the committee against any allegation of bias. The forms themselves will be treated in accordance with the statement of privilege on the other side of this page.

NATIONAL ACADEMY OF SCIENCES   NATIONAL ACADEMY OF ENGINEERING

INSTITUTE OF MEDICINE   NATIONAL RESEARCH COUNCIL

February, 1978

FIGURE 3. National Research Council Form "On Potential Sources of Bias." This version of the form was in use during the debate over _Toward Healthful Diets_. Reprinted by permission of the National Academy of Sciences.

P R I V I L E G E D

ASSEMBLY or COMMISSION	NAME
BOARD, DIVISION, or OFFICE	PRESENT EMPLOYMENT (title)
COMMITTEE	(organization)
SUB-UNIT	

(Above lines to be completed by cognizant office before form is sent to appointee)

1. REMUNERATIVE ORGANIZATIONAL AFFILIATIONS DURING LAST FIVE YEARS
   (if other than present employment shown above)

   (a) As an employee (state position)   (b) As a Director or Corporate Officer

   (c) As a consultant (more than five days in any year)

2. SOURCES OF RESEARCH SUPPORT OTHER THAN EMPLOYER (any source of more than
   $10,000 total in the last five years)

3. COMPANIES IN WHICH YOU OR YOUR SPOUSE OR MINOR CHILDREN HAVE FINANCIAL
   INTERESTS (any current holding with market value in excess of $10,000
   which also amounts to more than 10% of your or their total investments.
   Please do not list actual amounts.)

4. ADDITIONAL INFORMATION (see fourth paragraph on reverse side). If there
   are other circumstances in your background or present connections that in
   your opinion might reasonably be construed as unduly affecting your judgment in matters within the assigned task of the group to which you have
   been appointed, please describe them briefly.

Date	Signature

This statement is privileged to those offices whose proper business it is. It
may be released, on a privileged basis, to the head of an agency sponsoring
the study in which the committee is engaged, if that official so requests in
writing and if the Chairman of the National Research Council concurs. It will
not be otherwise released by the NRC or the agency except with the approval of
the individual completing the form.

the project and the tasks to be undertaken."[77] The booklet also sets forth the many limitations on sponsors: They cannot make final decisions on committee appointments or "engage in the oversight" of the project. They "are urged to attend the first meeting of the committee to present their perspectives" but may attend only open meetings and "have no role in the review process." Finally, they "may *assist* in developing a dissemination plan" (emphasis added) but the Academy retains "responsibility for handling the major public distribution" of reports.[78] Academy publications also describe the review procedures for evaluating and draft reports, stressing the rigor and objectivity of the process (see the accompanying text box). The authors of a draft "are not obligated to incorporate the changes suggested by reviewers," but "every point should be carefully considered, and if a particular change is not made, an explanation is to be provided in a response memorandum." Academy officials—for example, a "monitor" appointed by the report review committee (RRC) "in consultation with the RRC chairman"—determine "whether the authors have been responsive to reviewers' comments."[79]

Although one might wonder about the extent to which these schematic and probably somewhat idealized accounts of formal procedures capture the complex processes of organizational life, from a dramaturgical perspective a different issue emerges: How do these accounts contribute to impression management?[80] One answer, suggested by Steven Shapin and Simon Schaffer's analysis of the experimental narratives of the natural philosopher Robert Boyle, focuses on the role of these accounts in persuading outside audiences that Academy advice is credible. If outsiders cannot see the NRC process for themselves, if they cannot witness and evaluate the action directly, then they must be offered other reasons to trust its results.[81] These accounts, with their idealized treatment of Academy procedures, present a rationale for believing that its deliberations are objective and rigorous. But while Boyle's narratives used extensive descriptions and numerous illustrations to transform readers into "virtual witnesses" who perceived experiments almost as if they had seen them firsthand, the Academy's schematic accounts of its procedures do not even begin to give audiences the vicarious experience of having been there.[82] Even so, these accounts are both reassuring and difficult to challenge, since more detailed information is normally unavailable. Descriptions of the unobservable backstage, dramatically cast in the mold of a harmonious bureaucratic order, thus emerge as a means of convincing audiences of the intellectual and ethical integrity of the NRC process.

Review Criteria for National Academy of Sciences Reports

Since NRC reports cover a broad range of topics and appear in a variety of different forms, no uniform set of review criteria may be applicable to all reports. However, reviewers are usually encouraged to consider the following general questions:

1. Is the charge to the committee clearly described in the report? Are all aspects of the charge fully addressed? Does the committee go beyond its charge or its expertise?

2. Are the conclusions and recommendations adequately supported by evidence, analysis, and argument? Are uncertainties or incompleteness in the evidence explicitly recognized? If any recommendations are based on value judgments or the collective opinions of the authors, is this acknowledged?

3. Are the data and analyses handled competently? Are statistical methodologies applied appropriately? Are there any apparent errors in the data presented?

4. Are sensitive policy issues treated with proper care? For example, if the report contains recommendations pertaining to the reorganization of an agency or the creation of a new institutional entity, are the advantages and disadvantages of alternative options considered? If the report includes recommendations pertaining to budgetary or programmatic decisions, is the rationale for each fully explained?

5. Are the exposition and organization of the report effective?

6. Is the report fair? Is its tone impartial and devoid of special pleading?

7. Does the Executive Summary concisely and accurately describe the key findings and recommendations? Is it consistent with other sections of the report?

8. What other significant improvements, if any, might be made in the report?

Careful consideration of these questions at the outset of a study may be helpful to the committee in preparing its report and in avoiding subsequent delays in review.

SOURCE: National Academy of Sciences 1993, pp. 4–5. The text above is a verbatim quotation.

If this first answer focuses on persuading the audience, a second, complementary interpretation focuses on controlling the cast. In this view, these accounts help the Academy to create teams of performers who can put on an effective show. Descriptions of procedures not only depict idealized versions of the NRC process for outsiders; they also hold up role models, introducing prospective team members to idealized versions of such characters as "committee member," "sponsor," "reviewer," and "member of the NRC staff." These accounts thus provide guidelines for performers who are assuming these roles, suggesting what identities they should try to project, how they ought to comport themselves, and what they should expect from their teammates.

As an example of how the Academy's official descriptions of the NRC process contribute to impression management, consider *Getting to Know the Committee Process*, a 1996 NAS booklet intended for newly appointed committee members. It begins:

> You have been invited to work on an Academy project and may be wondering exactly what your role is as a committee member. This booklet is a brief introduction to the institution and is designed to give you a sense of the committee process.[83]

Later, it explains:

> Committees are expected to be evenhanded and to examine all evidence dispassionately. Although all interested parties should be heard and their views given serious and respectful consideration, one of the committee's primary roles is to separate fact from opinion, analysis from advocacy. Scientific standards are essential in evaluating all arguments and alternatives.[84]

For prospective committee members, such descriptions outline an identity to emulate, underlining the importance of objectivity to their role. For audiences, these statements provide reassurance that committees will consider diverse views, weigh them fairly, and work in an evenhanded, scientific way to separate fact from opinion. Such accounts thus tell team members how to perform and explain to outsiders why the characters who populate the invisible space inside the Academy can be believed.

Consider another example—this one from a section of the booklet for committees that describes the "*Role* of Staff" (emphasis added):

> Each committee is assisted in its work by highly qualified staff members who facilitate the work of the committee. . . .

Staff help to create the objective atmosphere in which the committee's deliberations take place. In addition, staff are responsible for ensuring that institutional procedures and practices are followed throughout the study, and that the study stays on schedule and within budget.

Staff members assist with many aspects of the report, including research, writing, integrating portions written by others, and providing consistent style and format. However, the conclusions and recommendations are those of the committee. Staff do not insert their personal conclusions or recommendations into the report.[85]

On the face of it, this account describes the division of labor between committee and staff, specifying the boundaries of responsibilities and a hierarchy of authorship. It clearly presents the Academy staff in a supportive role, while spotlighting the committee as star of the show. Staff "assist" the committee and "facilitate" its work. They may help to write or integrate the text, but they do not *author* reports or "insert their personal conclusions or recommendations" into them. Such statements thus assert that committees (with their visible expert credentials), not staff, are the *real* authors of reports—a formulation that is consistent with the Academy's policy of designating "the committee" as the "author of record."[86]

But, as the rather legalistic phrase "author of record" suggests, matters are more complex.[87] In writing of any kind, the designated "author" and the actors that performed the "work" need not match perfectly. (In fact, they need not match at all, as ghostwriters and plagiarists, among others, can attest.) Moreover, Academy reports are collaborative products: committee members, staff, and reviewers may all influence the evolution of the text. Finally, in collaborative writing projects, disagreements often emerge about who has contributed how much. It should come as no surprise, then, that in their offstage remarks, some Academy staffers suggest that the official line emanating from the front office downplays the extent of their influence over the evolution and content of reports.[88] But my point is not the unremarkable observation that there are sometimes discrepancies between the self-perceptions of staffers and the official accounts from the NRC executive office; analogous differences are found in all organizations. The point is that the official descriptions set forth norms of performance that make it inappropriate for staff, in their onstage role, to claim much credit for the content of a report. Put otherwise, these accounts specify the terms of dramaturgical cooperation—not the division of labor—between the committee and the staff. The objectives of the performance require the committee to emerge as the "author" and the staff to appear as a minor character. No matter how a staff member perceives his or her influence, it should remain largely behind the scenes.

As this discussion suggests, the Academy's descriptions of NRC procedures serve the complementary strategic functions of helping both to control performers and to persuade audiences (and, indeed, to achieve the latter in part by achieving the former). Ultimately, the Academy's accounts of its procedures not only constitute an idealized description of the NRC process and of the teams that prepare reports; these accounts also constitute the idealized identity of an objective space—a special institutional space that Academy procedures are intended to construct, a protected space, purged of vested interests, where qualified experts can deliberate privately in an unbiased manner about issues of vital national importance. Like the identities of the team members, the most important aspects of the identity of this space—its independence and objectivity—are enacted through the proper performance of procedures. By releasing descriptions of its procedures but keeping the action backstage, the Academy assures its audiences that they need not—and even that they should not—look behind the curtain.

LEAKS AND UNAUTHORIZED PERFORMANCES:
THE 1985 DRAFT OF THE RDAS

So far, we have analyzed the public performance embodied in *Diet, Nutrition, and Cancer*, examining how the narrative of the report creates a credible and unified voice and how negotiations and contingencies are concealed from public view. We have also considered two senses in which the Academy produces a backstage: by constructing barriers that limit the ability of its audiences to observe, influence, and criticize the process of report production, and by providing official "front-stage" descriptions of its "backstage" activities. Most of the time, these techniques seem to function without major disruptions, as they did with *Diet, Nutrition, and Cancer*. In this case, the Academy successfully presented a dramatic, univocal display of scientific authority, while walling off the private space in which it was prepared. Members of the audience may well wonder about the depth of a consensus or about the exactitude of official descriptions of backstage action, but information that might support alternative accounts is systematically rendered unavailable. However, the 1985 Draft of the Tenth Edition of the

Recommended Dietary Allowances is an unusual exception. In this case, disagreements within the team working to prepare the report became so unmanageable that the Academy's president canceled publication. Not only did the Academy fail to publish a report, but its normal modes of collective information control broke down. As the dispute progressed, participants began to leak internal documents and to talk to journalists about confidential matters, thrusting backstage information into public view. For this reason, the 1985 Draft offers an unusual opportunity to observe a breakdown in stage management. Analyzing how the Academy's system of closure performed under extreme stress provides insight into what this system accomplishes when it operates normally.

A Breakdown of Dramaturgical Cooperation

The Academy's stage-management techniques depend on dramaturgical cooperation among members of the teams who produce its reports. Sustaining a boundary between backstage and front stage requires team members to engage in ongoing collective work to control access to information. They must refrain from discussing their deliberations outside of the inner circle. They must impose the backstage/front-stage division on the many documents that they produce and use. Perhaps most important, they must maintain a theatrical self-consciousness attuned to the performative goals of the group and their roles within it. This is not to say that team members must be of one mind during the entire process of report production: on the contrary, they may disagree about many things without threatening stage management, so long as they continue to cooperate to put on the show, working as a team to keep their audience from observing things that might disrupt the performance.

The Academy's official rules of confidentiality present an idealized version of its system of information management, of course, not a description of its actual operation, and it would be truly astonishing if all team members performed their stage-management responsibilities flawlessly, never departing from their assigned roles.[89] But even given the inevitable contingencies of everyday practice, most teams seem to achieve reasonably tight control over information; the typical NRC report succeeds nicely in presenting a unified public performance and maintaining a relatively impermeable wall that preserves a private deliberative space long after publication.[90] The 1985 Draft is an unusual exception. As the project approached completion, intense controversy developed between the Committee on Dietary Allowances, which had written the draft, and various reviewers and Academy officials who took issue with its recommendations. Amid this increasingly bitter internal dispute, dramaturgical cooperation collapsed. Team members stepped out of their authorized roles, making the controversy public. Documents were leaked; Academy rules of confidentiality were violated; charges and countercharges were made in the media. Rather than collectively working to produce a public display of agreement, the team broke up into factions, which struggled to control how the nutrition community and the public would perceive their disagreements.

I cannot determine exactly when the leaks began, but the debate became a full-fledged public spectacle on September 23, 1985, when the *New York Times*, which had obtained a (previously) confidential draft of the report, published a front-page article on the subject.[91] Two weeks later, on October 7, the Academy announced its decision to cancel the report, and a flurry of controversy followed this news, while the Academy's leadership and the committee that had drafted the report struggled to define what had caused the cancellation and who was to blame. During this conflict, a variety of backstage information escaped containment. The Academy's injunction to limit public comments about unreleased reports went by the wayside: members of the committee and Academy officials alike described to journalists— often in conflicting ways—the nature of the dispute and the reasons the report had been canceled.[92] Participants leaked a number of documents, including not only the draft report but also bits of correspondence among people close to the report. News stories drawing on these statements and disclosures appeared in the *New York Times*, the *Los Angeles Times*, the *Washington Post*, *Time*, and *Science*, among other prominent publications.

Normally, the only published history of the production of an NRC report is the official account presented by the report itself. One of the effects—or better, one of the *goals*—of the Academy's confidentiality procedures is to limit the ability of outsiders to analyze its backstage activities. But in the case of the 1985 Draft, the breakdown in stage management loosened these constraints. The news coverage and leaked documents enabled outsiders to prepare accounts (albeit incomplete ones) of the backstage negotiations behind the report. Drawing on the fragmentary information that the news coverage, leaks, and public statements reveal, I have assembled a schematic—and admittedly incomplete—chronology of the negotiations about the 1985 Draft.[93] In producing this account, I have stripped away most of the contested interpretations in order to provide a relatively even-handed and uncontentious summary of what the available information suggests were the main events.

The 1985 Draft of the RDAs: A Schematic Chronology

1. A draft report is prepared.

   Summer 1980   A nine-member Committee on Dietary Allowances is appointed to revise the RDAs. Funding for the study is provided by the NIH.

   1980–85   The committee works to produce a comprehensive review of recommended nutrient levels based on current scientific evidence.[94] Its draft report suggests changes in the recommended levels of a number of nutrients; these changes included lowering the RDAs for vitamins A and C, and raising the RDA for calcium.[95]

2. The review process begins.

   Early 1985   Reviewers of the draft report suggest a number of changes. They object to the lower levels of vitamins A and C, given the possible role of these nutrients in preventing cancer, and they question the proposed RDA for calcium, which they deem to be too high. The levels of these nutrients is not the only controversial issue; the debate also encompasses the proper role of the RDAs in efforts to combat chronic disease, the place of data on the epidemiology of chronic disease in efforts to set RDAs, and several other matters.[96] Among those who criticize the draft are members of the Food and Nutrition Board (FNB), the committee's parent body. (The membership of the board rotates, so there was no overlap between the membership in 1980, when work on the report began, and 1985, when work was completed.)[97]

   March 18, 1985   One reviewer, D. Mark Hegsted, writes to the chairman of the FNB, Kurt J. Isselbacher, charging that the committee has approached its "task as a purely academic exercise and from a very limited perspective." Hegsted argues that rather than adopting an appropriate public health orientation, the committee has assessed nutrient needs from the narrow viewpoint of the nutritional biochemist. He predicts that publishing the report in its current form will lead to "congressional hearings, full discussion in the media, [and] accusations that the Food and Nutrition Board is either incompetent or insensitive to important issues, etc."[98]

April 1985   The chairman of the committee, Henry Kamin, writes Isselbacher and outlines the committee's response to the reviewers. Kamin reports that the committee has met several times and agreed to make many changes, including explaining its reasoning more fully, adding qualifications, tightening up the text, and lowering the RDA for calcium for postmenopausal women. However, Kamin says, the committee refuses to alter its numerical recommendations for vitamins A and C, contending that changes are unavoidable given its analysis of the scientific data. Kamin predicts that a revised draft will be completed in the coming weeks.

May 23, 1985   Kamin tells an audience in Chapel Hill, North Carolina, that he expects the report to be controversial: "I expect to spend more time, after the publication of the RDA's, ducking rotten tomatoes rather than catching roses."[99]

July 18, 1985   The *Los Angeles Times* reports that the previous week Helen A. Guthrie, a member of the committee, told the annual meeting of the Society for Nutrition Education that "the new RDAs, which should have already been released this month, are still undergoing a review process." Guthrie told the society that there would be a number of changes in the RDAs, but that they would not be announced until September, when the report would be released.[100]

3.   Academy outsiders attack the draft report.

August 13, 1985   Michael R. Lemov of the Food Research and Action Center (FRAC), a nonprofit group, writes Sushma Palmer, executive director of the FNB, asking the Academy to stop release of the proposed report. Lemov—who has somehow learned about the contents of the draft—argues that lowering the RDAs will adversely affect poor and nutritionally vulnerable people, because many organizations use the RDAs to design food assistance programs and diets for institutionalized populations. He calls on the Academy to develop a new, broader committee to review the report. (After the report was canceled, the question of whether such "pressure groups" as FRAC actually influenced the Academy became a controversial issue, to which we shall return in Chapter 4.)[101]

Summer 1985   Ongoing discussions between the reviewers and the Committee fail to settle the dispute. Numerous options are discussed, and some matters are resolved, but debate continues. For a time, the many disputed issues seem to find concrete expression in a more focused controversy about the appropriate levels for vitamins A and C. The Food and Nutrition Board unanimously agrees that the evidence does not justify changing several RDAs, especially those for vitamins A and C. The committee sticks to its original numbers.

4. The NRC chairman presses for a compromise.

August 15, 1985   Frank Press, the NRC's chairman, writes Henry Kamin in a effort to bring the dispute to closure. Academy procedures specify that the NRC chairman is responsible for making a decision when a committee and reviewers cannot reach agreement. Press informs the committee that he has been persuaded by the Food and Nutrition Board that the RDAs for vitamins A and C should not be lowered. He explains that he understands that the only remaining points of contention are the RDAs for those nutrients, and on the assumption that that is the case, he sets forth two options for ending debate:

The first option lays out a specific plan for altering the text. The report would present the points of view of *both* the committee and the Food and Nutrition Board. In the case of vitamin A, the report would include *two numbers*, the committee's number and the old RDA. Vitamin C would be handled the same way. A footnote, for which the Academy provided tentative wording, would explain the origins of the conflicting numbers:

> The two values given for vitamins A and C reflect different approaches to estimating nutrient needs for human health. The rationales for both are presented in Chapters 6 and 7. The lower numbers are those proposed by the present committee; the higher ones for children and adults are the same as those published in 1980. Until the relationship between the intake of these nutrients, health promotion, and disease prevention is better defined, the Food and Nutrition Board of the National Research Council recommends that the higher numbers be used because they confer a greater margin of safety.[102]

Finally, under the first option, Dr. Press would write a cover letter describing the NRC review process to accompany the report. The letter would explain that Press had asked the committee to give two numbers for each disputed nutrient, and that he had done so at the recommendation of the Food and Nutrition Board and the chair of the Commission on Life Sciences.[103]

The second option, which Press describes as an undesirable one, was far simpler: to cancel publication of the report.

5. The committee offers a counterproposal.

September 1985   Kamin writes Press, rejecting the proposed compromise. Kamin says that the committee objects to the proposed footnote, arguing that the phrase "health promotion, and disease prevention" lacks scientific content. He reports that the committee takes exception to the wording in which the Food and Nutrition Board "recommends" a value and the committee "proposes" one, because this wording would, in effect, overrule the committee's number.

Kamin also offers a counterproposal: let the report give a *single* number for vitamin A, the midpoint between the committee's recommendation and the old RDA. And give a single number, also the midpoint, for vitamin C. Kamin further proposes that the text explain the origins of these numbers, clearly stating that they stem from a compromise. The text should include a statement from the committee setting forth its views on vitamins A and C, along with a similar statement by the Food and Nutrition Board, giving its position.

6. The draft is leaked to the news media.

September 23, 1985   The *New York Times* publishes a front-page story that quotes from a leaked copy of the draft report. The article, which includes a table comparing the existing and "proposed" RDAs, begins:

> In a move with broad implications for American eating habits and food assistance programs, a committee of the National Academy of Sciences has drafted a report calling for lower recommended levels of some vitamins and minerals needed to maintain health. The authors of the report said that it was based on the best available scientific data. But some nutrition experts, including people asked by the academy to read the report as part of its internal review process, expressed concern. They said the report on the Government's recommended dietary allowances could be used by officials to justify further cuts in food stamps, school lunch subsidies and other feeding programs.[104]

Additional media coverage follows.

September 25, 1985   The Academy holds a "special, by-invitation-only meeting on the future of RDA's." At the meeting, Representatives of FRAC and other activists urge the Academy to obtain

comments from a broad-based group of scientists and
nonscientists on the RDAs.[105]

September 28, 1985   *Science News* reports that: "Committee chair
Henry Kamin, a professor of biochemistry of Duke University, in
Durham, N.C., refused this week to confirm or deny the allowance figures attributed to the committee report by the newspaper
[the *New York Times*]. He told *Science News* that the report,
scheduled for completion in November, is still in the Academy's
standard review process." Kurt J. Isselbacher, chair of the Food
and Nutrition Board, calls controversy over the report "premature," saying that "there is no final report yet, and all the
allowances are still under discussion."[106]

7. The Academy cancels publication.

October 7, 1985   The Academy's president, Frank Press, and Kurt J.
Isselbacher, chair of the Food and Nutrition Board, meet with
James Wyngaarden, the director of the National Institutes of
Health, to explain that the Academy will not publish the report.
In a public letter to Wyngaarden (excerpts of which are quoted
in media coverage), Press announces that the committee and the
reviewers have reached an "impasse."

> Despite months of discussion and deliberation, the committee and
> the reviewers were unable to agree on the interpretation of scientific
> data on several of the nutrients and consequently on RDAs for those
> nutrients. . . . Differences of opinion among committee members
> and reviewers extended to such issues as the appropriate data base
> for developing the RDAs, the adequate size of body stores for specific
> nutrients, and the advisability of modifying the definition of the RDAs.
> All these points of contention led to different conclusions about the
> allowance levels, which were reflected in a succession of drafts
> prepared in an unsuccessful attempt to reach consensus.[107]

8. Controversy continues.

October 1985–January 1986   Following cancellation of the report,
the controversy continues in the mass media, in letters to scientific
journals, and in private correspondence (some of which is leaked
soon after it is written). The media coverage conveys the impression of bitter infighting among people close to the report. For
example, the *New York Times* calls the dispute "an irreconcilable
conflict," and the *Washington Post* reports that the report "has
been postponed repeatedly because of disagreement between the
scientific panel and its independent reviewers."[108] Rather than

A Polyvocal Public Display

KURT J. ISSELBACHER (chairman, FNB): "I can assure you that neither the Kamin committee nor the Academy was influenced by pressure groups."[a]

ROBERT E. OLSON (former member, FNB): "The action of Frank Press, president of the National Academy of Sciences, to reject and suppress publication . . . is unprecedented, arbitrary and unwise. . . . No scientific arguments have been advanced against the facts or logic used by Dr. Henry Kamin's committee in arriving at the 1985 allowances."[b]

FRANK PRESS (NRC chairman): "Dr. Robert E. Olson's letter concerning my recent action on the 10th edition of the recommended dietary allowances ignores the single most important factor in my decision not to issue a report at this time. My decision was based on advice from scientific reviewers, including members of our food and nutrition board, which oversees the preparation of the R.D.A.'s, members of the National Academy of Sciences and other nutrition experts as competent as the panel that drafted the report."[c]

SUSHMA PALMER (executive director, FNB): "We were unable to resolve scientific differences."[d]

HELEN A. GUTHRIE (member, RDA committee): "The anonymous review committee had some recommendations for modification. We agreed on everything but vitamins A and C. We simply couldn't reach agreement on these two nutrients or they did not accept our compromise. So they decided not to publish anything at all."[d]

a unified and univocal performance, the media coverage depicts a multivocal controversy featuring disagreement not only about what levels of nutrients should be recommended but also about why the report was canceled, whether pressure groups had influenced the Academy, and whether a compromise might have been possible (see the accompanying text box).

9. The Academy initiates a new RDA study.
    June 1987   A new panel, a subcommittee of the Food and Nutrition

HENRY KAMIN (chairman, RDA committee): "If you ask me, the real issue is not with A and C. . . . The academy rejected the report because they feared controversy. They panicked. The whole thing is bizarre and represents a misunderstanding and a collapse to social pressures. The issues are not issues of science."[d]

JAMES A. OLSON (vice-chairman, RDA committee): "The scientific basis for lowering the vitamins is that previous recommendations were based on certain assumptions we no longer feel are valid."[d]

KAMIN: "We were not terribly far apart. I can't think that anyone would think no progress was being made. The academy may well deny it, but I think they were afraid that our results would be controversial. . . . It makes me very angry. I think this is a poor way of doing science."[e]

PALMER: "The reason for not issuing a report is scientific. The academy has nothing to gain or lose. We're a scientific organization, not a political one."[d]

KAMIN: "[The failure of the Academy to provide concrete reasons for rejecting the report] led me to think that they might not have even read the document . . . and that there is enormous confusion and incompetence at the National Academy of Sciences."[d]

SOURCES:
[a] Eliot Marshall, "The Academy Kills a Nutrition Report," *Science*, Oct. 15, 1985, p. 421.
[b] Robert E. Olson, letter to the editor, *New York Times*, Oct. 26, 1985, p. 26.
[c] Frank Press, letter to the editor, *New York Times*, Nov. 9, 1985, p. 26.
[d] Rose Dosti, "Requirements for Vitamins A and C Disputed," *Los Angeles Times*, Oct. 31, 1985, p. 33
[e] Warren E. Leary, "Academy of Sciences Says It Won't Release Nutrition Findings," Associated Press, Oct. 7, 1985

Board, begins work to prepare a revised edition of the RDAs. The 1985 Draft serves as a starting point for the new committee.
October 1989   The Academy publishes the tenth edition of the RDAs. The panel that wrote the 1985 Draft is acknowledged in the preface.[109]

Let us stop the clock at this point. We could go on to describe the lawsuit that Victor Herbert, one of the members of 1985 RDA committee, filed against the Academy for copyright infringement in 1990. (Herbert alleged that the Academy had appropriated some of his writings, which he had drafted as a member of the committee, including them without permission in the revised RDAs published in 1989. The federal courts ruled against Herbert.)[110] But the chronology laid out above—*if* we can trust it—tells us a good bit about the backstage negotiations surrounding the 1985 Draft. What a different account this chronology gives us about these negotiations from the one *Diet, Nutrition, and Cancer* reveals about its own history! How much more detail this sketchy chronology—even with its many gaps—provides about the world of the backstage! Instead of the invisible but objective world described in official Academy publications, the chronology reveals fragments of a disorderly and contentious process. We see disputes about the interpretation of evidence, charges of incompetence, and accusations of caving in to vested interests. We see intractable conflict between committees and reviewers. We see an effort to reach a compromise that looks less like a candid exchange of scientific views than like hardball bargaining and brinkmanship. In short, the chronology presents an account of the closed space of Academy deliberations that is radically different from that depicted in the institution's official statements. Viewed in this light, the Academy's official accounts of the backstage appear to offer a misleading gloss on a set of stories that are much more interesting and complex.

But before we conclude that the above chronology provides a behind-the-scenes look at the negotiations surrounding Academy reports, before we conclude that we have finally seen the backstage, we should reflect on an important issue: to what extent can we consider this chronology a credible account of the negotiations surrounding the 1985 Draft and the backstage world of the Academy? Even though the chronology offers fascinating details, we know that it is based on sources that provide incomplete and inconsistent evidence and interpretations. Moreover, the gaps in those sources do not appear in random places. Like the documentary record of the Iran-Contra hearings analyzed by Michael Lynch and David Bogen, the news accounts and leaked documents do not constitute a collection of evidence that is somehow "above" the controversy and is therefore capable of providing independent insight into the objective facts about it.[111] On the contrary, the controversy *produced* the record—but not as a mere residue of documents that simply accumulated. Instead, a struggle to shape the public record was an integral part of the action. The collapse of dramaturgical cooperation prevented the normal NRC process from containing negotiation backstage, and rather than working together to stage a unified report, the team split into factions that battled to control the public presentation of the dispute. Thus, the Academy leadership, as the box on p. 78 shows, argued that it canceled the report for "scientific" reasons, whereas the committee blamed pressure group politics for this outcome. Leaks—and other disclosures about activities that the Academy's confidentiality procedures normally keep backstage—became a central means of conducting this battle.[112] The protagonists in the dispute selectively released bits of once-confidential information, providing the news media with material to incorporate into public accounts of the debate over the report. Thus, the record of the dispute, and the gaps that remain in it, took shape as the competing protagonists issued strategically crafted statements and disclosed carefully selected details to journalists and other Academy outsiders. In short, the news coverage and the leaks were the upshot of a struggle about how the "backstage" action would be represented on the "front stage," and this contest shaped both the record underlying the chronology and the gaps in it. (We shall return to this struggle to "emplot" the cancellation of the 1985 Draft in Chapter 4.)

These problems, of course, are not unique to this chronology or this episode; all histories, as Lynch and Bogen point out, are profoundly shaped by the efforts of the participants to control the documentary record and thereby influence what can be known and said about them.[113] But the central point is not only that the chronology above—like all historical accounts—emerged via a complex social process in which the protagonists of history worked to shape perceptions of the events that they enacted. The point is that the Academy's techniques of stage management shape what audiences can observe even when (as we can now see) they *partially* fail. Even in cases where leaks bring accounts of the backstage into public view, analysts and audiences can only acquire the most limited and contestable information. The above chronology is a case in point. Not only are there reasons to harbor doubts about its accuracy and completeness, but even if one were to grant that it provides useful details about the history of the 1985 Draft, one must recognize that the negotiations surrounding most Academy reports are almost certainly more collegial, less protracted, and more successful. Information about Academy deliberations is contained, not only by procedures of confidentiality, but also by the logic of a situation in which any revelations that emerge during controversial episodes remain arguably of dubious relevance to more "normal" backstage action. Even when information leaks out, the Academy retains the epistemological high ground with respect to knowledge about its inner workings.

Unauthorized Performances

Analysts who wish to examine the negotiations surrounding Academy reports can only observe incomplete and potentially misleading accounts, such as official Academy descriptions of the NRC process or the unauthorized disclosures that emerge when dramaturgical cooperation breaks down. But even if the Academy's techniques of information control prevent us from obtaining satisfactory information about the backstage, the case of 1985 Draft tells us much about the role of stage-management practices in creating authorized voices that speak with scientific authority on the front stage. To present a univocal performance, a team must contain its differences, enclosing them spatially, socially, and textually so that audiences cannot observe them. In the case of the 1985 Draft, the Academy lost its ability to manage the stage tightly, and leaks and unauthorized disclosures propelled open displays of conflict into the nation's leading newspapers. Rather than a carefully controlled drama of unity, the episode produced an unpresentable "succession of drafts" and a polyvocal public spectacle.

The transformation of the 1985 Draft into an unpublished "nonreport" underlines the potential fragility of the negotiations that (if they succeed) create what ultimately becomes the final *text* of the report, while simultaneously assembling the network that becomes, in a sense, its *author*. The two aspects of these negotiations—doing the "text work" and building this network—are inextricably linked, and for an advisory report to emerge, they must reach a common solution.[114] Until the final "sign-off" authorizes its release, the report—an evolving assemblage of text and author—can in principle still break apart, failing to agree about what "it" should say; the multiple, conflicting texts, the "succession of drafts" may never converge into a single, final version. In the case of the 1985 Draft, the negotiations failed and the planned assemblage fragmented. (We cannot see into precisely how many pieces it broke. Committees tend to gain solidarity around their reports, and they may end up perceiving the reviewers as "the enemy"; however, at times, individual committee members who are unhappy with a draft report may attempt to use the review process to reopen issues.) The link between the committee and the Academy was formally severed; what had once been the "Committee on Dietary Allowances NRC-NAS" began to refer to itself as the "1980–85 RDA Committee"; and the text was condemned forever to remain a draft, since without the Academy's authorization, a committee can only produce a manuscript, not author a report. "Reports," an Academy brochure explains, "are the product of the institution, not of the committee alone."[115] The director of the National Institutes of Health, which had commissioned the 1985 Draft, concurred, saying that the NIH cannot accept an NRC report that lacks the Academy's endorsement and approval.[116] Thus, in the case of the 1985 Draft, the text, instead of being made to speak with one voice, fell apart and was rendered mute. The team that attempted to prepare the report, instead of being united behind (and by) the text, split into factions that ended up blaming each other for the report's demise. No authorized report emerged and unauthorized performances produced a public display of disunity.

CONCLUSIONS

The Academy's stage-management practices are central to the process through which it produces credible science advice. This chapter has used the dramaturgical perspective to examine the means of information control that the Academy uses to construct authoritative reports. The analysis explores the role of stage management in producing an authorized voice that can speak with scientific authority. The Academy's regime of information control is designed to achieve a strict separation between the roles of performer and audience, creating a theater of scientific authority based on limited audience participation.

Our analysis of *Diet, Nutrition, and Cancer* illustrates how this system of stage management operates. As a performance, this report is carefully packaged in a way that allows the audience to view only part of the activities that produced it. The Academy's procedures for preparing reports establish a set of spatial, temporal, and social barriers to divide the process into front stage and backstage. The official performance is spatially packaged between the covers of a book. This neatly bounded object presents the univocal narrative depicted by Figure 1, but other spaces associated with the report cannot be directly observed by the reader. Stage management allows the Academy to constrain what its audiences can perceive, suppressing details about backstage deliberations that observers might use to fashion alternative accounts. The polyvocal world of frank discussion and evolving drafts is thus enclosed, making the official, univocal narrative harder to challenge for lack of information. At the same time, the Academy's official accounts of the backstage—which it presents as an objective space, purged of vested interests, from which truth can emerge—reinforce the front-stage performance.

Of course, no system for enclosing information is immune to unauthorized disclosures, and, as we have seen above, Academy insiders and others sometimes breach the social, spatial, and temporal boundaries that regulate access to the backstage. In the case of *Diet, Nutrition, and Cancer*, the Academy managed to prepare a report, to create an authorized voice, to maintain dramaturgical cooperation, and to construct an invisible backstage that audiences could only "access" through tightly regulated, official accounts. In the case of the 1985 Draft, however, the Academy achieved none of these things. Negotiations broke down, and no report was published, no author emerged, and a collapse of dramaturgical cooperation led to confidential documents and information that normally would be contained being widely circulated. In their efforts to prosecute their divergent points of view, the protagonists in the dispute selectively released bits of information from the officially private backstage, providing the news media with material from which to fashion public accounts of the debate over the "controversial report." The breakdown in stage management prevented the Academy from staging a single, univocal performance—such as *Diet, Nutrition, and Cancer*—that enacted a drama of unity and credibility. Instead, the upshot of the struggle was a confusing collection of conflicting statements.

Most of the time, the Academy's process for producing reports is more successful—although critics of the NRC on occasion charge that this process sometimes produces only the most watered-down "consensus" statements.[117] But when the negotiations are successful (as they were in the case of *Diet, Nutrition, and Cancer*), when a report is "finalized," when the last team members sign off on the ultimate draft, the author *and* the text simultaneously solidify. The report finds its voice and at the same time defines the author(iz)ing network that stands behind its voice. The credibility of this network, dramatically displayed in a narrative that draws together many sources of scientific authority (Fig. 1), is reinforced by modes of information control that sequester contingency and negotiation backstage, thus restricting the ability of audiences to produce their own alternative accounts of the process of report production.

By applying these techniques and working to build a report that presents the narrative summarized in Figure 1, the teams that prepare reports enact what one might call the basic drama of Academy advice: a performance about how a committee of experts, appropriately selected by the prestigious National Academy, entered a special institutional space—carefully insulated from the contaminating influences of interested audiences—where experts can partake in a "candid exchange of views" and "vigorous internal debate"; a story of how these experts reviewed the literature, collected testimony, weighed the evidence, and wrote a report that withstood rigorous peer review; a story of why the reader should consider the report to make a credible claim to the cultural authority of science. A rhetoric of procedures and techniques for shaping what audiences can witness helps to underwrite this story, restricting the gaze of the audience, and, at the same time, presenting sanitized accounts of the hidden action that the audience cannot directly see. In these ways, the Academy presents itself as a trustworthy and objective advisor, leaving contingency backstage and allowing its reports and recommendations to emerge as fully formed, unified performances.

CHAPTER 3

Attacking Advisory Reports

Advisory reports cast themselves as embodying a narrative of scientific authority, and to reinforce this impression, they control information that might bring contingencies into view and display the backstage as a place of objectivity. But audiences need not accept these performances uncritically. Officials and publics, who do not always find these dramas moving, may respond with indifference or skepticism. Reports may encounter suspicious readers, who pour over their texts, searching between the lines for hints of backstage controversy, clues about compromises, signs that conclusions have been watered down. Moreover, in controversial areas, well-organized critics — who seek to present reports in a new, unflattering light — often step onto the stage. How do these critics package their messages for public display? How do they manage the delicate problem of challenging prestigious science advisors, such as the Academy, without discrediting themselves? And under what circumstances do the critics succeed in upstaging a report's performance and stealing the show?

This chapter uses a dramaturgical perspective to undertake an analysis of the critical reception of science advice. During polarized controversies, reports often face adversaries who seek to produce as damaging a critique as possible (within the limits imposed by the situation).[1] These critics — whether individuals or organizations — are likely to be familiar with a range of rhetoric useful for dramatizing and deconstructing cultural authority; many are seasoned "operatives," experienced in the ways of mass media and Washington and equipped with significant resources, such as skilled political professionals.[2] For such critics, challenging a report is a creative endeavor in which they assess what kind of attack they can convincingly "pull off." Their comments, whether embodied in text or delivered in live interaction, constitute performances, in which they strike poses and make arguments with an audience in mind, subject to the constraints and opportunities that flow from the materials at hand.[3] Although the elements of convincing performances are complex and contextually specific, there are clearly some minimal requirements for successfully creating a situation in which the critic of an advisory report can score a valid point. The critic must present a credible persona, must convincingly render the report as deficient in some consequential way, and must meet these requirements on a stage already occupied by other performers (such as the team that produced the report), who may or may not choose to respond.

To analyze these performative contests between advisors and critics, this chapter compares the strategies that critics used to attack *Diet, Nutrition, and Cancer*, the 1982 report examined in Chapter 2, and *Toward Healthful Diets*, the short report questioning the scientific basis of recently issued advice on diet and chronic disease that the Food and Nutrition Board prepared in 1980.[4] As one might expect in the contentious world of diet and health recommendations, neither report was greeted with a uniform response. In keeping with its authors' intent, some observers presented *Toward Healthful Diets* as an authoritative debunking of much of the nutrition reformers' advice, especially regarding cholesterol, fats, and heart disease.[5] More often, observers framed the report as evidence that the "last word" on diet and heart disease was not yet in.[6] Likewise, many actors treated *Diet, Nutrition, and Cancer* as an authoritative, credible account. Many observers repeated the report's recommendations without critical comment, and some health advocates incorporated them into anticancer meal plans and recipes.[7] Among policymakers and in the research community, *Diet, Nutrition, and Cancer* played a significant role in consolidating interest in using diet to prevent cancer.[8]

But each report also became the focus of dispute. Proponents of dietary change relentlessly attacked *Toward Healthful Diets*, and the mass media by and large treated it as controversial.[9] Its publication provoked the Food and Nutrition Board's Consumer Liaison Panel to sever relations with the board in protest, and the report became the topic of two congressional hearings.[10] Commenting on *Diet, Nutrition, and Cancer* grew into a small industry. Meat and dairy groups, in particular, objected to its recommendations. Reports *on* the report were prepared by two cabinet-level federal agencies (the DHHS and the USDA); by the Congressional Research Service; by the Council for Agricultural Science and Technology (CAST); and by an epidemiological consulting firm hired by two meat industry groups.[11] Several of these reports, especially those of CAST and the USDA, criticized aspects of *Diet, Nutrition, and Cancer.* Finally, the General Accounting Office prepared a report entitled *National Academy of Sciences' Reports on Diet and Health — Are They Credible and Consistent?* that looked at both *Toward Healthful Diets* and *Diet, Nutrition, and Cancer.*[12] As we shall see, the critics of *Toward Healthful Diets* did much more damage to that report's claims to authority than did the critics of *Diet, Nutrition, and Cancer.* After examining how critics challenged each report, the chapter compares their attacks and analyzes the conditions that account for this outcome.

ATTACKING "TOWARD HEALTHFUL DIETS"

As advisory reports go, *Toward Healthful Diets* was a low-budget production, prepared for only $10,000 and just 24 pages long. In contrast, *Diet, Nutrition, and Cancer* cost about $1 million and took 478 pages. Yet despite these differences, the two reports used similar performative techniques to stake their claims to cultural authority. Like *Diet, Nutrition, and Cancer, Toward Healthful Diets* cast itself as the result of an objective, rational process of expert deliberation, creating a show in which many actors appeared to speak in unison. Any disagreements and negotiations that might disrupt the public performance were relegated to an invisible backstage region. At the same time, the Academy's generic accounts of its orderly, rule-governed procedures helped bolster the authority of the reports. But the proponents of dietary change did not accept this story passively; they attacked the report in news media and in congressional hearings. And they were anything but timid. Drawing on leaks to the media that exposed troubling details about the activities backstage, the critics harshly denounced the report.

Reconcentrating Distributed Authorship

Academy reports are supposed to reflect the objective and considered judgments of qualified scientists *in general*, not represent the narrow views of idiosyncratic individuals or groups. The credibility of advisory reports stems from the network over which authorship of the claims they contain is distributed (see Fig. 1). Thus, one strategy that critics of *Toward Healthful Diets* used to attack the report was to reconcentrate authorship by retelling the story of what went on backstage. An article by Daniel S. Greenberg, a long-time observer of science policy and the editor of *Science &*

Government Report, a Washington-based newsletter, provides an example.[13] Using the investigative reporter's technique of delving into the story behind the story, Greenberg gathered a set of resources that allowed him to contradict the report's narrative. He drove a wedge between the NAS, a "venerable institution that, in effect, serves as the nation's supreme court of science," and the "small group in the academy" that wrote the report. To "the astonishment and dismay of many people in and around the Academy," this small group "cunningly dropped [the report] on the public."[14] He proceeded to concentrate authorship even further. The report was

> produced by the organization's Food and Nutrition Board, a voluntary, 15-member group that is among the 800 or so boards, committees and panels through which the academy carries out its advisory duties. With membership determined within the academy — there's no accountability to outside authorities — the food board, like many expense-paid-trip-to-Washington committees, tends to be dominated by a few members who pay close attention, while the rest defer to their energy and specialized knowledge.[15]

Narrowing authorship still further, Greenberg identified Alfred E. Harper and Robert E. Olson as the "key figures" in preparing the report and went on to say: "One board member told me in a telephone interview, 'I just wasn't paying as much attention as I should have. I left it to the others.' "[16]

By using interviews to "reach" backstage, Greenberg thus shifted the locus of authorship from a distributed network of actors (such as that shown in Fig. 1) first to a "small group in the academy," then to a "15-member group," then to "a few members who pay close attention," and finally to two "key figures."[17] In a few deft moves, Greenberg created a new story in which the team that produced the report no longer spoke with a unitary voice. The voice of the report — really the voice of two "key figures" — was created through cunning manipulation of a voluntary group that was not paying sufficient attention. The report only appeared to speak for the entire network; actually, some team members had, in effect, been silenced.

Attacking the Committee's Composition

Not only did critics reconcentrate authorship, they also redefined the key characters in the report's story. Consider the "the Food and Nutrition Board." The report casts the board as the voice of scientific expertise: its main role is to state which dietary recommendations rest on a "sound scientific foundation."[18] But critics defined the board as lacking relevant expertise, repeatedly pointing out that there were no epidemiologists or cardiologists on the committee.[19] For example, at a news conference held by the Chicago Heart Association, Dr. Jeremiah Stamler, chair of the American College of Cardiology's committee on prevention of cardiovascular diseases, argued that the board fundamentally misunderstood the methodology of biomedical science:

> I'm sure most of you are aware that one of . . . [the report's] key authors, Dr. Olson from St. Louis, on television yesterday stated that the report was based on a review that excluded the epidemiological literature. Now anybody who knows the scientific process realizes that research tackling a tough disease problem must bring to bear every weapon that medicine has to offer in its research armamentarium . . . including the epidemiologic method, the animal experimental method, the clinical investigative method, the autopsy method. . . . Thus, to ignore the facts about the population distribution of disease is a gross scientific error. . . .
>
> Dr. Olson, in saying that he ignored the epidemiological data is testifying to his ignorance. I say this to you publicly and for quotation. I regret to say that about a colleague, but it needs to be said.[20]

Critics also defined the board as unbalanced, consisting of scientists who represented marginal, rather than mainstream, views. James S. Turner, chair of the Consumer Liaison Panel that resigned to protest the report, wrote in a letter to the Academy's president, Philip Handler, which was made public:

> We can only conclude that the Board is dominated by a group of change-resistant nutrition scientists who share a rather isolated view about diet and disease. This perspective is maintained through the Board's self-perpetuating election process whereby current members elect new members and can insure that its attitudes will not be challenged.[21]

Greenberg made similar charges:

> Though the academy piously states that those who prepare its reports are chosen "with regard for an appropriate balance," no one associated with the scientifically dominant view that a link does exist [between cholesterol, fat, and heart disease] was included on the committee.[22]

Attacking the Report's Representation of Scientific Knowledge

Following another line of attack, critics tried to break the links between the report and current scientific knowledge. The report was frequently taken to task for ignoring epidemiologic evidence, and critics also identified many other putative deficiencies in the interpretation of evidence.[23] The Center for Science in the Public Interest (CSPI), a consumer group, charged that the report's "arguments against lower fat diets suffer from omission of important facts, misrepresentation of research findings, and an unattainable and inconsistently applied standard for evaluating the evidence at hand."[24] CSPI elaborated that the report "ignores a wealth of knowledge gleaned from experimental studies with laboratory animals" and that it "overlooked" important research on humans, such as studies of migrating populations.[25] Charges that the report misrepresented the degree of scientific uncertainty were also prevalent, especially concerning the link between heart disease and diets high in fats and cholesterol. Critics also commented on the small size of the report; it was a "brief report,"[26] a "20-page polemic, decked out as a scientific statement."[27] The implication, clearly, was that such a short document could not adequately represent the literature.

Attacking Academy Procedures

Critics also attacked the Academy procedures used to prepare *Toward Healthful Diets*, arguing that the institution had failed to follow its usual methods for constituting well-balanced committees.[28] Critics assailed the review process, charging it was conducted in an "irresponsible manner."[29]

> Two of the three outside scientists chosen to review the report are not atherosclerosis experts. The third is a vocal proponent of the view that diet should not be changed to reduce the risk of heart disease. His work was heavily cited in the report.[30]

Adding New Characters

In their most dramatic move, critics of *Toward Healthful Diets* pulled off a surprising twist in the plot: they added new characters to the story of the report — the meat, egg, and dairy industries — and thus transformed a tale of disinterested science into a story of conflict of interest. The news media revealed that several members of the Food and Nutrition Board had received funding or consulting fees from the dairy industry, from the nation's largest cheese manufacturer, and from the Egg Board, a commodity group within the USDA.[31] As one headline put it, "Food Firms Helped Fund Diet Report: Scientists Had Financial Ties with Industries."[32]

A variety of critics pounded home the conflict-of-interest theme. "The board and some of its members have been funded by food companies whose sales might suffer from large-scale changes in eating habits, so the appearances are not right," the *New York Times* declared.[33] "Representative Fred Richmond of New York, chairman of the House Agriculture Subcommittee on Domestic Marketing, Consumer Relations and Nutrition, even suggested that lobbyists for the food industry — particularly meat, dairy and egg producers — 'must have been at work here,' " *Time* magazine observed.[34] Writing in *Science*, William Broad reported that Michael Jacobson of the Center for Science in the Public Interest had said that the board included two "food company executives" and several "paid consultants of the food industry," adding: "Jacobson notes that the NAS diet report was financed by funds paid to the NAS by the 80 food companies represented on the board's Industry Liaison Panel."[35]

Samuel S. Epstein, M.D., a professor at the University of Illinois Medical Center, wrote in a letter to the *New York Times*:

> Skepticism of the report in part expresses general recognition that the membership of the Food and Nutrition Board reflects persisting and generally undisclosed special interests. Dr. Harper, chairman of the N.A.S. panel, consults for Kraft, the meat industry and others. Dr. Robert Olson, author of the heart-disease section of the report, is a consultant to the egg, dairy and other food industries.[36]

Often the conflict of interest charges were presented not as an assertion but in the form of a question: had improper influence occurred? An exchange at a news conference held by the Chicago Heart Association provides an example:

> REPORTER: Dr. Stamler, in your view, what's really behind this report, what are the real motives?
> DR. STAMLER: In this area I do not like to talk about views. First of all, like you, I possess no scientific instrument which measures sincerity or motivation, therefore I can't comment on that aspect. The only living thing I can deal with is objective facts. The *New York Times* article by Jane Brody, a very responsible and able science writer, noted that this report was immediately greeted by spokesmen for the egg, meat, and dairy industries. That's in yesterday's *New York Times* as a stated fact. Whether there's any relationship between what the Food and Nutrition Board did and special private interests, I have no way of knowing, but I think it's a valid question.[37]

By adding new characters to the story, critics raised the question of whether the food industry was implicitly one of the authors of the report, thereby undermining its objectivity. They thus suggested that the backstage world of the Academy — at least in this case — might not be a space for disinterested deliberation but a site for influence peddling.

Rewriting the Story: Transforming the Plot

If we consider the panorama of charges that various critics of *Toward Healthful Diets* made in light of Figure 1, we see that attacks were aimed, with almost systematic precision, at all of the main nodes and links of the narrative that advisory reports use to claim cultural authority. Obviously, not everyone who challenged *Toward Healthful Diets* endorsed all of these charges; in particular, some distanced themselves from the charges of industry influence.[38] However, viewed as a whole, these charges formed a coherent *package* that constituted a searing attack on the report's self-presentation. By concentrating authorship, by questioning the review process and appointment procedures, by charging that the report inadequately covered the literature, by adding new, unauthorized characters to the story, critics radically rewrote the report's story of what had happened backstage. In effect, the critics aimed to transfer authorship of the report from a network like the one in Figure 1 to a new network — an assemblage composed, not of "scientific entities," such as experts, evidence, and disinterested inquiry, but of "political" ones, such as philosophical and financial biases, omissions, poor procedures, and conflicts of interest (Fig. 4). According to the critics, *Toward Healthful Diets* only appeared to be true to the narrative it publicly displayed. The report merely posed as legitimate science advice: in reality it was a masquerade, a political polemic "decked out" (in Greenberg's words) as a scientific statement.[39]

Of course, the critics who built this counternarrative were not unopposed; the report had allies as well as enemies. *Toward Healthful Diets* was welcomed by the meat and dairy industries, who praised it as an example of "sound science."[40] The Food and Nutrition Board vigorously defended itself, reasserting its scientific identity, and charging the critics with injecting politics into science.[41] To the suggestion that the report was based on an incomplete review of the literature, the board replied that it had in fact reviewed 400 references on diet and heart disease, although it had chosen not to cite most of them.[42] The board's chair, Alfred E. Harper, countered the charges of industry influence, saying that scientists "value their scientific prestige more highly than their consulting dollars."[43] Philip Handler, the Academy's president, appeared twice on Capitol Hill to defend the report and the integrity and "impressive and impeccable" credentials of the Food

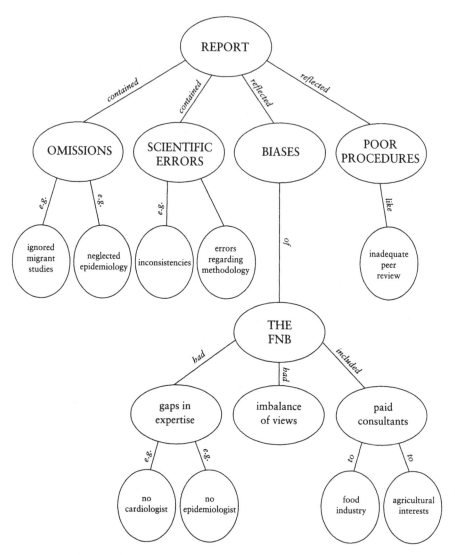

FIGURE 4. The Critics' Counternarrative

and Nutrition Board.[44] A column in the *Wall Street Journal* suggested that the hearings held by Representative Fred Richmond, one of the report's harshest critics, were an attempt "to take a respectable scientific and medical dispute and turn it into a scandal hunt."[45]

Even so, in this climate of leaks and innuendo, the Academy's public defense of the report openly exposed matters that, from the point of view of enacting a compelling performance, might better have been left backstage. At the congressional hearings, a confusing story emerged about how the USDA had originally planned to commission the Food and Nutrition Board to conduct a more comprehensive study of dietary guidelines for the U.S. population. However, believing the board to be biased against nutrition reform, the Consumer Liaison Panel apparently urged USDA officials to halt the study or take steps to guarantee balance and involve consumers.[46] After the USDA abruptly withdrew its promise of financial support, Handler explained, the board decided to undertake on its own initiative the low-budget effort that produced *Toward Healthful Diets*. To conduct this small-scale study, the board appointed a panel from its own membership. But because the board was already in place, no event triggered the usual Academy procedures for scrutinizing its committees. The Academy therefore did not reexamine the panel to ensure that it was suitable for its new task, and no new checks for balance or reviews of potential sources of bias were performed. This "previously unrecognized gap" in Academy procedures, Handler conceded, contributed to an "*appearance* of conflict" of interest. (He stressed that "appearances, and only appearances, have been offended in this instance.") Handler also said that in hindsight he might have added to the panel "an ardent proponent of cholesterol avoidance" or an epidemiologist or biostatistician.[47] To some extent, these explanations reinforced an impression that critics sought to foster: that *Toward Healthful Diets* had been improperly prepared.

Overall, the critics of *Toward Healthful Diets* were quite successful, and they severely damaged the report's credibility. The public spectacle following its release left in its wake two conflicting representations of the report: one version — the report's original performance — matched the standard narrative of science advice (Fig. 1), the other presented the critics' rewritten version of the story (Fig. 4). Both of these versions of the story circulated during the broader public debate over diet and health. The critics' counternarrative did not gain complete hegemony, but it was picked up in the media and widely disseminated. The report became indelibly marked with the adjective "controversial," which significantly tarnished its image of authority.

ATTACKING "DIET, NUTRITION, AND CANCER"

Why did the critics of *Toward Healthful Diets* enjoy this degree of success? Before considering this question, let us look at the case of *Diet, Nutrition, and Cancer*. This report, as we shall see presently, suffered much less damage at the hands of its critics after its publication in 1982. Because the attacks on *Diet, Nutrition, and Cancer* enjoyed relatively limited success, they are of considerable interest for purposes of comparative analysis. How, then, did critics challenge *Diet, Nutrition, and Cancer*? Were their strategies and arguments structurally similar to those that critics used on *Toward Healthful Diets*? Did they try to rewrite the story of the cancer report completely? Or did they gravitate toward other lines of attack?

Attacking the Committee's Composition

Just as critics charged that the committee that prepared *Toward Healthful Diets* had omitted key disciplines, so too some critics of *Diet, Nutrition, and Cancer* charged that it failed to represent pertinent areas of expertise. But while the critics in each case made structurally similar arguments, the dramatic force of the attacks differed. Critics of *Toward Healthful Diets* faulted the Food and Nutrition Board for neglecting "core" areas of biomedicine, such as epidemiology and cardiology. In contrast, most critics of *Diet, Nutrition, and Cancer* pointed to weakness in "applied" areas closely linked to agriculture and food production, rather than in "core" areas of biomedical science. The importance of these putative gaps in expertise may not have been transparently obvious to audiences. Critics of the cancer report therefore faced the burden of persuading people that these gaps mattered.

In its official review of the report, the USDA wrote that the committee lacked expertise in "food technology, animal science or dietary guidance,"[48] leading it to neglect how differences in food-processing techniques, which vary greatly among countries, can produce variations in the chemical composition of similar foods. A properly constituted committee, the USDA suggested, would have recognized that epidemiological data collected in foreign countries might not apply to the United States: "Lack of attention to the details of processing in countries where the cancer incidence is elevated, and even to the kinds of food involved, has implicated erroneously a wide variety of wholesome foods. These include pickled vegetables such as sauerkraut and cucumbers as well as cured and smoked meat."[49]

Meat industry groups made similar arguments, charging that the report's advice to minimize consumption of smoked and pickled foods unfairly indicted American products, such as hot dogs and bacon, that were prepared in ways completely different from the methods used in the countries studied.[50]

Beyond noting the lack of food technology, animal science, and dietary guidance experts, few critics questioned the committee's expertise. Robert E. Olson (of *Toward Healthful Diets*) was an exception, and he attacked the committee aggressively.

> As regards the composition of the 13-member Committee on Diet, Nutrition, and Cancer, . . . four identified themselves with the subject of nutrition (Campbell, Gussow, Kritchevsky, and Mertz) but only one (Campbell) of these admitted any involvement in research activities relating diet to carcinogenesis; two were cancer epidemiologists (Kolonel and Miller); four were molecular biologists (Cairns, Prival, Slaga, and Wattenburg); and two were specialists respectively in the kidney and gastro-intestinal tract (Berliner and Broitman). No clinical oncologist or food scientist was a member. The chairman, Dr. Grobstein, lists his interests as developmental biology and biomedical technology assessment. Though distinguished in some ways, I do not consider this group a strong or balanced committee to be asked to undertake a critical appraisal of the subject of diet, nutrition, and cancer.[51]

Olson thus replaced "the committee" with the people who made it up, splitting a unitary actor into a list of persons who could be criticized both individually (for lack of relevant expertise) and as a group (for lack of balance). In a sense, Olson's attack inverted the procedure by which the Academy had created "the committee," making it into *less*, not more, than the sum of its parts. Such comprehensive challenges to the committee's expertise were rare, however, and won little media coverage.[52]

Charging Conflict of Interest: Redefining Roles

Conflict of interest was not a major theme in the attacks on *Diet, Nutrition, and Cancer*, and suggestions of improper influence were both unusual and circumscribed. A few critics suggested that the committee might have been led too far, perhaps against its own better judgment, by the requirements of its contract with its funder, the National Cancer Institute, which had instructed the Academy to issue appropriate dietary recommendations where warranted. Alfred E. Harper drew on phrases from the cancer report to ask:

> What motivated [the Diet, Nutrition, and Cancer committee] . . . to make recommendations on the basis of beliefs when it had concluded that "the data base is not yet adequate for firm recommendations to be made"? Was it because of its assumption that "the public often demands certain kinds of information before such information can be provided with complete

certainty"? Was it because, as noted by [the Academy's president] Frank Press, there is "a pervasive desire to adopt 'preventive' measures against chronic diseases"? Was it because it had agreed to provide the National Cancer Institute with recommendations as part of the contract under which the report was prepared?[53]

Elsewhere, Harper questioned whether the Academy should accept "contracts that require recommendations for the public on controversial issues," arguing that the Academy and its committees "should determine whether recommendations are appropriate, not the grantor."[54]

These suggestions of inappropriate influence contrast sharply with the corresponding charges that critics made about *Toward Healthful Diets*. In the earlier case, critics used allegations of food-industry involvement to rewrite the story of the report dramatically, suddenly introducing brand-new characters — such as meat and dairy producers, who had not figured in the report's self-presentation. The sensational revelations, wrapped in the rhetoric of the exposé, produced a surprising twist in the plot. In contrast, Harper's charge that the NCI might have exerted undue influence over *Diet, Nutrition, and Cancer* never succeeded in twisting the plot. Rather than revealing new, illegitimate characters, Harper's attack required redefining an existing character, the NCI, and transforming it from a source of appropriate funding into a source of bias. Although it is clearly possible to effect such a transformation, there is little doubt that to do so poses challenges. For example, given the NCI's public purpose of combating a dreaded disease, the claim that an NCI contract had led a committee to err on the side of safety might appear less troubling than the claim that narrow private interests, such as the food industry, had improperly influenced committee deliberations. Ultimately, then, the conflict of interest charges aimed at *Diet, Nutrition, and Cancer* were not only less common but also less intense than those directed at *Toward Healthful Diets*.

Highlighting Uncertainty

Critics of *Diet, Nutrition, and Cancer* developed a number of lines of attack that the enemies of *Toward Healthful Diets* tended not to employ. One of these strategies emphasized that the data on diet-cancer relationships were incomplete and sometimes contradictory. Claims of scientific uncertainty are often used to build or undermine specific arguments, and in many contexts, actors deploy uncertainty to justify action (or inaction).[55] In the case of diet and health, the debate had already been framed in such a way that perceptions of uncertainty tended to strengthen the position of opponents of dietary change: why recommend changes if the evidence to justify them was soft? Thus, critics of *Diet, Nutrition, and Cancer* could weaken support for the report's dietary advice by placing uncertainty under the spotlight. For example, a few days after the report was released, C. W. McMillan, an assistant secretary of agriculture and former trade association executive in the beef industry, told a national food policy conference that:

> The NAS report . . . made recommendations based on uncertain and incomplete scientific evidence, as the Academy took great pains to point out repeatedly throughout the text. I don't fault NAS for its efforts. To the contrary, I commend the scientists that labored over this study for their diligence and concern for the American people. They did the best they could with the data available to them.[56]

These arguments allowed critics to undermine confidence in the report's conclusions without attacking the scientists who wrote it or challenging the Academy directly. Indeed, as the above example shows, a critic pursuing this line of attack can actively commend the committee for contending with inadequate evidence and for honestly reporting the limitations of the data. Through this strategy, the authority of the report was turned upon itself.

Constructing a Context of Disagreement

Advisory reports gain much credibility from the notion that they reflect a scientific consensus. Critics of *Diet, Nutrition, and Cancer* worked to undermine the report's univocal performance by emphasizing disagreement in the scientific community. They framed the report not as the authoritative, scientific view of diet and cancer, but as one opinion from a range of conflicting perspectives. To spotlight scientific disagreement, critics often juxtaposed the report, or statements from it, with conflicting claims. This general theme took several specific forms. In one of the most common, critics presented the report as merely the most recent of several conflicting Academy reports on the same topic. These accounts treated different Academy committees as if they were the same organization or different "branches" of the same institution. Meat and dairy groups started using this strategy immediately following the publication of *Diet, Nutrition, and Cancer*. The American Meat Institute (AMI), for example, "challenged the report" in a news release, saying that it was "based on insufficient evidence and in conflict with other recent reports issued by the Academy."[57] A coalition of nine meat, poultry, egg, and dairy organizations asked the NAS's president, Frank Press, "immediately" to name "a special task force within the Academy . . . to clarify the grossly divergent views of the Academy and its branches" — a reference to the fact that *Toward Healthful Diets* had argued there was "no basis" for recommending that people alter consumption of such macronutrients as fat, whereas *Diet, Nutrition, and Cancer* had offered interim dietary guidelines.[58] And the National Meat Association (NMA) issued a news release complaining about the "almost steady stream of contradictory statements" — such as *Toward Healthful Diets* and *Diet, Nutrition, and Cancer* — "coming from the scientific community" about diet and cancer.[59]

Staging disagreements among Academy reports offered a quick and dirty way to foster the impression that the report was surrounded by controversy. The Council for Agricultural Science and Technology (CAST) produced a much more elegant display of conflict: CAST asked a variety of natural and social scientists to prepare short reviews of *Diet, Nutrition, and Cancer*, then published them in a report titled *Diet, Nutrition, and Cancer: A Critique*, which it distributed to the news media and on Capitol Hill. At the front of the 80-page booklet, CAST listed the names and affiliations of the 47 reviewers, or "Task Force Members"; then, following a "Summary" and "Overview," it devoted 70 pages to presenting each and all of the individual reviews. These statements, which took widely varying positions, appeared in alphabetical order, and CAST made no effort to reconcile the comments or to develop a joint pronouncement. This literary form, which CAST explained it had adopted because the participants were "unlikely" to agree on a single statement, was extremely well suited to making controversy visible.[60] Inverting the consensus logic of Academy reports — in which backstage negotiations produce a single, unified voice — the CAST report brought 47 discordant voices to the center stage. One might well think of the CAST report as an example of a "dissensus report," a literary technology for displaying disagreement.[61]

CAST not only developed a literary form that dramatized controversy; it also argued explicitly in the "Overview" to its report that scientists disagreed about diet and health. Like many other critics of *Diet, Nutrition, and Cancer*, CAST used boundary work to divide up the scientific community, discursively constructing categories of scientists who differed in their "philosophy" of nutrition advice.[62] CAST described three categories:

Nonrecommenders "hold the opinion that the role of scientists is to discover the facts and to set forth alternative public uses of these facts and the probable consequences of such uses, but to avoid making recommendations of public policy." In this view, not scientists but "persons designated by society" should make policy.

Hesitant recommenders "are willing to make recommendations of public policy based upon science when the recommendations are backed by evidence that meets scientific standards."

Recommenders "are willing to accept less than rigorous evidence as a basis for recommendations if they perceive a need for prompt use of existing scientific knowledge in the public interest or for other reasons."[63]

In applying these categories to the debate over *Diet, Nutrition, and Cancer,* CAST argued that the committee that produced that report represented the "recommenders," whereas the committee that wrote *Toward Healthful Diets* represented the "hesitant recommenders."[64] CAST went on to present the view of the "hesitant recommenders," devoting about four times more space to their arguments than to the views of the "recommenders."[65]

CAST's way of delineating its categories of scientists is strategically interesting. It defines the "hesitant recommenders" as occupying the middle ground between the "nonrecommenders" at one extreme and the "recommenders" at the other.[66] Moreover, CAST places the authors of *Toward Healthful Diets* in the "hesitant" category, thus defining them as moderates, rather than as extreme nonrecommenders, the designation that critics of that report in effect used. CAST does not identify any reports or individuals as representing the category of nonrecommenders. Most important, CAST links the hesitant recommenders to an insistence on "rigor" and on meeting "scientific standards." Recommenders, however, are "willing to accept less" — a phrase that clearly implies that their views are less scientific.

Dividing the Performance

The enemies of *Toward Healthful Diets* had nothing good to say about their target, but many critics of *Diet, Nutrition, and Cancer* praised parts of the report while condemning others. These critics defined *Diet, Nutrition, and Cancer* not as a single, unified performance but as a show with several parts: the main "body" of the report, the "Executive Summary," and the "interim dietary guidelines." (*Diet, Nutrition, and Cancer* consists of eighteen chapters, and the executive summary, which is Chapter 1 of the report, contains a section called "Interim Dietary Guidelines.") By spotlighting the divisions between these parts of the text, the critics depicted them as separate entities—distinct performances aimed at different audiences. Similarly, they highlighted the difference between "the report itself" and the "news release" about it. The critics portrayed the "body" of the report (a.k.a. "the actual report," and "the text") as its most "scientific" part, presenting it as an authoritative literature review for scientists. In contrast, they presented the executive summary, the guidelines, and the news release as aimed at broader publics. These critics praised the "body" of the report, yet strongly condemned the executive summary, guidelines, and the news release. The problem was important, they charged, because the "parts most exposed to the public, convey greater conviction than does the text."[67] Media messages lacking an adequate scientific foundation thus might be communicated to large audiences, adversely affecting food producers for no good reason.

The USDA review of *Diet, Nutrition, and Cancer* provides an example. After calling the report "a thoughtful and carefully considered review of the current scientific literature" and "an authoritative source for many years to come," the agency continued in a much more critical vein:[68]

> Summaries and conclusions in the body of the NRC report are very carefully worded and indicate uncertainties and gaps in the information base. . . . The Executive Summary, however, does not show so clearly the limits of knowledge within which the Committee developed its conclusions. And the press release, which provides the only information most of the public would have received about the report, is even less tentatively worded. These changes in emphasis can easily result in a perception by the public that the interim dietary guidelines are much less "interim" and are more firmly established than the Committee intended.[69]

A number of other critics developed similar attacks on the executive summary. CAST, for example, argued that "the numerous reservations and qualifications that accompanied most of the findings reported in the text tended to disappear in the 'Executive Summary' and the news release."[70]

This general pattern of attack continued in the USDA's discussion of the guidelines.[71] Commenting on the advice to minimize consumption of salt-cured and smoked foods, the agency argued:

> The dietary factors implicated are alcohol drinking, high intakes of pickles and moldy foods possibly containing mycotoxins or N-nitroso compounds, trace mineral deficiencies and the consumption of very hot beverages. None of these factors relates to the processed food products made in this country. . . . Thus, the generalization in the guidelines has unfairly implicated wholesome and nutritious foods. (This implication is not made by the report itself.)[72]

The USDA was by no means the only critic that praised "the report" while attacking "the guidelines."[73] After calling *Diet, Nutrition, and Cancer* a "monumental publication," useful for future research, A. M. Pearson, a professor of food science and human nutrition, reproached the committee, saying it had "ignored its own cautious statements" about the limits of the evidence when it advised lowering fat intake.[74]

The USDA used a parallel strategy to attack the news release, charging that it unfairly named American meat products as hazardous:

> The news release was a straightforward case of distortion, particularly in its examples of salt-cured or pickled and smoked foods to be avoided. These foods — sausages, smoked fish and ham, bacon, bologna and hot dogs — are simply not associated in the United States with elevated rates of esophageal and stomach cancer, and nowhere does the actual report claim that they are.[75]

Other critics made similar arguments.[76] The president of the American Meat Institute (AMI), C. Manly Molpus, requested a "written acknowledgement" from the Academy that the news release was "erroneous." Molpus was incensed because the news release told people to avoid precisely those foods that AMI members produce:

> The part of the news release which recommends eating very little sausage, ham, bacon, bologna and hot dogs is unsupported by the study. . . . If examples of specific products are used . . . in the future, it seems appropriate to refer to products cited in the literature, namely, salted pickles, smoked and pickled mutton, and singed sheep heads and feet.[77]

As these examples show, the critics of *Diet, Nutrition, and Cancer* sliced the report into several pieces that could be contrasted and attacked. The Academy responded with arguments aimed at defending the report's unity. NRC officials pointed out that the executive summary and guidelines had never been intended to stand apart from the rest of the report. A single committee had written the entire text, which constituted a single document, and the executive summary, the guidelines, and the other seventeen chapters had been reviewed as a whole. The Academy also defended the news release, saying that the committee chairman and appropriate NRC staff had approved it.[78]

Even so, the critics' arguments drew indirect support from the widespread perception that science is frequently distorted in popular forums.[79] Their boundary work divided the report into more and less "popular" parts. In effect, the critics separated the main show (the "body" of the report) from a brief epilogue (the executive summary and the guidelines) prepared for a broader audience. They also depicted the news release as a lowbrow sideshow. The critics thus cast the "popular" parts of the show as danger-ously misleading *retellings* of the original scientific story. This strategy allowed critics to pursue a divide-and-conquer strategy that used the "sci-entific" authority of the main report to undermine the "popularized" parts. Redefining the boundaries of the performance thus enabled the critics to challenge the Academy without taking on the burden of developing a "tech-nical" critique of the parts of the report that they deemed most scientific. At the same time, this line of attack targeted precisely those messages that, owing to their potential to impact food marketing, most worried industry groups.

Changing the Plot: Major Rewrites and Minor Revisions

The critics who challenged *Diet, Nutrition, and Cancer,* as we have seen, tended to pursue several lines of argument, such as highlighting uncertainty, constructing disagreement, and charging that the actual report had been dis-torted as its story was retold. Critics also attacked the committee for lack of expertise in food technology, and several individuals suggested that the NCI contract might constitute conflict of interest. Considering these attacks as a whole clearly shows that, overall, the assault on *Diet, Nutrition, and Cancer* was much less aggressive than the one on *Toward Healthful Diets.*

Comparing the reception of these two reports demonstrates that critics use a wide range of techniques to undermine science advice. The ways to challenge advisory reports, it appears, can be arrayed along a spectrum, with different strategies ranked according to how extensively they aim to change the narrative that underwrites authoritative advice. At one end of the spec-trum lie efforts to rewrite the drama of a report completely; these attacks aim at nothing less than a wholesale transformation of the plot. At the other end of the spectrum are arguments that propose comparatively minor revi-sions in the story. The contrast between rewriting and revising clearly defines a dimension in rhetorical space, not a binary distinction. The issue here is not to pinpoint the precise position that each argument occupies on this spectrum; the goal is rather to call attention to the range of rhetorical options that critics may select. Confronted by a report's performance, crit-ics can weigh which accusations they can "make stick" and which are likely to rebound on them, damaging their own credibility. Depending on their assessments of what kinds of performances they themselves can likely pull off, they can attempt to rewrite the story of the report completely or to push for more limited revisions.

Opting for a radical rewrite, the critics of *Toward Healthful Diets* undertook a no-holds-barred assault on the report's objectivity and balance, on its omission of critical evidence, and on the integrity of the people and procedures that produced it. In contrast, the critics of *Diet, Nutrition, and Cancer* attempted to revise and qualify the story of the report. They placed the report in an unflattering context of uncertainty. They positioned it as part of a controversy, orchestrating displays of discordant views. They used divide-and-conquer arguments to detach targets, such as the news release or the executive summary, from its central narrative (Fig. 5). Thus, rather than seeking to supplant the original performance with a radically new one (Fig. 4), the critics of *Diet, Nutrition, and Cancer* worked to undermine it in more circumscribed ways.[80]

THE FATE OF THE REPORTS

In contrast to the attack on *Toward Healthful Diets*, which virtually upstaged the report, the assault on *Diet, Nutrition, and Cancer* was (by a variety of measures) much less successful. The assault on the cancer report never grew into a fully articulated, well-integrated, self-reinforcing counternarrative of the type that so damaged *Toward Healthful Diets*. Instead of attempting to overthrow the central narrative of the report, the critics of *Diet, Nutrition, and Cancer* chose to snipe away at its edges. Moreover, the most aggressive attacks on *Diet, Nutrition, and Cancer* reached smaller audiences, appearing only in publications with limited circulation, such as the CAST report, whereas the charges against *Toward Healthful Diets* received prominent play in the national media. But what accounts for these contrasting outcomes? Why did the critics of the two reports adopt different strategies? Why did the media coverage of the critics' charges differ? How, in short, can one understand the fate of these reports? Clearly, many contingencies shaped the answers to these questions. Nevertheless, the fate of each report, I suggest, was heavily influenced by its dramatic strength and by the public identities of its critics.

Narrative Strength and Dramaturgical Cooperation

Did the reports, to begin with, differ significantly in their own strength as performative displays? Were there features of *Toward Healthful Diets* that

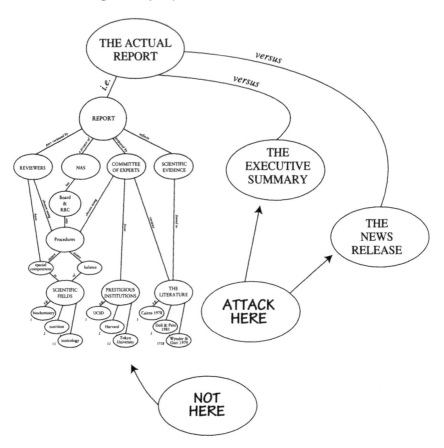

FIGURE 5. Divide-and-Conquer Strategies

left it particularly exposed to attack? Although each report presented itself using similar literary and staging techniques, the strength of the delivery differed. As we saw in Chapter 2, the team that prepared *Diet, Nutrition, and Cancer* nicely staged a drama of cultural authority, drawing together many actors and resources and creating a persuasive text and credible author. As a public performance, the report displayed many artfully selected details about the participants in its production, the large volume of data and expertise that underwrote it, and the careful procedures that certified its authority.

In the case of *Toward Healthful Diets*, this story was much less fully articulated. For one thing, by all possible counts, *Diet, Nutrition, and Cancer* was far and away the more impressive assemblage. It was 20 times longer than *Toward Healthful Diets*; it cost 100 times as much money to produce; and it cited 33 times as many references. Moreover, this comparatively grand array of resources was directed exclusively at cancer, whereas *Toward Healthful Diets* addressed not only cancer but also cardiovascular disease, obesity, hypertension, and diabetes. Still more important, the team that produced *Diet, Nutrition, and Cancer* created a much more convincing display of unity. It conducted more inclusive and extensive backstage negotiations, holding more meetings and workshops, consulting more experts, and drawing together more people (from both inside and outside the Academy). As a result, *Diet, Nutrition, and Cancer* enjoyed the support of a network that was both more tightly integrated and more encompassing than the network that backed *Toward Healthful Diets*.[81]

When *Toward Healthful Diets* was publicly released, critics exploited the weaknesses in its performance. Disputes among actors close to the report contributed to a partial breakdown in dramaturgical cooperation, enabling critics to breach the sanctity of the backstage and bring unauthorized accounts of its history into full public view. Leaks and interviews with "people in and around the Academy" provided fodder for exposés that sharply conflicted with the narrative of orderly procedures, allowing critics to create an atmosphere of scandal.[82] The resignation of the Consumer Liaison Panel dramatically displayed the lack of unity. Pointing to the odd history of the report, not to mention the charges of industry influence, critics raised unsettling questions: Had the normal Academy reviews been adequately performed? Had bias and error slipped through the cracks? Philip Handler's assertion — that "appearances, and only appearances, have been offended in this instance" — may have been empirically correct; no smoking gun ever demonstrated foul play.[83] But from a dramaturgical perspective, Handler's claim is, at best, a weak fall-back position; indeed, in a sense, it is entirely beside the point. After all, *the* critical test of a performance is whether it creates the desired appearances. One need not accept all the charges against *Toward Healthful Diets* to conclude that crucial defects in its performance eased the task of challenging its cultural authority.[84]

In contrast, because the team that produced *Diet, Nutrition, and Cancer* built a more inclusive and integrated network, the critics of that report were unable reach behind the curtain and reveal shocking departures from the official story. Lacking the props to object forcefully to the report's account of the backstage, these critics had to find ways to attack the visible parts of the performance. But how could they approach this task? To prepare a detailed critique of the entire report, a 478-page document with some 1,700 references, posed severe practical problems. To identify "omissions" in the study, for example, was no mean feat. Indeed, the American Meat Institute and the National Live Stock and Meat Board hired an epidemiological consulting firm, Epistat Associates, to "determine whether the NAS report was based on a thorough review of the epidemiological literature." The firm was specifically asked to look for scientific studies that the committee had failed to cite.[85] Ultimately, Epistat concluded that the literature review had indeed been thorough. Charges of omissions did not emerge.[86] In contrast, the critics of *Toward Healthful Diets* quickly identified "omissions" and charged that the report rested on an incomplete and misleading review of the literature. Unlike the meat industry groups, the Chicago Heart Association and the Center for Science in the Public Interest did not face a massive literature review that they had to ignore, address, or praise; they could readily examine the 24-page document, scrutinize its 52 references, and select targets.

As a performance, *Diet, Nutrition, and Cancer* enjoyed a number of advantages over the earlier report. Its staging techniques, which were backed by more complete dramaturgical cooperation, successfully resisted efforts to rewrite its account of the backstage. Critics who sought to contest the claims in its text directly faced serious obstacles owing to the size and comprehensiveness of the document. The strength of the performance thus constrained its critics, who opted for low-cost lines of attack. Dennis T. Gordon, a researcher from the Department of Food Science and Nutrition at the University of Missouri, put the matter bluntly: "To do a completely thorough job of reviewing *Diet, Nutrition, and Cancer*," he wrote, "would require close examination of the published reports cited to determine what they do and do not show."[87] Like many others, Gordon declined to criticize the "actual" report, focusing his complaints on the news release:

> I see no major fault with the report. . . . Only after doing all the work and reading all the materials, as this committee has, would I offer more specific comments. The major problem that has developed is in the transition from a scientific report to a press release. I think the committee should be asked to restate its findings and recommendations.[88]

The Public Identities of the Critics

Flaws in the delivery of *Toward Healthful Diets* go a long way toward explaining its critical reception. Conversely, the stronger performance of *Diet,*

Nutrition, and Cancer suggests why that report fared better. But differences in the reports were only part of the explanation for the outcomes in these cases. On average, the critics of *Toward Healthful Diets* possessed public identities that better equipped them to persuade audiences to accept their claims of cultural authority than did the critics of *Diet, Nutrition, and Cancer.*[89]

What were the public identities of the performers who criticized each of the NAS reports? Table 4 displays some illustrative examples of the public identities of critics who attacked each report. (These examples are drawn from such stylized forms as official titles of persons, names of organizations, and the brief identifying phrases that appear in mass media accounts.)[90] Despite some clear exceptions, the table shows that in the aggregate, the critics of *Toward Healthful Diets* had "calling cards" more strongly linked to high-status areas of science and medicine than did the critics of *Diet, Nutrition, and Cancer.* For example, the American Heart Association is better equipped to claim the cultural authority of science in matters of health than is the American Meat Institute. This pattern persists when one compares the organizational and disciplinary affiliations of individual scientists from each group of critics. Many critics of *Toward Healthful Diets* were associated with "core" areas of biological science and medicine, such as biochemistry, cardiology, and epidemiology. A number of critics of *Diet, Nutrition, and Cancer* also possessed public identities that connected them to the "core" of biomedical science. But many others were linked to fields, such as animal science, food science, meat science, and poultry science, that bear some stigma as "applied" disciplines more closely affiliated with agriculture and food production than with core areas of medicine and biology.[91] This is not to say that these "applied" disciplines are in fact any less scientific; my purpose is not to engage in my own boundary work about the limits of science, but to point out the effects of boundary work that has already been accomplished.[92] Stereotypes about the character of disciplines have concrete consequences. Meat science is in a poor position to challenge, say, molecular genetics for the right to speak about matters pertaining to the biology of cancer. Medicine — which today is sometimes seen as a monopolistic industry rather than an altruistic profession — may encounter cynicism when it claims the moral legacy of an age-old, sacred commitment to serving the patient; however, it is less likely to do so than would a pious pronouncement about the selfless dedication of ham and sausage makers to the cause of public health.[93]

TABLE 4
Comparison of the Public Identities of the Critics of Two Academy Reports

Critics of *Toward Healthful Diets*	
Person/Organization	Titles or Identifying Details
American Heart Association	
Dr. Donald M. Berwick	"of the Harvard School of Public Health"[a]
Center for Science in the Public Interest	
Consumer Liaison Panel to the FNB	
D. Mark Hegsted, Ph.D.	administrator, USDA Human Nutrition Center
Dr. Robert Levy	"director of the National Heart, Lung and Blood Institute, a division of the National Institutes of Health."[b]
J. Michael McGuinnis, M.D.	deputy assistant secretary for health, DHHS
Dr. James Schoenberger	professor and chairman, Department of Preventive Medicine, Rush-Presbyterian-St. Luke's Medical Center; President-Elect, American Heart Association
Dr. Jeremiah Stamler	Dingman Professor of Cardiology and chairman, Department of Community Health and Preventive Medicine, Northwestern University Medical School; chairman, Committee on Prevention of Cardiovascular Diseases, American College of Cardiology
D. Robert Wissler	Donald N. Pritzker Distinguished Service Professor of Pathology, University of Chicago

(continued)

Public identities are not permanently fixed, of course, and they may be reshaped by events or performers. During the controversy over the Academy reports, events modified the public identities of some of the key players. For example, during the debate over *Toward Healthful Diets*, the reputations of Robert E. Olson and Alfred Harper were damaged by allegations and innuendo suggesting that the food industry had influenced their scientific judgments. Despite the absence of proof and their efforts to defend their integrity, their public identities were altered. As a result, during the debate about *Diet, Nutrition, and Cancer*, science journalists and other informed

TABLE 4 *(continued)*

Critics of *Diet, Nutrition, and Cancer*	
Person/Organization	Titles or Identifying Details
American Meat Institute	
Council for Agricultural Science and Technology	
Dr. Alfred E. Harper	"professor of nutrition and biochemistry at the University of Wisconsin and chairman of the Academy's Food and Nutrition Board. . . . In addition to his academic work, Dr. Harper says, he derives about 10 percent of his income from 'industry consultantships,' mainly for Pillsbury, producer of many bakery and other products, and Kraft, the nation's largest purveyor of cheese products."[c]
National Broiler Council	
National Cattlemen's Association	
National Live Stock and Meat Board	
National Meat Association	
National Milk Producers Federation	
National Pork Producers Council	
National Turkey Federation	
Robert E. Olson, M.D., Ph.D.	Alice A. Doisy Professor and chairman, Department of Biochemistry; professor of medicine, St. Louis University School of Medicine
United Egg Producers	
Milton L. Scott, Ph.D.	Jacob Gould Schurman Professor of Nutrition, Emeritus, Cornell University
Dr. George Wilson	"American Meat Institute vice president for scientific affairs."[d]

NOTE: The table displays illustrative examples of the names and titles of critics of *Toward Healthful Diet* and *Diet, Nutrition, and Cancer*. In some cases, short quotations from major news outlets indicate how journalists publicly identified them in articles about the reports.

SOURCES:

[a] "A Few Kinds Words for Cholesterol," *Time*, June 9, 1980, p. 51.

[b] Jane Brody, "Experts Assail Report Declaring Curb on Cholesterol Isn't Needed," *New York Times*, June 1, 1980, p. 1.

[c] Marian Burros, "Prudent Diet and Cancer Risk," *New York Times*, June 23, 1982, p. C1.

[d] Victor Cohn, "Reshaping the Nation's Diet; Drastic Changes Urged to Avoid Cancer," *Washington Post*, June 17, 1982, p. A1.

observers were likely to view Olson and Harper as partisans for a point of view, rather than neutral scientists. Indeed, in some contexts, their consulting relationships with food producers continued to be noted alongside the scientific aspects of their public identities.[94]

This argument about the relative ability of different actors to claim scientific credibility in public arenas is, quite deliberately, stated in terms of dramatic resources, not actual levels of scientific expertise. Put otherwise, my argument does not rest on claims about the actual technical capabilities or moral properties of the actors, only on cultural expectations about them.[95] Nevertheless, these expectations matter. The observers of public spectacles draw on them to help them decide whom to believe. Journalists and other important gatekeepers use public identities to decide what is news and to package events into stories that reach millions.[96] Public identities also shape the performances of potential critics, who consider their own identities, and those of their opponents, when they determine whether, where, and how to attack. The critic who lacks the cultural weight to strike a body blow is likely to try some form of rhetorical jujitsu. Commending a report for pointing out the limitations of the data on which it is based provides a means to use its own cultural authority against its conclusions. Positioning a report in a field of controversy offers a way to direct the cultural authority of one group of scientists against another. Charging that popularizers have distorted a more nuanced message avoids the hardest targets, yet strikes the claims that reach the largest audiences. The public identities of the critics, like the dramatic strength of the reports themselves, played a crucial role in shaping the reception of these reports.

CHAPTER 4

The Character of the National Academy of Sciences

The debates over the NAS reports on diet and health provoked vigorous questioning of the very nature of the Academy: If these reports were the work of the most prestigious scientific organization in the country, why were they surrounded by controversy? Were the "deficiencies" of these reports merely the visible symptoms of more fundamental problems? Could policy-makers count on the Academy to provide objective, reliable advice? Had the public been misled about the character of the Academy? Or were misguided attacks on the NAS reports impugning the integrity of a venerable scientific institution and, even more ominously, undermining the authority of science itself?

This chapter explores how the debates over the NAS reports on diet and health became, more profoundly, battles about whether the Academy was a trustworthy advisor to government and a responsible guardian of the cultural authority of science. In other words, these debates became a site in which the Academy's public identity came under sharp attack. In Chapter 2, we treated its public identity as an unproblematic social fact, something the Academy could use to help shore up its reports. Now, however, it is time to consider how the Academy defends its identity when its character is questioned. To address this issue, I examine the public debate over its decision not to issue the 1985 Draft of the Tenth Edition of the Recommended Dietary Allowances. On one level, as we saw in Chapter 2, the cancellation of the 1985 Draft resulted from the failure of the team preparing the report to resolve conflicts over the text, which precipitated a breakdown in dramaturgical cooperation and public exposure of the dispute. But this very general story begs questions of greater social and moral significance, such as why the NAS halted publication and who was to blame, the 1980–85 RDA committee, which had written the draft report, or the Academy leadership, which had canceled it. More generally, the cancellation of the report raised awkward and potentially discrediting questions about the character of the Academy. Had Academy procedures functioned properly in this case, or had the systems intended to guard the integrity of the Academy's work failed? Was the report flawed, or had the Academy "suppressed" a sound scientific report for "political" reasons? Was the cancellation necessary to preserve the Academy's credibility, or did the episode signal that public trust in the Academy was undeserved?

As these questions suggest, the dispute over the 1985 Draft became an event that demanded a social accounting. The dispute was a threat to the social order surrounding Academy advice, a threat that required explanation, judgment, and action. But clearly, such events do not arrive ready-made on the public stage: performers must give them narrative structure, fitting them into stories that define the identities of the characters and inscribe events into plots.[1] Moreover, in an agonistic forum — such as a mass-mediated controversy — actors attempt to rebut competing stories, constructing stylized narratives and deploying techniques of information control to present their versions of events and preempt alternative accounts.[2] Thus, in the aftermath of the cancellation of the report, the Academy and the 1980–85 RDA committee struggled to emplot the dispute in very different ways, offering sharply conflicting accounts of what had happened backstage. The central issue in this theatrical contest was the moral character of the Academy, which the committee sought to discredit and the Academy sought to defend. The debate over the report's cancellation thus became a dynamic struggle to define not only the nature of backstage events but also the very identity of the Academy.

This chapter analyzes the performative techniques that the protagonists in this debate used to emplot "backstage" action for public display and thereby to construct the character of the Academy. My central concern is exploring how "what happened" backstage — and the moral meaning of those "events" — were defined through the process of being theatricalized.[3] The chapter begins with a brief overview of the public debate over the cancellation. It then develops a detailed analysis of several key texts in this debate, including the Academy's announcement that the report would not be published and an attack on the decision by Henry Kamin, chair of the RDA committee, that appeared as a letter to the editor in *Science*. Through a comparative analysis of these performances, the chapter explores how the protagonists emplotted the action and gave it dramatic form. The analysis reveals each text to be an extremely stylized drama that not only reinforces its performer's claims and preferred identity but also becomes a site for defining the nature of the Academy, its place in the social order, and its relations with the outside world.

THE PUBLIC DEBATE OVER THE DEMISE OF THE 1985 DRAFT

The cancellation of the 1985 Draft provoked a bitter public debate. As noted in Chapter 3, proponents of nutrition reform objected to a number of aspects of the draft, including its lowering of the RDAs for vitamins A and C. Its authors, who shared the outlook of the committee that wrote *Toward Healthful Diets*, disagreed with the reformers' arguments, and the draft became the subject of negotiations at the highest level during the spring and summer of 1985.[4] Even given the leaks discussed in Chapter 2, I cannot determine exactly when debate about the report spread beyond the Academy to include actors other than committee members, reviewers, and Academy officials, but there is little doubt that this had begun to happen by August. Nor is it possible to determine when negotiations finally broke down.[5] But although many details of the discussions inside the Academy remain behind the curtain to this day, the debate became a public controversy following the announcement, on October 7, 1985, of the decision to cancel the report, and a flurry of controversy followed this news, as we saw in Chapter 2.

In their public performances following the decision to halt publication, the Academy leadership and the 1980–85 RDA committee struggled to define what caused the cancellation and who was to blame. The Academy framed the decision as an appropriate resolution of a regrettable situation. The committee and its supporters, on the other hand, framed the cancellation as an illegitimate intrusion of politics into science that required a reassessment of the Academy's identity. To the Academy, the decision was the inevitable result of following proper institutional procedures. To the committee and its supporters, it was a portentous development that signaled an end to the Academy's commitment to defending science against political pressure. My analysis of this struggle focuses on three key texts, written by principal protagonists in the dispute:[6]

    1. *The Academy Announcement.*   The Academy's most definitive account of its decision appeared in letter from the NRC's chairman, Frank Press, to James B. Wyngaarden, director of the National

Institutes of Health, which had funded the RDA study. This letter, which the Academy immediately made public, announced and explained the decision. It is the most detailed presentation of the Academy's version of events publicly available. The letter was quoted in the mass media and reprinted in its entirety in the *Journal of the American Dietetic Association.*[7]

2. *The Kamin letter.* This extended public attack on the Academy's decision was written by Henry Kamin, chair of the 1980–85 RDA committee, and published as a letter to the editor of *Science*, the nation's most broadly based scientific journal. Kamin's letter was occasioned by a news article by a science writer, Eliot Marshall. Alongside Kamin's letter, *Science* published a letter by Robert Olson (also examined below) attacking the Academy's decision.[8]

3. *The NRC Chairman's reply.* Press's response to the Marshall article and Kamin and Olson letters, published alongside the letters in *Science.*[9]

THE ACADEMY'S ANNOUNCEMENT: A DRAMA OF ORDER

At first glance, the Academy's announcement might appear to be a straightforward description of how and why the NRC chairman decided to cancel the report. But read from a dramaturgical perspective, the letter emerges as a carefully crafted piece of real-life political theater, produced for display under the public spotlight and aimed at shaping public understanding of the episode. The incompleteness of the available records (which, of course, stems largely from the Academy's information-control practices) precludes an examination of the process that shaped the letter, but this limitation does not imply that we cannot analyze the letter as a public performance, for there is little doubt that the Academy approached the task of announcing the cancellation in a theatrically self-conscious manner. Like others schooled in the mass-mediated politics of late-twentieth-century Washington, D.C., Academy officials are well versed in the arts of public communication, and the front-page coverage that the *New York Times* gave the leaked report can only have underlined the delicacy of the situation. Not only did Academy officials have every reason to anticipate that the decision to cancel would be vetted under the glare of publicity, but the leaks and publicity had also partially defined the symbolic terms in which one might expect key audiences, such as journalists, to interpret the decision (e.g., as a result of "pressure" on the Academy).[10] My claim is not that the Academy approached the task of justifying its decision cynically but that it viewed the announcement as a matter that required careful attention to managing information and impressions.

The Academy announcement, as we shall see, presents an intense drama about the maintenance of social order, but the theatricality of Press's letter is easily obscured by its bureaucratic style and formal language. To bring the plot to the fore, I have therefore taken the liberty of repackaging the announcement as a play in three acts by rearranging the original text, supplying stage directions, adding a Greek chorus, and providing literary annotations. My interpretation is supported by verbatim quotations from the letter itself. The play allows me to develop several voices for exploring the structure of the plot, the nature of the author's voice, the rhetorical techniques that construct that voice, and the modes of information control woven through the letter (e.g., what it does not reveal). This analytic method, obviously an interpretive one, serves to highlight aspects of the letter that are important to my dramaturgical analysis, providing a means of examining the strategies of self-presentation that the Academy used to defend its character. Readers who wish to probe the plausibility of my interpretation are invited to compare the play with the original letter, which is reprinted in the Appendix.[11] The letter consists of about 1,600 words (140 lines). All quotations from the original letter are identified by line number.

A LETTER FROM THE CHAIRMAN: A PLAY IN THREE ACTS

*Dramatis Personae**

THE CHAIRMAN: The NRC's chairman, occupant of the highest post in the Academy complex.**

THE COMMITTEE: The Committee on Dietary Allowances, which is overseen by the Food and Nutrition Board, whose parent body is the Commission on Life Sciences.

THE REVIEWERS: A group of scientific reviewers, some of whom are members

* The Chairman, the Committee, and the Reviewers are the main characters. Note the hierarchy of authority among them.

** The author of the play does not name the Chairman, even though historical documents clearly show that the letter that served as the basis of the play was signed by Frank Press, who was then chairman of the National Research Council. This obviously deliberate omission of the name has a significance that will grow clearer as the drama progresses.

of the Food and Nutrition Board and some of whom were appointed by the National Research Council.

NUTRITION-RELATED ORGANIZATIONS: These include numerous government agencies, nonprofit organizations, the health services sector, and the food industry.

THE MEDIA

THE PUBLIC

THE SCIENTIFIC COMMUNITY AT LARGE

CHORAGOS: Leader of the Chorus.

CHORUS

Note: Throughout the play, The Chairman, Choragos, *and* The Chorus *are the only characters who speak. All others silently mime their actions.*

Act I

Constitution Avenue in Washington, D.C.* At center stage, a stately building, The Academy, with large doors and many windows, all of which are shut. Outside, The Public and The Media *go about their business, paying little attention to the Academy.* Nutrition-Related Organizations (*hereafter* The Organizations) *are busy implementing their programs. The Scientific Community at Large quietly works at a laboratory bench.*

The doors and windows open, revealing many offices inside. People work at computers, read, hold meetings. An organizational chart is prominently displayed.**

CHORUS: High authority must attend
to the serious matter at stake.
From Chairman to Director
this message is dispatched.

CHORAGOS: What have we here? Malice and satire?
Can one treat a bureaucrat's letter
as if it were a play?

CHORUS: *Satire?* No! The drama is a tool.
It helps us hear the meaning of his words.
This does not mock the Chairman.
It just brings his voice to life.[†]

The Chairman, *who cannot be seen, begins from inside the building.*

---

* The location is not coincidental and reflects the importance of science to the modern state.

** The original letter does not contain an organizational chart or any other figures or tables.

[†] At this point, the author of the play uses the Chorus to clarify for the audience the intent of the drama, which (his other writings suggest) he does not regard as a derisive attack on the Academy, or on the Chairman personally, but as an analytic device.

CHAIRMAN [*as if giving a tour to visiting dignitaries*]: "The National Research Council works by establishing a panel of experts specifically to examine an issue and to prepare a report based on analysis of all data relevant to that issue." (42–44)

CHORUS: The Chairman speaks of order,
of a rational, technical world.
Rules govern action.
Experts weigh the facts.

CHAIRMAN: "Although the Research Council gives serious consideration to the judgment of its expert committees, a key element in the completion of reports is review by scientific experts outside the study group. This review proceeds under the auspices of the Research Council's Report Review Committee in conjunction with a scientific unit that oversees the work of the expert committee."* (44–48)

CHORUS: Regular procedures. Methodical review.
Committees in their rightful place.
Hierarchy. Oversight. Control.

CHAIRMAN: "This process ensures that all scientifically valid interpretations of the data are considered and that the conclusions and recommendations follow clearly from the evidence presented. This process of checks and balances and judgments at multiple levels was designed to guard against the promulgation of the view of one group of scientists that may be unwarranted in the considered judgment of another group of equally capable scientists."** (48–54)

CHORUS: Protect us from the narrow mind!
Defend against the expert
who seizes more than he is due!
Post guards to keep out error!

CHAIRMAN: "Thus, the review process enables the National Research Council to minimize errors and to enhance the credibility of its reports by achieving a broader consensus than may be derived by a single group of experts." (54–56)

A pause.

CHORAGOS: Our subject is the RDAs. Why all the fuss?

CHAIRMAN [*introducing a new subject*]: "The RDAs are based on a comprehensive analysis of scientific evidence. They represent the best scientific judgment

---

* The present tense, which dominates the Chairman's discussion of the Academy, conveys the sense that this orderly state of affairs is a permanent and essential feature of the institution's very nature.
** This sentence, with its momentary departure from the present tense, invokes the language of "checks and balances" to suggest that the NRC represents a system, not unlike the U.S. Constitution, that was consciously *designed* for the explicit purpose of protecting against the illegitimate use of power.

derived from examination of results of experimental studies in animals and humans, including nutrient balance studies and biochemical measurements, as well as food consumption patterns and epidemiological observations." (13–17)

> CHORUS: Grounded in good science. Formally defined.
> Products of this world of order: the RDAs.

CHAIRMAN [*with legalistic precision*]: "The allowances have traditionally been defined as 'the levels of intake of essential nutrients considered, in the judgment of the Committee on Dietary Allowances of the Food and Nutrition Board on the basis of available scientific knowledge, to be adequate to meet the known nutritional needs of practically all healthy persons.' " (8–12)

"Yet the RDAs are themselves *estimates* of nutrient allowances based on certain assumptions and may change as the underlying science progresses." (17–18)

> CHORUS: Science advances. Knowledge grows. Revision is rational.

CHAIRMAN [*proud of this record*]: "Over the last four decades, successive editions of the RDAs have incorporated new knowledge and expanded from recommendations on 9 nutrients and energy in 1941 to include 17 nutrients, energy, and 'safe and adequate dietary intakes' for 12 additional vitamins and minerals in 1980." [*He pauses.*] (18–22)

"Originally designed to serve as a guide for planning and procuring food supplies for the nation, the RDAs have acquired multiple uses. They have been voluntarily adopted as the cornerstone for a variety of nutrition-related activities undertaken by government agencies, industry, academia, and the health services sector." (87–90)

The lighting outside the Academy increases slightly, revealing The Organizations *to be referring to the RDAs as they perform their missions.*

CHAIRMAN: "For example, the RDAs are used by government agencies as guides for planning and procuring food supplies related to federal food assistance and other programs, as a basis for meal planning for population subgroups, as a reference point for evaluating dietary intake from national food consumption surveys, as a component of food and nutrition education programs, and, more recently, as a basis for nutrition labeling of foods and dietary supplements." (90–96)

> CHORUS: Order is contagious and it spreads throughout the world.
> The strength of the Academy proliferates outside.
> Science and system build credible claims.
> The RDAs, no mere numbers, are tools to standardize action.
> They stabilize not just nutrition but society as well.
> How else to coordinate our complex world?[12]

CHAIRMAN: "In the private sector, the uses of the RDAs extend to food fortification, the formulation of food products, and competitive marketing." (96–97)

A pause.

CHORAGOS: Internal order. Reliable knowledge.
A standardized world.
But if harmony prevails,
if order spreads from inside out,
then why this letter
written in grave tones?

A spotlight falls on The Committee, *which is hard at work at a conference table.*

CHAIRMAN *[in a matter-of-fact tone]*: "The present committee began work on the 10th edition of the RDAs in 1980."* (57–58)

A calendar is projected on the stage. Its pages flip, indicating the passage of five years.

"When the draft report was subjected to the Research Council's rigorous process of review, many of the committee's conclusions and recommendations did not gain the full support of the reviewers." (58–60)

CHORAGOS: Tell the tale and do not spare the facts.

CHAIRMAN *[with self-conscious neutrality]*: "The committee had proposed modifications of the RDAs for many nutrients, whereas reviewers" *[he interrupts himself to make an important point]* "including members of the Food and Nutrition Board — the unit responsible for oversight of the committee — " *[returning to his earlier tone]* "whereas reviewers . . . in general concluded that changes in existing RDAs are warranted for only a few of these nutrients." (64–67)

"Differences of opinion among committee members and reviewers extended to such issues as the appropriate data base for developing the RDAs, the adequate size of body stores for specific nutrients, and the advisability of modifying the definition of the RDAs."** (67–70)

Arguments, which the actors silently mime, break out in the Academy and slowly grow heated. The Committee and The Reviewers *confront each other only through intermediaries. Several people who begin as observers of the debate find themselves getting caught up in it.*

CHORAGOS: And where, sir, do *you* stand in this debate? Outside?

---

* At this point, as the Chairman shifts topics from the Academy to the RDA affair, he also shifts into the past tense. Thus, he no longer speaks about the unchanging essence of the Academy but about a specific, temporally situated episode.
** Through his persistent use of the past tense, the Chairman helps signal his ultimate intention to call the controversy closed and move on.

CHAIRMAN [*working at being evenhanded*]: "In general, the committee believed it sufficient [*the slightest trace of skepticism creeps into his voice*] to base its conclusions on a reexamination of previously considered evidence and some new data using criteria and assumptions it considered to be the most valid." [*The skepticism vanishes.*]   (77–79)

"Most reviewers believed, however, that modifications to the RDAs are justified only in the face of compelling new evidence — not merely as a result of a reinterpretation of existing data based on assumptions that may be no more valid than those applied previously. The reviewers concluded that the evidence presented did not fully justify the committee's conclusions for several of the nutrients."*   (79–84)

The Organizations *begin to detect the argument under way inside the Academy. Some appear concerned.*

CHORAGOS: This dispute appears quite troublesome.
What mischief makes for this debate?

CHAIRMAN [*in a reassuring, almost complacent manner*]: "It is not uncommon for scientists to disagree over certain issues, such as the association between nutrient intake and health, for which new data are constantly emerging, and the data set is never complete."   (23–25)

"Indeed, competent scientists may use different, equally defensible assumptions and physiological indexes of good health and arrive at divergent conclusions and recommendations."**   (29–31)

CHORUS: Differences are normal, not simply to despise.
Debate itself does not suggest
the NRC has failed.

CHAIRMAN: "The resolution of such differences of opinion necessitates the involvement of an impartial, authoritative group of scientists whose opinion is highly regarded and whose judgment the public views with confidence."
(32–34)

CHORUS: By virtue of its expertise, procedures, and techniques,
its reputation well deserved as fair and wise,
place trust in the Academy to end disputes!

---

* In this passage, the Chairman positions himself as a neutral reporter, who describes in turn what each side said. However, the terms he uses to characterize the Committee's arguments imply that he believes it was unduly satisfied with its own idiosyncratic criteria and assumptions. He thus sets the stage for his ultimate judgment.
** The Chairman's return to the present tense at this point shifts the state of affairs he describes back into the unchanging world of the permanent present. Scientific disagreement is thereby rendered part of the natural order of science, not the surprising result of institutional problems in the NRC. Indeed, in the lines below, not only is the existence of disagreement made to seem normal but it becomes a reason that the NRC is needed.

CHAIRMAN *[proudly]*: "Since its establishment in 1863, the National Academy of Sciences, and, later, the National Research Council have, through their committees, been able to meet this need very successfully in a multitude of studies of national importance. The institution's commitment to impartiality and scientific excellence is reflected in our recent reports on nutrition, such as those on the association between diet, nutrition, and cancer; the public health implications of the nation's meat and poultry inspection program; the importance of nutrition in medical education; and the carcinogenic potential of cyclamate." (34–41)

CHORAGOS: A record long and recent, one cannot but commend. Yet what happened in this case?

CHAIRMAN *[tired and grave]*: "Despite months of discussion and deliberation, the committee and the reviewers were unable to agree on the interpretation of scientific data on several of the nutrients and consequently on RDAs for those nutrients." (60–63)

In the backrooms of the Academy, discord increases.

"All these points of contention led to different conclusions about the allowance levels, which were reflected in a succession of drafts prepared in an unsuccessful attempt to reach consensus." (70–73)

Inside the building, someone slams his fist on the table. A telephone crashes into the receiver. Near the back, a person who cannot be clearly seen hands a package to The Media. *It is a draft of the report!*

CHAIRMAN *[notably displeased]*: "One of these drafts unfortunately found its way to the media and has clouded the issue in the public's eye because of the tentative numbers that were quoted." *[The word "unfortunately," a frankly evaluative term that is almost out of character for* The Chairman, *is charged with suppressed anger.]* (73–75)

The Media *rush around the stage, carrying television cameras, speaking into microphones, distributing newspapers. A commotion spreads among* The Public *and* The Organizations. The Scientific Community *looks up from the lab bench. Telephones ring. People scurry about. One man leaps onto a soapbox and begins miming an impassioned speech. Faces look puzzled, worried, angry.*

Curtain

Act II

The same. The commotion continues, making the threat of disorder palpable. All action abruptly freezes and the stage is left in silence. After a moment the stage goes dark. When light returns, the Academy doors are shut. Outside, The Media, The Public, *and* The Organizations *remain frozen exactly as before.*

CHORUS: Trouble in the Academy
threatens the world outside.

Action must be taken.
The solution must be found.
To render rational judgment
is the Chairman's solemn task.

The doors open. Inside, the furniture is now arranged in a manner reminiscent of a courtroom. The Chairman sits at an elevated bench. The Committee and The Reviewers, seated at separate tables, face him. A spotlight illuminates The Chairman, who strikes a gavel and begins to speak. Everyone else remains perfectly still.*

THE CHAIRMAN *[tired, but resolute]*: "After exhaustive deliberation over the last 6 months, I have concluded that the National Research Council will be unable to issue the 10th edition of the *Recommended Dietary Allowances* at this time. My decision, as Research Council Chairman, is based on the recommendations of our Food and Nutrition Board and its parent body, the Commission on Life Sciences."**   (1–5)

CHORUS: Consultation, consideration, deliberation, judgment.
The highest official has resolved this case.

CHORAGOS: But was the judgment right? Let us wait to hear his reasons.

CHAIRMAN *[as if beginning a long explanation]*: "Our decision not to issue a report of the RDAs at this time stems primarily from an impasse that resulted from . . . scientific differences of opinion between the committee, scientific reviewers appointed by the Research Council, and additional reviewers from the Food and Nutrition Board."† (25–28)

---

* The play's author clearly intends the courtroom layout not as a literal depiction of the actual process followed at the Academy, but as the physical expression of the *stance* that the Chairman takes as the official authorized to mediate among the parties, attempt to settle the dispute, and, if necessary, impose a resolution.

** Several points must be made about this passage. First, these two sentences use first-person singular pronouns, which appear nowhere else in the letter and evoke a Truman-esque, the-buck-stops-here, personal ownership of the decision. But even as the Chairman accepts full responsibility, his reference to his official position in the Academy clearly signifies that he acted not as a lone individual but as the authority duly charged with resolving such matters. As if to underline this point, he notes that before reaching a judgment he consulted with appropriate other NRC officials.

The second point is of historical as well as literary interest: the Chairman does not indicate precisely when the decision to cancel the report was made. Consequently, we cannot know whether this resolution was reached before or after the leak of the draft report. How the leak was related to the decision, if indeed it was, remains unclear.

† At this point, the Chairman begins to describe the reasons for his decision. Interestingly, in his account, human agents, such as the Committee or the Reviewers, do not cause the

CHORAGOS: But if the cause was an impasse, what tipped the judgment to one side?

CHAIRMAN: "Some of the reviewers' concerns about adequate justification for change derived from their recognition of the RDAs' potentially vast impact on public health. . . . [Their] wide applications suggest that modifications to the RDAs must be based on a strong rationale and a comprehensive analysis of scientifically corroborated, persuasive evidence; they should reflect concurrence of scientific opinion."* (85–86, 98–100)

CHORUS: The burden of proof must rest
on those who propose a change.

CHAIRMAN: "Furthermore, reviewers suggested that unless scientific evidence indicates otherwise, the recommendations for *nutrient intakes* — the RDAs — must be consistent with recommended *dietary guidelines* for the maintenance of good health." (110–12)

He pauses.

"Other events contributing to our decision not to issue a report now include the deepening understanding of the interplay between nutritional factors and health, especially the importance of these factors in the aging process and in susceptibility to chronic diseases." (101–4)

CHORAGOS: It's well known that events change situations.
When science grows it's surely no one's *fault*!
But are the Fates to blame for this disaster?
Or should we call forth villains to account?

CHAIRMAN: "Neither the present committee nor the committee responsible for the previous edition was specifically asked to consider these issues. Nonetheless, the reviews of the report strongly suggest that the scientific developments in the past 5 years relating nutrition to health should be considered and that a more comprehensive approach is now warranted for assessing nutrient intake to satisfy 'the known nutritional needs of practically all healthy persons' in the United States." (104–10)

---

decision; the proximate cause is an "impasse," which, in turn, stems from "scientific differences of opinion." Although the Chairman ultimately sides with the Reviewers, he never explicitly blames the Committee for the impasse. Instead, as we see below, he outlines various factors that he considered, such as the gravity of the Reviewers' concerns, the changing nature of nutrition science and policy, and the need for broad rather than narrow analysis.

* Note how the Chairman positions the Reviewers as advocates of health, a core value in contemporary American society.

"Thus, although the committee followed the charge given to it in 1980, it became apparent that its primary focus on the avoidance of nutritional deficiencies may be neither sufficient nor appropriate."* (112–15)

CHORUS: A limited charge, loyally followed.
Blameless defeat meets joyless victory.

CHAIRMAN [*summing up*]: "For all these interrelated reasons, the National Research Council has concluded that the publication of the next edition of the RDAs warrants a more encompassing analysis of data pertaining to nutrients and health by a new committee specially constituted to address these issues." [*He strikes the gavel.*] (125 – 28)

Curtain

Act III

The doors of the Academy are closed. Outside, The Media, The Public, The Organizations, *and* The Scientific Community *are still frozen exactly as they were.*

CHORUS: The Chairman has acted. Rationality prevails.
Order is restored.

The doors open. The courtroom furniture is gone and the interior is again in its original state. Normal business proceeds inside. The Chairman's voice is heard, but once again he cannot be seen.

CHAIRMAN [*calmly*]: "In the weeks to come, our Food and Nutrition Board, in consultation with the National Institutes of Health, will consider various options and will make recommendations to the Research Council accordingly."** (128–30)

"Whatever course of action is taken, the next report concerning the RDAs

---

* The complex ambiguities of the Chairman's treatment of blame for this episode should be noted. At times, the Chairman strikes a pose of complete evenhandedness. At times, he hints that the Committee stubbornly resisted reasonable criticism. At times, he attributes a causal role to events that were clearly outside the Committee's control. At times, he positions the Committee as "narrow" (which he freights with a negative valence) rather than "broad" or "encompassing." Yet the Chairman also points out that the Committee followed its charge, providing it with an extremely strong defense, given that acting in accordance with one's formal instructions is a cardinal duty in a bureaucracy. Surely, the fact that scientific progress made the charge obsolete cannot be held against the Committee. The Chairman's words about blame are thus potentially consistent with a variety of interpretations. The Academy thereby avoids attacking the Committee directly or contending that it was culpable, yet leaves open the option of — and indeed lays the groundwork for — doing so in the future.
** The future tense is prominent in this Act, which is the only place in the play where it appears. It serves to direct the audience away from an episode that is now conclusively over and toward a future in which order again prevails in the Academy and the world of nutrition.

will, like all our reports, be prepared, reviewed, and published in accordance with [the] Research Council's highest standards. We are confident that it will represent the best scientific judgment on matters of nutrient intake and health — issues that have an enormous impact on public health." (131–35)

"Until a new report is issued, the only National Research Council recommendations in effect are those contained in the ninth edition of the RDAs, which was published in 1980." (136–38)

As The Chairman *speaks,* The Public, The Media, The Organizations, *and* The Scientific Community *begin to unfreeze. Worry and anger vanish from their faces. Confidence replaces confusion. Harmonious business resumes.*

CHAIRMAN: "The public and the scientific community at large should rest assured that there is no cause for concern and that they may continue to place confidence in the RDAs that have been in effect for the past 5 years."* (138–40)

All of the characters on the stage naturally drift into precisely the same positions that they occupied at the instant the play began.**

Curtain

By repackaging the Academy announcement as a play, I have tried to unpack the way the letter inscribes the demise of the 1985 Draft in a narrative about the maintenance of social order. It is a tale of breach, crisis, redress, and reintegration that follows, to a striking degree, the narrative structure of the social dramas described by Victor Turner.[13] The Chairman's profoundly normative story recounts how the internal order of the Academy, embodied in its smoothly functioning procedures, allows it to transform controversy into consensus, producing reliable knowledge and enhancing the order of the outside world. When disorder appears in the form of an intractable dispute, the Academy ultimately proves robust enough to respond to this challenge: the Chairman takes strong action and order is restored. Interestingly, even the disorder surrounding the intractable dispute appears to be rather orderly. All of the actors (at least within the Academy) appear to perform more or less as they should. There is no hint of malfeasance or incompetence; the characters

---

* As we have seen, the internal order of the Academy, the credibility of its advice, the reliability of the RDAs, and the order in the world of nutrition are all linked. The restoration of order entails restoring confidence at all these levels.

** At the end of the play, the problem of the intractable dispute is solved and the episode is closed. The deliberate, studied consideration of appropriate next steps signals the return to normalcy within the Academy. The nutrition community can continue as before. Public concern is unwarranted. Inside and outside the Academy, the social order has been restored.

are not fools or villains; no one seeks to transform expertise into illegitimate power or to corrupt science with bias. The Academy's institutional machinery does not break down. Indeed, in the Academy's announcement, the RDA episode is not a symptom of more profound problems, but a demonstration of how well its procedures function even in exceptionally difficult situations.

To be sure, the Chairman's letter gently suggests that the committee may have been too stubborn or too committed to a narrow view of the RDAs, but any such criticisms are muted. After all, the Committee has followed its charge — a cardinal duty in a bureaucracy. Indeed, everyone in the Academy (the Chairman, the Food and Nutrition Board, the Reviewers — even the Committee!) seems to have followed the scripted roles that appear in the Academy's official accounts of its backstage operations. The leak to the media represents the only bona fide departure from proper procedures. (The Chairman marks this exception with the word *unfortunately*. Nothing else in the letter merits such a frankly evaluative word; the impasse is not called *regrettable*, the failure to reach consensus is not labeled *unfortunate*, no developments are said to be *unfavorable, distressing, disturbing, troubling,* or *outrageous.*) Only the leaker, who the Academy did not or could not publicly identify, broke the rules.

Even though the cancellation of an NRC report is a rare event, the Academy announcement casts it as completely normal, framing it as a logical consequence of the situation, not an aberration: The Academy successfully contained the problem posed by an "unsuccessful attempt to reach consensus." A true institutional breakdown — publishing an unsound report — was successfully averted. The Academy, the Chairman assures us, performed as it should.

THE KAMIN LETTER

The chair of the 1980–85 RDA committee, Henry Kamin, inscribed the same events in a very different plot. Whereas the Academy contended that its decision stemmed from its commitment to providing reliable science advice, Kamin argued that the episode pointed to serious institutional problems in the Academy — problems that signaled an end to its ability to offer credible nutrition advice. In short, Kamin argued that the Academy had suppressed a sound scientific report for political reasons; the cancellation was thus an ominous instance of politics contaminating science.[14]

An important methodological tenet in science and technology studies is the principle of symmetry, which calls for using the same analytic tools to examine all sides of a controversy. Accordingly, the analysis now develops a detailed reading of how the Kamin letter emplots the action and defines the identities of the characters. In this case, however, I shall stick to conventional prose, rather than adapting the letter for the stage (two plays in one chapter might grow tedious). Like the Academy announcement, the Kamin letter is highly stylized, and it could easily be transformed into a melodrama about defending Science against Politics. (A play based on it might be set in the Middle Ages and called *Treason in the Castle*, or perhaps *Barbarians at the Gates*. In the dark world it portrays, ignorant hordes, pretenders, and unfaithful courtiers vastly outnumber the guardians of truth. But rather than continue this sketch, I shall leave the task of repackaging the Kamin letter as a play to exercise the interested reader.) The full text, which consists of about 1,100 words, appears in the Appendix. Quotations are indicated in the notes by line number.

Kamin's Story

Let us begin with a brief summary of the basic story of the Kamin letter. The tale unfolds as follows:

1. The RDA committee, which sought to provide "the best science possible," produced a solid, scientific report.[15]

2. "Misguided" critics pressured the Academy to alter the report.[16] These critics attacked the report with erroneous arguments. Among the critics' complaints was the incorrect charge that the report was systematically reducing the RDAs. The critics also objected because the draft report sought to lower the RDAs for vitamins A and C, a move that the critics opposed for policy reasons.

3. The RDA committee, dedicated to upholding scientific principles, resisted these political demands. The committee, appropriately, remained open to modifying the report in response to "valid scientific critiques." Quite properly, it also refused to make changes based on "hunches, personal preferences, public relations, fear of controversy, or criteria of whether they support or question existing programs."[17]

4. In an act of cowardice, the Academy canceled the report, despite the absence of sound scientific reasons for doing so.

5. The conduct of the Academy in this case is so troubling that it calls into question its integrity as an institution.

The Moral Stakes

Kamin's letter casts the events surrounding the 1985 Draft as a struggle between science and nonscience, or, in more traditionally theatrical terms, as a melodramatic conflict between good and evil. Let us consider the normative framework he uses to position characters and their acts in this sharply defined moral space. Kamin's normative framework relies on a sharp distinction between the "scientific" and the "nonscientific," especially between science and policy. For Kamin, the central moral issue is the need to maintain the purity of science, and he frames the episode as a "conflict between those who wish to give the best science possible — a viewpoint identified with the RDA committee — and those who appear to be injecting policy considerations into scientific judgments."[18] The Academy leadership and other critics of the RDA committee fall into the policy-motivated category. In contrast, the RDA committee was dedicated to maintaining the integrity of science.

The Kamin letter is overtly normative, providing explicit moral instruction to both scientists and policymakers, the two most important general categories of actors in the story. The social order of science and of policy depends on maintaining the proper relationship between science and policy:

> scientists should give the best advice they can and should not twist their science to meet the needs or desires of policymakers, constituencies, or special interest groups. The product of the latter attitude is both bad science *and* bad policy. Who are we on the RDA committee to make the judgment that present policies are necessarily correct? Or wrong? Good administrators recognize this. . . .[19]

Good scientists and good administrators alike recognize that science and policy are separate endeavors that must not be confused. Science can inform policy, but policy should not contaminate science.

The Characters: Heroes and Villains

The Kamin letter features a diverse cast of characters:

"Eliot Marshall"   The *Science* reporter who wrote the article that occasioned the Kamin-Olson-Press exchange. Marshall's article strongly suggests that policy considerations influenced the Academy, and Kamin calls it "informative," "generally correct," and "valuable in identifying the issues."[20]

"those who oppose our committee's draft"   This group is guilty of "the major errors and misconceptions."[21]

"those who wish to give the best science possible"   The RDA committee and its allies.[22]

"The RDA committee" (also referred to as *"we"*)   When preparing the report, the RDA committee attempted to provide "the best science possible." In the debate surrounding drafts of the report, the RDA committee also displays an appropriate openness to evidence, remaining "totally flexible" about modifying its recommendations in response to "sound and documented science." Kamin consistently portrays the RDA committee as objective.[23]

"those who appear to be injecting policy considerations into scientific judgments"   The opponents of the RDA committee.[24]

"National Academy of Sciences president Frank Press"   Not only does Press cancel the report, but in Kamin's hands he also appears to be guilty of duplicity: "If, as National Academy of Sciences president Frank Press says, there are substantial 'scientific differences of opinion,' then surely they could have been expressed in the language of documented science. But these 'scientific' reasons have not emerged despite repeated requests on the part of the RDA committee."[25]

"Michael Lemov of the Food Research and Action Center"   Lemov, a leading critic of the draft report, cites "the 'shocking' possibility that reducing the RDA's would mean 'less food and more hunger for millions of people' in food programs." Kamin presents this claim as without merit.[26]

"D. Mark Hegsted"   In the Kamin letter, Hegsted, a well-known nutrition scientist and advocate of nutrition reform, plays the leading villain and Kamin refers to a number of his misdeeds:

Hegsted "accuses" the RDA committee of approaching its "task 'as a purely academic exercise and from a very limited perspective' " and "seems to imply" that it is "insensitive to the impact" of its changes on policy.[27]

Hegsted writes a letter that "may have . . . frightened the Academy." His letter "makes grave warnings about bad public relations, controversy, congressional hearings, and so forth — that the public would be confused and the Academy embarrassed."[28]

Hegsted is "a long-time critic of RDA's" — a phrase that suggests he may be biased against them.[29]

Hegsted makes erroneous statements about previous Academy reports, incorrectly alleging that the 1985 Draft would "undercut" *Diet, Nutrition, and Cancer*. "Our RDA's have no inconsistencies with the 1982 report, but may be inconsistent with the publicity-induced mythology that surrounds it," Kamin contends. In any case, even if there *were* inconsistencies, "must all scientists, 'speak with a single voice'?" Because Hegsted seems to think so, he emerges as an agent of orthodoxy.[30]

"critics" of the RDA report   Owing to its placement in the letter, this term clearly includes Hegsted and Lemov, but it may also extend to other unnamed people and groups. The critics are "misguided on several grounds":

"(i) The RDA's have not been systematically 'reduced'; we made no effort to impose a direction of recommendation for the 29 or so nutrients covered. Some are up, some are down, and a few are unchanged. We simply went nutrient by nutrient, giving each the best value we could.

"(ii) It is ridiculous, on the basis of the few RDA's 'leaked,' to predict overall cost or food pattern, and my own guess is that there would be little if any effect."[31]

"Betty B. Peterkin, acting administrator of the Human Nutrition Information Service of the U.S. Department of Agriculture"   Peterkin helps refute the critics. Kamin quotes her statement that the "possible effects of changes in RDA for a few nutrients . . . on food assistance programs [have] been greatly exaggerated."[32]

Kamin casts Peterkin as a "good administrator" who appreciates the importance of maintaining the purity of science: "Peterkin writes of her 'whole-hearted support of [our] view that the Recommended Dietary Allowances should represent the best advice scientists can give and should not be affected by policy considerations. . . .' "[33]

"the present Academy administration"   The current administration considers the report *Toward Healthful Diets* to be a "fiasco." In fact, the report "is by no means dead, since the issue it raised is a strategic one: would the public be better served if the advice to decrease fat intake were to be strongly targeted to those at risk or diffused throughout the entire population?"[34]

"the present nutritional establishment at the Academy"   A group that may not be capable of providing "impartial scientific advice."[35]

"Philip Handler's administration"   Kamin portrays the Handler administration, which immediately preceded that of Frank Press, as a guardian of the integrity of science. It defended *Toward Healthful Diets* "vigorously."[36]

"the Academy"   The Kamin letter uses this term to refer to the Acad-

emy under Press's leadership, which appears unwilling to stand up for scientific principles. The Academy "can act timorously and be frightened away by hints of controversy, 'bad' image, public relations, and other nonscientific considerations, such as fear of 'giving confusing signals to the public.'"

The Academy also dealt inappropriately with the committee: "Its responses, thus far, have consisted in extolling its review procedures and systematically avoiding direct discussion of the scientific justification of its objections to the actual points at issue — the proposed RDA's for vitamins A and C. Our attempts to reopen serious discourse on these issues have been unsuccessful over a period of months. We remain open to such discourse. . . ."[37]

As the letter draws to a close, Kamin presents the consequences of the Academy's present weaknesses as truly ominous: in its "attempt to avoid controversy," the Academy "has forced attention on more serious questions: the capability of the present nutritional establishment at the Academy to give impartial scientific advice and the Academy's fundamental integrity as a defender of the scientific process."[38]

Perhaps most striking about the above inventory of characters is the ease of separating them into sharply defined, opposing categories of heroes and villains (Table 5).[39] The RDA committee, Peterkin, and Philip Handler's administration are among the heroes. Hegsted, Lemov, Press, and the current Academy leadership are among the villains. Thus, in keeping with the melodramatic genre, the characters of the Kamin letter fall neatly into two camps, good versus evil, as they struggle over the central moral issue: defending objective science from interested politics.

The Scene: Science Besieged

Beyond examining the characters, it is useful to consider the scene of the Kamin drama. In what kind of space does the action occur? The story takes place in a world where science is under attack. Science is surrounded by nonscientific forces. Pressure groups encircle it, and its loyal followers must protect it from policymakers, constituencies, and special interests that seek to compromise its purity. In short, Kamin's letter describes a society in which science is besieged.[40] Worse still, the Academy — which is supposed to be "a defender of the scientific process" — has fallen under the control of bad leaders. In the past, the Academy had been strong; Handler defended *Toward Healthful Diets* "vigorously." But the present Academy leadership and

TABLE 5
Heroes and Villains in Henry Kamin's Drama

Heroes	Villains
The RDA committee	D. Mark Hegsted
Philip Handler's administration	Michael Lemov
Betty B. Peterkin of the USDA	Frank Press
"those who wish to give the best science possible"	"those who oppose our committee's draft"
"Philip Handler's administration"	"those who appear to be injecting policy considerations into scientific judgments"
	"critics" of the draft RDA report
	"the present Academy administration"
	"the present nutritional establishment at the Academy"

SOURCE: Kamin 1985b. For full text, see Appendix B.

NOTE: Listed in order of appearance.

nutritional establishment are weak. Thus, not only is the Academy being attacked from outside, it is also threatened from within.

The Olson Letter

The Kamin letter was not the only text to treat the story of the 1985 Draft in these terms. Other prominent critics of the Academy's decision developed similar melodramas. Robert E. Olson's letter to *Science* provides an example that merits brief consideration.[41] Like Kamin, Olson features outsiders, such as "nutrition activists, sociologists, lawyers, and some zealous scientists," who generate "social and political pressure." Like Kamin, Olson morally objects to the idea that nonscientific pressures "should be able to nullify a sound scientific report." Like Kamin, Olson attacks Frank Press, questioning the legitimacy of the cancellation. ("Chairmen of the National Research Council," Olson wrote, "have occasionally taken exception to NRC reports, but if the science has been acceptable, as it seems to be in the case of the report of the 1985 RDA committee, they have not banned them.") Like Kamin, Olson criticizes the Academy's nutrition establishment, suggesting that its connections to federal programs aimed at dietary change might constitute "conflict of interest."[42] Finally, like Kamin, Olson closes his letter with an ominous statement about the integrity of the Academy:

> the failure to publish the 1985 RDA Committee's report by the NAS is unprecedented, unjustified, arbitrary, and unwise. There are no valid scientific arguments against publication of this report. The rejection of the report by the Academy, presumably because of social and political pressure, is a frightening harbinger of the future. The Academy is supposed to be the highest shrine in America for the protection of good science against these very pressures.[43]

In short, Olson and Kamin both describe a world in which the integrity of science is under assault, the Academy leadership is weak or corrupt, and the prospects for the future look alarming.

THE DRAMAS COMPARED

The Academy announcement and the Kamin letter do not merely make opposing arguments; they also describe very different worlds. In many respects, the contrast could not be more striking. The Academy's announcement presents the cancellation as a legitimate means of maintaining social order. The Kamin letter frames the cancellation as an illegitimate action that threatens science and the social order. But these two accounts of the episode do not simply tell different versions of the "same" story; they paint vastly different portraits of the Academy, the backstage space where its reports are prepared, and its relationship to the social order.

One way to highlight the contrasts between these worlds is to compare the characters that populate them. At times, characters in the two dramas have the same name yet differ greatly. A good example is "the RDA committee." A steadfast defender of scientific integrity in the Kamin letter, the committee is just another expert committee in Chairman Press's account. In other cases, characters that are prominently featured in one drama are entirely absent from the other. Hegsted, Lemov, and Peterkin all play notable roles in the Kamin drama. Yet none of them make even a cameo appearance in the Academy announcement. Neither do "nutrition activists, sociologists, lawyers, or zealous scientists" (to use Olson's words). Nor does anyone else who seeks to inject "policy considerations into scientific judgments." On the other hand, the reviewers, who play a major role in the Academy announcement, are completely missing from the Kamin letter.[44] Olson mentions the reviewers only once; the NRC chairman refers to them nine times.[45]

The characters of these dramas also differ greatly in the kinds of acts they perform. Many of the figures in Kamin's letter behave in ways that express overt conflict or exhibit their individual psychology or failings. Lemov objects to a "shocking" possibility. Hegsted "accuses" the committee and "makes grave warnings." The Academy becomes "frightened" and acts "timorously." But in Chairman Press's account, the characters (who generally are bureaucratic entities, not individuals) execute impersonal, organizational functions: they appoint, deliberate, review, or recommend.[46]

What sort of characters inhabit the world outside of the Academy? In the chairman's account, the characters in the outside world include NIH Director James Wyngaarden, the public, the media, government agencies, industry, academia, the health services sector, the private sector, the scientific community, and the National Institutes of Health. Almost without exception, these figures are cast as *users* of knowledge generated by the Academy. Influence — in the form of sound scientific advice — flows from inside the Academy outward, contributing to the orderly operation of the wider world. There is no hint that influence might possibly flow in the opposite direction. The principal threat in the chairman's announcement is the danger that weak advice might wreak havoc beyond the Academy. But in the Kamin letter, matters seem nearly reversed. The world outside the Academy is populated by policymakers, constituencies, and special interest groups who seek to influence the Academy's conclusions. Although some "good administrators," such as Peterkin, are wise enough to oppose efforts to pressure the Academy, the opponents of the committee's draft succeed in persuading the Academy to twist the science. Influence flows from the outside world into the Academy, threatening the social order with the prospect of "bad science *and* bad policy."

If we direct our gaze inside the Academy, what sorts of characters do we encounter? In the chairman's account, most characters are officially chartered entities, with the hierarchical relationships among them duly noted (Table 6). In the Academy announcement, these entities behave properly, performing their organizationally sanctioned roles as they should. (Recall that even the committee followed its charge.) The only clear breach of appropriate conduct is the leak, and its source is not specified. In Kamin's account, however, the inside of the Academy looks rather different. The Academy houses a number of villains who have abandoned their sacred commitment to protect the integrity of science. The good guys who once occupied leadership positions have been replaced, and the change has effected a moral transformation of the Academy. "Philip Handler's administration" was better than "the present nutritional establishment" precisely because it was willing to defend good science — as embodied in *Toward Healthful Diets* — vigorously. In contrast, Chairman Press's letter conveys the impression that the orderly rationality of the Academy is a stable feature of its character, which is not significantly altered by changes in personnel.

The chairman's account also systematically downplays the influence of individual people. Indeed, the letter makes no mention at all of individuals, with two exceptions — James Wyngaarden, to whom it is addressed, and Frank Press, who signed it. The names Wyngaarden and Press each appear once (in the salutation and signature lines, respectively). The first two sentences of the letter also use first person singular pronouns when Press takes Trumanesque responsibility for the decision.[47] In the Kamin letter, individuals are both more numerous and more significant. But more telling than this quantitative difference is the qualitative contrast in the nature of the characters. The classic sociological distinction between the *person* and the *office* that the person holds is useful here. For Press, the Academy is a world of offices. Individuals are irrelevant. Offices matter. People are merely the temporary occupants of institutional positions, and organizational scripts seem to govern their activities. Thus, the Academy presents itself as the embodiment of procedures that are both more powerful and more permanent than those who perform them.[48]

Kamin portrays the Academy very differently. Individuals are not interchangeable parts but are manifestly capable of influencing institutions. The individuals in Kamin's account leave distinct personal marks on the institution. The NRC of "Philip Handler's administration" differed from the NRC of "the present Academy administration." Frank Press is a different sort of chairman from those of the past, for he alone (to use Olson's words) has taken the "unprecedented, unjustified, arbitrary, and unwise" step of banning a report to which he took exception.

And what of institutional procedures, the central source of stability in the world of the chairman's drama? Kamin refers to them exactly once. The Academy's responses, he writes,

TABLE 6

Comparison of the Characters in Chairman Press's Letter
and the Kamin Letter

The Chairman's Letter	The Kamin Letter
SPECIFIC INDIVIDUALS	
James Wyngaarden	Eliot Marshall
Frank Press	Frank Press
	D. Mark Hegsted
	Michael Lemov
	Betty B. Peterkin
	Philip Handler
	James Wyngaarden
	Henry Kamin
SPECIFIED ORGANIZATIONAL ENTITIES	
National Research Council	the committee
Research Council Chairman	National Academy of Sciences
Food and Nutrition Board	Food Research and Action Center
Commission on Life Sciences	the Human Nutrition Information Service of the USDA
committees of the National Research Council's Food and Nutrition Board	the Academy
Committee on Dietary Allowances of the Food and Nutrition Board	previous RDA committees
the committee	the present Academy administration
reviewers appointed by the Research Council	Philip Handler's administration
reviewers from the Food and Nutrition Board	"the present nutritional establishment at the Academy"

(continued)

so far, have consisted in extolling its review procedures and systematically avoiding direct discussion of the actual points at issue — the proposed RDA's for vitamins A and C. Our attempts to open serious discourse on these issues have been unsuccessful over a period of months.

Kamin thus betrays considerable skepticism about the efficacy of Academy procedures — at least when implemented by the present nutritional establishment. The Academy may praise the virtues of procedures, but talk of procedures may only be talk. When executed by the wrong people,

TABLE 6 *(continued)*

The Chairman's Letter	The Kamin Letter
SPECIFIED ORGANIZATIONAL ENTITIES	
National Academy of Sciences	
the Research Council's Report Review Committee	
the reviewers	
National Institutes of Health	
CATEGORICALLY DEFINED ENTITIES	
scientists	"those who oppose our committee's draft"
the public	"those who wish to give the best science possible"
experts	"those who appear to be injecting policy considerations into scientific judgments"
the media	critics [of the report]
government agencies	scientists
industry	policymakers
academia	constituencies
the health services sector	special interest groups
the private sector	good administrators
the scientific community	the public
	other nations

SOURCES: Press 1985a and Kamin 1985b. For full texts, see Appendixes A and B.

NOTE: Within each category (e.g., specific individuals, etc.), characters are listed in order of appearance in the original letters.

procedures cannot guarantee that serious scientific matters will be properly addressed.

Many other contrasts emerge from comparing these dramas:

In Press's letter, the Academy is strong. Its track record is impressive, its procedures are robust, its advice is sound. Its ability to bring this difficult matter to closure demonstrates its institutional strength.

In Kamin's letter, the Academy is weak. Its porous boundaries cannot resist contaminating pressures and its leadership lacks resolve or integrity.

The Academy announcement frames the decision-making process as adjudication; it is a tripartite process in which the Academy bureaucracy, personified by the chairman, mediates between, and ultimately decides between, two groups, the committee and the reviewers.

The Kamin letter frames the decision-making process as a direct confrontation between two groups, with no judge standing outside. One of these groups is "scientific," one "unscientific." In the chairman's letter, the competing groups and the judge are all "scientific."

In the chairman's letter, the cancellation of the report was a legitimate matter of "science."

In Kamin's account, the decision was an illegitimate intrusion of "policy" into science.[49]

In the chairman's letter, it is appropriate for the Academy to consider the uses of its advice on the world outside.

In the Kamin account, to consider impacts on the world outside is tantamount to twisting science.

The Academy's account is the story of an isolated incident that temporarily interrupts the normal state of affairs. The orderly world of the Academy is temporarily disrupted by a disorderly event, but the problem is neatly contained, paving the way for an orderly future.

The Kamin letter is a story of decline. Not only is science besieged, but one of its great institutions has lost its resolve or even fallen into enemy hands.

Table 7 summarizes the differences between the two dramas. Because these accounts contrast so sharply, it might be tempting to think that they share no common features. But to conclude this would be to overlook the fact that they also share some fundamental similarities. Both accounts present policymakers as profoundly dependent on sound advice, stressing the importance of maintaining its quality. A central theme in the chairman's account is the need to prevent the publication of unreliable advice. Kamin, too, insists on the need for good science, which is an essential input to good policy. Thus, each account is premised on the notion that the maintenance of proper social order *within* science is necessary to produce impartial, reliable science advice, and, at the same time, trustworthy science advice is essential to the maintenance of social order *outside* of science. However, these highly stylized accounts emphasize different threats to order, painting very different portraits of the world of the backstage as they dramatize their competing assessments of the true character of the Academy.

TABLE 7
The Dramas Compared

The Academy's Announcement	The Kamin Letter
The dispute is between two scientific groups (the committee and the reviewers).	The dispute is between one scientific group (those who seek to provide the best science) and one nonscientific group (those who seek to inject policy considerations into science).
The decision to cancel was a matter of science.	The decision to cancel was a matter of policy.
The Academy bureaucracy adjudicates between the disputants.	There is no third party to adjudicate between the disputants.
The decision to cancel is made inside the Academy.	Outsiders participate in the Academy's decision.
The Academy is strong; its boundaries are firm.	The Academy is weak; its boundaries are porous.
The Academy is surrounded by users of its advice. Influence flows from inside the Academy out.	The Academy is surrounded by pressure groups that seek to alter its advice. Influence flows into the Academy from outside.
The actors inside the Academy uniformly behave properly.	Some actors inside the Academy behave improperly.
The Academy is a world of procedures and offices. Individuals appear only as the occupants of institutional posts.	The Academy is a world of persons. Individuals leave their personal mark on institutions.
The Academy is stable over time.	The Academy may change significantly when the administration changes.
The cancellation was a normal consequence of an unusual situation.	The cancellation was abnormal and unprecedented.
Procedures are powerful.	Talk of procedures may only be talk.
The cancellation was necessary to preserve the social order.	The cancellation constitutes a breach of the social order.
The episode is an isolated incident. The future looks good.	The episode signals troubled times ahead. The future looks ominous.

THE CHAIRMAN'S REPLY

The Kamin and Olson letters fiercely attacked the Academy's self-presentation, claiming that the idealized image of the Academy no longer matched its true character and that its words did not match its deeds. How did the

Academy respond to these serious charges? The answer appears in our third and final key text, NRC Chairman Frank Press's letter to the editor of *Science* replying to Kamin and Olson. In his response, Press made four main moves:

1. *Denying the charges.*   Press restates and rejects Kamin and Olson's charges and reiterates the Academy's official explanation of the cancellation:

> Eliot Marshall's article in the 25 October issue implies and Kamin and Olson in letters in this issue assert that the recent action of the National Research Council on the Recommended Dietary Allowances (RDA's) was governed by policy considerations, pressure from special interest groups, and a fear of controversy. In fact, our decision was based on advice from scientific reviewers, including members of the Food and Nutrition Board and the Commission on Life Sciences, which oversee the preparation of the RDA's; members of the National Academy of Sciences; and other nutritionists as scientifically competent as the panel that drafted the report.[50]

2. *Claiming that the report did not pass scientific peer review.*   In the original Academy announcement, Press uses the language of "impasse" (the committee and the reviewers were "unable to agree," there were "differences of opinion," they took "different scientific approaches").[51] His reply to Kamin and Olson, however, uses the language of failure:

> It was the judgment of these reviewers that the RDA panel's suggestions for modifying the recommended levels for certain nutrients were not justified by the scientific evidence presented. The panel was apprised of these detailed criticisms — over 130 pages in all. However, the panel's responses satisfied neither its parent unit — the Food and Nutrition Board — nor the officers of the National Research Council.[52]

Later, Press argues:

> Despite months of deliberation and discussion, the panel's draft did not pass the scientific peer review and achieve the standards expected of Research Council reports.[53]

3. *Presenting the NRC as orderly and rule-governed.*   Like the original Academy announcement, Press's reply depicts the NRC as a place of rational, impersonal, objective procedures:

> To ensure accuracy, completeness, and balance in interpretation of scientific data, every Research Council report is reviewed by specifically appointed inde-

pendent scientific experts and any professional unit that oversees the work of the panel.[54]

And:

> All Research Council professional units are periodically examined for balance of expertise and viewpoints. The current Food and Nutrition Board is a broadly constituted, well-balanced group of experts from academia and the public and private sectors.[55]

As in the Academy announcement, the individuals that occupy Academy offices are not named (with the exception of Press, who appears as the author of the letter). The only individuals named are Marshall, Kamin, and Olson.

4. *Undermining the credibility of Kamin and Olson.*   Press questions Kamin's account of the discussions within the NRC:

> Regrettably, the flexibility claimed in Kamin's letter was not apparent during lengthy discussions between him and various representatives of the Research Council in intensive efforts to resolve certain differences of scientific opinion. The suggestion that the RDA's for vitamins A and C were the pivotal points for my decision is misleading.[56]

His attack on Olson is even more damning:

> Robert Olson was neither a part of the panel nor party to the review process. His letter contains unverified assertions about the NRC's decision, selective citations, faulty characterization of the review process, and unjustified attacks on members of the Food and Nutrition Board.[57]

Finally, Press suggests that Kamin and Olson are rejecting peer review:

> Kamin, Olson, and others who take issue with the Research Council's process of decision-making appear to reject the most basic tenet of American science — the peer review process.[58]

These four moves, which I have presented separately, in fact fit together into an integrated rebuttal of Kamin and Olson's contention that the Academy had gone seriously astray: not only, according to Press, was it untrue that the Academy had twisted science to meet the needs of policy, but the individuals who asserted this were not credible, the report had been canceled for purely scientific reasons, and the Academy continued to exemplify disinterested scientific rationality.

In Press's reply to Kamin and Olson, the Academy once again casts itself as the personification of impersonal procedures. But the reply departs in important ways from the original Academy announcement. A story of impasse is replaced by one of failure to pass peer review; differences of opinion are reframed as lack of rigor; blame is sharpened and focused. The stubbornness of the committee emerges more clearly, and Kamin enters the story as an inflexible individual. Olson appears as a purveyor of unjustified, ad hominem attacks. Through these means, Kamin and Olson, the people who deny that the Academy is a world of procedures, are depicted as untrustworthy commentators. Press's reply thus blends a tale of untrustworthy individuals into the Academy's original story of orderly procedures, a recasting of the drama that allows the Academy to dismiss Kamin, Olson, and their criticisms. The Academy should be trusted; its critics should not.[59]

CONCLUSIONS

The leaks and public displays of disunity that accompanied the cancellation of the 1985 Draft raised doubts about whether the backstage world of the Academy markedly differed from the orderly, rule-based system that its official accounts describe. To understand how the Academy defends its character in such situations, this chapter has taken a detailed look at three central texts in the struggle over the cancellation of the report. The analysis explores the techniques that the main protagonists — the NAS leadership, on the one hand, and Kamin (and Olson), on the other — used to emplot the action and develop compelling accounts of events. As we have seen, the critics and the NAS leadership cast the Academy in starkly different terms (Table 7). The extreme stylization of their accounts is not an artifact of my analysis but stems from the means that the protagonists, as theatrically self-conscious actors, used to produce their performances. The point of this analysis is not just that these accounts compress ambiguous and complex events into simple and streamlined stories. Nor is it merely that the opposing images of the Academy that emerge from this process are caricatures. The point is that the techniques of emplotment examined above are central to creating, contesting, and maintaining the public identity of the Academy as a character in the drama of public life.

The Academy's efforts to emplot events in a narrative consistent with its everyday self-presentation provide an example of an attempt to achieve what we might call "discursive containment" — the use of narrative devices to recapture embarrassing leaks and unfortunate spectacles within a storyline that is consistent with a performer's everyday self-presentation. Discursive containment, with its re-presentation of potentially discrediting events in minimally discrediting ways, works hand in hand with other information-control practices.[60] The Academy's normal confidentiality procedures, not to mention its legal ownership of the draft report, allowed it to halt publication despite the committee's objections, to negotiate with the NIH about next steps, and to limit public access to a great deal of information. Thus, even after dramaturgical cooperation broke down and leaks made aspects of the dispute public, the Academy was able to maintain control over many important documents, thereby constraining the kinds of investigations that interested parties could conduct. The Academy thus sought to defend its character by simultaneously restricting access and channeling the perceptions of observers through its own carefully formulated accounts. Clearly, the success of the Academy as a source of authoritative science advice is inextricably connected to its ability to define its public persona in ways that protect it from challenges to its scientific and moral integrity. For this reason, the narrative devices and information-control techniques that the Academy uses to construct and defend its character are not mere epiphenomena but are indispensable to its performance.

CHAPTER 5

Conclusion

Science advice plays a crucial, if underappreciated, role in the politics of contemporary societies. Governments find expert advice to be an indispensable resource for formulating and justifying policy and, more subtly, for removing some issues from the political domain by transforming them into technical questions. Nevertheless, the authority of science advice is often problematic. Science advisors frequently encounter challenges to their objectivity and expertise, and struggles over the credibility of expert advice play a pivotal role in many policy arenas. Previous studies, however, pay little attention to the social machinery that advisory bodies use to construct and maintain their credibility. This book has developed a dramaturgical perspective for examining this machinery and has used it to conduct a comparative analysis of the struggles over three controversial National Academy of Sciences reports. This exercise not only illuminates the operation of the Academy — an important source of high-quality advice in many policy domains — but also illustrates how the investigation of stage management can yield more general insights about the role of information control in constructing the authority of expert knowledge.

The Academy's significant contributions to U.S. government rest on its credibility, and this book has examined the interactive process through which the credibility of its advice is produced, challenged, and sustained. The analysis shows that stage management and struggles over the enclosure and disclosure of information play a central role in shaping the fate of Academy reports. The Academy's techniques of information control, which aim to achieve a sharp separation between front- and backstage, operate on both "sides" of the boundary that they are designed to maintain. Practices that regulate access to information create the backstage, a "space" defined via confidentiality procedures that manage the flow of persons, speech, and documents. Means of information control are also built into the texts that the Academy presents on the front stage. Its reports display univocal narratives of expert agreement, concealing details about backstage deliberations that might undermine the appearance of unity. In addition, while working to prevent audiences from observing the backstage directly, it publicly presents authorized descriptions of it. These accounts — in keeping with the Academy's presentation of self — portray the backstage as a world populated by disinterested characters, regulated by impersonal procedures, and separated from contaminating interests. The official accounts thus assure outsiders that the objectivity of the NRC process is grounded in procedures that guarantee expertise, independence, and balance.

This system of stage management plays a central role in creating authoritative reports. When it is successful, as it was in the case of *Diet, Nutrition, and Cancer*, the Academy produces very compelling performances. Stage management helps the Academy draw its teams together, creating a single, collective voice while disciplining the individual voices of team members, whose authority to speak is circumscribed according to organizationally imposed spatial, temporal, and social boundaries. These practices also contribute to the Academy's ability to constrain the voices of its audiences. Its system of stage management creates a particular kind of performance, one that offers only limited opportunities for members of the audience to participate in the production. (As a point of contrast, consider avant-garde theatrical experiments that deliberately blur the boundaries between performers and audiences.) In addition, making the backstage unobservable except through the Academy's stylized, and arguably sanitized, accounts restricts the ways in which members of the audience can authoritatively "talk back" to a report. The Academy's system of stage management is thus not merely a mechanism to regulate the flow of information but also a means of structuring the relations between experts and publics — or, more deeply, of *constituting* performers and audiences with particular capabilities (and enforced inabilities) of speech and perception.

But, as the nutrition reports show, the Academy's system of stage management does not always function perfectly. Members of the teams that produce Academy reports sometimes resist the institution's efforts to discipline their actions and manage their voices, and, on occasion, they leak information from the officially closed world of the backstage. Moreover, the Academy's audiences need not accept its reports at face value, and, in controversial areas, critics may attempt to upstage its advice. They may choose to attack in many different ways — for example, by highlighting uncertainty, staging disagreements among experts, charging bias, or attacking committees for lack of balance — but some lines of attack, as we have seen, entail "rewriting" the core narrative of Academy reports, whereas other, less aggressive attacks target such "retellings" of that story as executive summaries, news releases, and media coverage. In developing lines of attack, critics are sometimes aided by Academy insiders who leak information, helping them "reach" backstage and rework its boundaries. When critics cannot exploit flaws in a performance or take advantage of incomplete dramaturgical cooperation, they may still come up with inventive strategies to undermine reports without reaching backstage; the polyvocal "dissensus report" that the Council for Agricultural Science and Technology (CAST) used to criticize *Diet, Nutrition, and Cancer* is a good example. Many contingencies shape the battles over science advice, and clearly, their dynamics cannot be deterministically predicted. But, as the comparative analysis of the reception of *Toward Healthful Diets* and *Diet, Nutrition, and Cancer* suggests, the narrative strength of reports, the degree of dramaturgical cooperation achieved, and the public identities of the critics play a crucial role in shaping outcomes.

The credibility of the Academy as an advisory body also depends on its ability to respond effectively to challenges to its integrity as an advisor to government and a guardian of science. In the case of the 1985 Draft, leaks, breakdowns in dramaturgical cooperation, and public displays of disunity provoked questions about the moral character of the Academy. Such "events," to be sure, are not objective occurrences that simply happen and possess self-evident meanings; their significance is constructed as the protagonists in these evolving social dramas work to fit them into storylines consistent with their self-presentations. In the case of the 1985 Draft, the Academy's critics emplotted events in a melodrama that presented the institution as besieged, fragile, and guided by a weak or corrupt leadership. The Academy, in contrast, worked to emplot events in a story of crisis, redress, and reintegration: when an intractable dispute threatened to disrupt the moral order, the NRC's chairman took action, and order was restored. By inscribing events within this stylized story, the Academy sought to recompose its character, mitigating the impact of potentially discrediting disclosures by containing them discursively.

To summarize, this study has examined the reports of diet and health as a means of analyzing the Academy's system of stage management and efforts to disrupt it. In each case, the Academy maintained control of the stage to varying degrees. *Diet, Nutrition, and Cancer* was the most influential of the three reports, and in this instance, the Academy retained rather tight control of the stage. In contrast, *Toward Healthful Diets* was partially discredited, as critics exploited weaknesses in its execution and drew on disclosures about the backstage to rewrite the narrative of the report. The 1985 Draft, clearly the least successful of the three, produced a polyvocal public spectacle rather than the unified narrative that the Academy seeks to enact. Comparing the outcomes and the struggles that produced them has revealed how central stagecraft — and attempts to disrupt it — are to the Academy's techniques for producing reliable advice and helping to resolve public issues.

More generally, this study suggests that struggles over the enclosure and disclosure of information play a far more important role in stabilizing (and destabilizing) scientific texts and knowledge than most work in science and technology studies has recognized. Stage management is a technology of closure, and local systems and conditions that shape collective modes of information control are an important part of the social processes that shape the production of knowledge. This book shows how dramaturgy can provide new and useful insights about how scientific texts achieve authority in public arenas. Struggles over information control are not something that analysts of science and technology can afford to ignore, because they are a prominent feature of knowledge production in precisely those organizational contexts, such as states and corporations, where extremely consequential decisions are routinely made.

Finally, the analysis presented above suggests that the recent national debate about lack of openness at the Academy has been framed in overly simplistic terms. Champions of transparency have sometimes romanticized openness, without adequately considering the merits of confidential processes or fully recognizing the ubiquity and inevitability of information control. (Allowing outsiders to observe meetings, for example, may lead performers to displace sensitive activities further "backstage.") For their part, defenders of the status quo have at times seemed to suggest that the Academy's current system is the only conceivable one for accomplishing the goal of producing reliable, independent advice, and some have cast the threat posed by openness in nearly apocalyptic terms.[1] My argument sug-

The Academy Announcement

1   After exhaustive deliberation over the last 6 months, I have concluded that
the National Research Council will be unable to issue the 10th edition of the
Recommended Dietary Allowances at this time. My decision, as Research Council
Chairman, is based on the recommendations of our Food and Nutrition Board and its
5   parent body, the Commission on Life Sciences.

Beginning in 1941, committees of the National Research Council's Food
and Nutrition Board have periodically reevaluated the Recommended Dietary
Allowances (RDAs). The allowances have traditionally been defined as "the levels of
intake of essential nutrients considered, in the judgment of the Committee on Dietary
10   Allowances of the Food and Nutrition Board on the basis of available scientific
knowledge, to be adequate to meet the known nutritional needs of practically all
healthy persons."

The RDAs are based on a comprehensive analysis of scientific evidence.
They represent the best scientific judgment derived from examination of results of
15   experimental studies in animals and humans, including nutrient balance studies and
biochemical measurements, as well as food consumption patterns and epidemiological
observations. Yet the RDAs are themselves *estimates* of nutrient allowances based on
certain assumptions and may change as the underlying science progresses. Over the
last four decades, successive editions of the RDAs have incorporated new knowledge
20   and expanded from recommendations on 9 nutrients and energy in 1941 to include 17
nutrients, energy, and "safe and adequate dietary intakes" for 12 additional vitamins
and minerals in 1980.

It is not uncommon for scientists to disagree over certain issues, such as
the association between nutrient intake and health, for which new data are constantly
25   emerging, and the data set is never complete. Our decision not to issue a report of the
RDAs at this time stems primarily from an impasse that resulted from such scientific
differences of opinion between the committee, scientific reviewers appointed by the
Research Council, and additional reviewers from the Food and Nutrition Board.
Indeed, competent scientists may use different, equally defensible assumptions and

30 physiological indexes of good health and arrive at divergent conclusions and
recommendations.

The resolution of such differences of opinion necessitates the involvement
of an impartial, authoritative group of scientists whose opinion is highly regarded and
whose judgment the public views with confidence. Since its establishment in 1863,

35 the National Academy of Sciences and, later, the National Research Council have,
through their committees, been able to meet this need very successfully in a multitude
of studies of national importance. The institution's commitment to impartiality and
scientific excellence is reflected in our recent reports on nutrition, such as those on the
association between diet, nutrition, and cancer; the public health implications of the

40 nation's meat and poultry inspection program; the importance of nutrition in medical
education; and the carcinogenic potential of cyclamate.

The National Research Council works by establishing a panel of experts
specifically to examine an issue and to prepare a report based on analysis of all data
relevant to that issue. Although the Research Council gives serious consideration to

45 the judgment of its expert committees, a key element in the completion of reports is
review by scientific experts outside the study group. This review proceeds under the
auspices of the Research Council's Report Review Committee in conjunction with a
scientific unit that oversees the work of the expert committee. This process ensures
that all scientifically valid interpretations of the data are considered and that the

50 conclusions and recommendations follow clearly from the evidence presented. This
process of checks and balances and judgments at multiple levels was designed to
guard against the promulgation of the view of one group of scientists that may be
unwarranted in the considered judgment of another group of equally capable
scientists. Thus, the review process enables the National Research Council to

55 minimize errors and to enhance the credibility of its reports by achieving a broader
consensus than may be derived by a single group of experts.

The present committee began work on the 10th edition of the RDAs in
1980. When the draft report was subjected to the Research Council's rigorous
process of review, many of the committee's conclusions and recommendations did not

60 gain the full support of the reviewers. Despite months of discussion and deliberation,
the committee and the reviewers were unable to agree on the interpretation of
scientific data on several of the nutrients and consequently on RDAs for those
nutrients.

The committee had proposed modifications of the RDAs for many

65 nutrients, whereas reviewers, including members of the Food and Nutrition Board—the
unit responsible for oversight of the committee — in general concluded that changes in
existing RDAs are warranted for only a few of these nutrients. Differences of opinion
among committee members and reviewers extended to such issues as the appropriate
data base for developing the RDAs, the adequate size of body stores for specific

70 nutrients, and the advisability of modifying the definition of the RDAs. All these
    points of contention led to different conclusions about the allowance levels, which
    were reflected in a succession of drafts prepared in an unsuccessful attempt to reach
    consensus. One of these drafts unfortunately found its way to the media and has
    clouded the issue in the public's eye because of the tentative numbers that were
75 quoted.

       Many of the reviewers and committee members used somewhat different
    scientific approaches to the task. In general, the committee believed it sufficient to
    base its conclusions on a reexamination of previously considered evidence and some
    new data using criteria and assumptions it considered to be the most valid. Most
80 reviewers believed, however, that modifications to the RDAs are justified only in the
    face of compelling new evidence — not merely as a result of a reinterpretation of existing
    data based on assumptions that may be no more valid than those applied previously.
    The reviewers concluded that the evidence presented did not fully justify the
    committee's conclusions for several of the nutrients.

85   Some of the reviewers' concerns about adequate justification for change
    derived from their recognition of the RDAs' potentially vast impact on public health.
    Originally designed to serve as a guide for planning and procuring food supplies for
    the nation, the RDAs have acquired multiple uses. They have been voluntarily
    adopted as the cornerstone for a variety of nutrition-related activities undertaken by
90 government agencies, industry, academia, and the health services sector. For
    example, the RDAs are used by government agencies as guides for planning and
    procuring food supplies related to federal food assistance and other programs, as a
    basis for meal planning for population subgroups, as a reference point for evaluating
    dietary intake from national food consumption surveys, as a component of food and
95 nutrition education programs, and, more recently, as a basis for nutrition labeling of
    foods and dietary supplements. In the private sector, the uses of the RDAs extend to
    food fortification, the formulation of food products, and competitive marketing.
    These wide applications suggest that modifications to the RDAs must be based on a
    strong rationale and a comprehensive analysis of scientifically corroborated,
100 persuasive evidence; they should reflect concurrence of scientific opinion.

       Other events contributing to our decision not to issue a report now
    include the deepening understanding of the interplay between nutritional factors and
    health, especially the importance of these factors in the aging process and in
    susceptibility to chronic diseases. Neither the present committee nor the committee
105 responsible for the previous edition was specifically asked to consider these issues.
    Nonetheless, the reviews of the report strongly suggest that the scientific
    developments in the past 5 years relating nutrition to health should be considered and
    that a more comprehensive approach is now warranted for assessing nutrient intake to
    satisfy "the known nutritional needs of practically all healthy persons" in the United

110   States. Furthermore, reviewers suggested that unless scientific evidence indicates
otherwise, the recommendations for *nutrient intakes*—the RDAs—must be consistent
with recommended *dietary guidelines* for the maintenance of good health. Thus,
although the committee followed the charge given to it in 1980, it became apparent
that its primary focus on the avoidance of nutritional deficiencies may be neither
115   sufficient nor appropriate.

A recent workshop sponsored by the Food and Nutrition Board to
discuss future editions of the RDAs reinforced the importance of the RDAs, the need
to broaden their scope, and the need to enhance their utility by considering new
methodological approaches and multiple applications. The Food and Nutrition Board
120   intends to pursue these recommendations. The Board believes that both the scientific
community and the public would be served better by guidelines that are broadly based
on diverse but pertinent scientific evidence, including that on diet-related chronic
diseases, and that incorporate new methods that permit the characterization of health
risks associated with different levels of nutrient intake.

125   For all these interrelated reasons, the National Research Council has
concluded that the publication of the next edition of the RDAs warrants a more
encompassing analysis of data pertaining to nutrients and health by a new committee
specially constituted to address these issues. In the weeks to come, our Food and
Nutrition Board, in consultation with the National Institutes of Health, will consider
130   various options and will make recommendations to the Research Council accordingly.

Whatever course of action is taken, the next report concerning the RDAs
will, like all our reports, be prepared, reviewed, and published in accordance with
[the] Research Council's highest standards. We are confident that it will represent the best
scientific judgment on matters of nutrient intake and health—issues that have an
135   enormous impact on public health.

Until a new report is issued, the only National Research Council
recommendations in effect are those contained in the ninth edition of the RDAs, which
was published in 1980. The public and the scientific community at large should rest
assured that there is no cause for concern and that they may continue to place
140   confidence in the RDAs that have been in effect for the past 5 years.

SOURCE: Press 1985a.

The Kamin Letter

1   Eliot Marshall's article "The Academy kills a nutrition report" (News and Comment, 25 Oct., p. 420) is informative, generally correct, valuable in identifying the issues, and clear in its designation of which individuals and groups are identified with which viewpoint. Marshall attributes the major errors and misconceptions, correctly, to those who oppose our committee's

5   draft of the 10th edition of the Recommended Dietary Allowances (RDA's).

    The major issue is the conflict between those who wish to give the best science possible — a viewpoint identified with the RDA committee — and those who appear to be injecting policy considerations into scientific judgments. If, as National Academy of Sciences president Frank Press says, there are substantial "scientific differences of opinion," then surely they could have

10   been expressed in the language of documented science. But these "scientific" reasons have not emerged despite repeated requests on the part of the RDA committee.

    Adverse policy effects are predicted by D. Mark Hegsted (a long-time critic of RDA's who is cited in Marshall's article). Hegsted accuses us of approaching our task "as a purely academic exercise and from a very limited perspective," and seems to imply that we are insensitive to the

15   impact of our changes on policy. Michael Lemov of the Food Research and Action Center is quoted as citing the "shocking" possibility that reducing the RDA's would mean "less food and more hunger for millions of people" in food programs.

    These critics are misguided on several grounds. (i) The RDA's have not been systematically "reduced"; we made no effort to impose a direction of recommendation for the

20   29 or so nutrients covered. Some are up, some are down, and a few are unchanged. We simply went nutrient by nutrient, giving each the best value we could. (ii) It is ridiculous, on the basis of the few RDA's "leaked," to predict overall cost or food pattern, and my own guess is that there would be little if any effect. This is confirmed by Betty B. Peterkin, acting administrator of the Human Nutrition Information Service of the U.S. Department of Agriculture, who writes me:

25   "The possible effects of changes in RDA for a few nutrients . . . on food assistance programs [have] been greatly exaggerated. RDA changes, since the development of the school lunch meal pattern in the 1940's, the poverty formula in the 1960's, and the food stamp standard in the early 1970's have *not* affected the dollar-related aspects of these standards.

    But the most important reason for rejecting these arguments is that scientists should give

30 the best advice they can and should not twist their science to meet the needs or desires of
policymakers, constituencies, or special interest groups. The product of the latter attitude is both
bad science *and* bad policy. Who are we on the RDA committee to make the judgment that
present policies are necessarily correct? Or wrong? Good administrators recognize this, and
Peterkin writes of her "wholehearted support of [our] view that the Recommended Dietary
35 Allowances should represent the best advice scientists can give and should not be affected by
policy considerations. . . ."

Hegsted, in the 18 March letter cited by Marshall, makes grave warnings about bad public
relations, controversy, congressional hearings, and so forth — that the public would be confused
and the Academy embarrassed. His allegations that our report would "undercut" the 1982
40 Academy report *Diet, Nutrition, and Cancer* are incorrect. Our RDA's have no inconsistencies
with the 1982 report, but may be inconsistent with the publicity-induced mythology that
surrounds it. Even if this *were* true, must all scientists "speak with a single voice"? If the
credibility of the Academy rides upon resistance to change, then it is a far weaker institution than
one would have thought.

45 Another misconception is that the RDA's are "minimal." The change in the wording of the
definition was actively encouraged by the Food and Nutrition Board (FNB) to sharpen the
distinction between the quantitative "nutrient" approach of the RDA's and the qualitative
"dietary pattern" approach of a "Diet and Health" project the FNB was planning; we were
making room for "their" place on the turf. But this does not justify the use of the term
50 "minimal"; our goals, including generosity of safety factors, were the same as those of previous
RDA committees, and we state explicitly that "the committee can cite no additional benefits of
increasing intakes of nutrients beyond the quantities recommended for persons consuming a
normal mixed diet of foods from a variety of biological sources."

What may have happened is that Hegsted's letter frightened the Academy. His use of the
55 term "fiasco" in referring to the report *Toward Healthful Diets* is correct only in that it is so
considered by the present Academy administration; Philip Handler's administration defended it
vigorously. The report is by no means dead, since the issue it raised is a strategic one: would the
public be better served if the advice to decrease fat intake were to be strongly targeted to those
at risk or diffused throughout the entire population? The question is a serious one and is not going
60 away.

But the Academy can act timorously and be frightened away by hints of controversy, "bad"
image, public relations, and other nonscientific considerations, such as fear of "giving confusing
signals to the public." Its responses, thus far, have consisted in extolling its review procedures
and systematically avoiding direct discussion of the scientific justification of its objections to the
65 actual points at issue — the proposed RDA's for vitamins A and C. Our attempts to reopen serious
discourse on these issues have been unsuccessful over a period of months. We remain open to
such discourse; as I wrote in my 29 October letter to James Wyngaarden, "I have often stated that
no values are final until the book is in print, and we have been totally flexible in modifying our
values for other nutrients in response to valid scientific critiques. But critiques must be based

70   upon sound and documented science, and not upon hunches, personal preferences, public
relations, fear of controversy, or criteria of whether they support or question existing programs. . . .
We remain open to such [scientific] criticism, but in its absence the NAS should withdraw its
objections to these chapters."

Future reports will provide the history of how our committee failed in its attempts to find
75   a common scientific language with the Academy. But it is clear that in its attempt to avoid
controversy over two numerical values (values that fall comfortably within the range of
recommendations of other nations), the Academy has forced attention on more serious questions:
the capability of the present nutritional establishment at the Academy to give impartial scientific
advice and the Academy's fundamental integrity as a defender of the scientific process.

SOURCE: Kamin 1985b

Chapter 1

1. See, e.g., Brickman et al. 1985 and Jasanoff 1990.
2. Latour 1993.
3. See, e.g., Nelkin 1979, 1984, and 1992.
4. See ibid.; Dickson 1984. On patient rights, see Rothman 1991. On feminist critiques, see, e.g., Haraway 1989 and Keller 1995. On lay experts, see Epstein 1996.
5. Brickman et al. 1985; Jasanoff 1990, 1992, 1995, and 1997.
6. Ibid.; see also Yearley 1991 on the epistemological limits of environmental science.
7. See, e.g., Nelkin 1979, 1984, and 1992; Noble 1984; Sclove 1995; Winner 1980 and 1986.
8. Shapin and Schaffer 1985, p. 343. Indeed, some analysts perceive in these doubts a crisis of modernity; see, e.g., Ezrahi 1990, Beck 1992, and Latour 1993.
9. The topic of credibility is central to the agenda of science and technology studies, as Shapin 1995 forcefully argues.
10. Cultural authority—like the closely related concepts of epistemic authority and cognitive authority—concerns the ability to make compelling assertions and judgments about the nature and meaning of the world. On the epistemic authority of science, see Gieryn 1999. On cognitive authority, see Barnes and Edge 1982, p. 2. On cultural authority, see Starr 1982, pp. 13–17; and on authority in general, see Weber 1978. As Gary Downey notes, "the credibility of scientists in the public domain is at once a culturally-structured and a contextually-variable phenomenon"—thus, particular scientists or advisors may find their credibility challenged by audiences who accept the background cultural assumption that science is a privileged source of authoritative knowledge; see Downey 1988, p. 26.
11. On quantity and quality of advice, see Golden 1995. Another well-developed theme, sometimes captured under the rubric "the politics of expertise," concerns the tension between objectivity and politicization. However, research on the politics of expertise has done more to undermine the notion of a sharp divide

between scientific facts and social values than to scrutinize the means that advisors use to produce advice and acquire and preserve credibility.

12. This argument, for example, is frequently made by science advisors themselves.

13. Bimber 1996.

14. B. L. R. Smith 1992.

15. A significant exception is Jasanoff's work (e.g., 1990, 1992), which makes pathbreaking moves in this direction, such as her treatment of boundary work.

16. See, e.g., Bimber 1996 and B. L. R. Smith 1992.

17. On dramaturgy, see Goffman 1959, 1961a, 1961b, 1963b, and 1974; see also Burke 1989 and Gusfield 1989. Much of Goffman's work is directed at developing a truly social (as opposed to psychological) account of the self, and his writings focus on face-to-face interaction; for a discussion, see Waksler 1989. Goffman's theoretical vision is by no means limited to the individual, however, and dramaturgical concepts can be applied to social actors other than individuals.

My theoretical approach is also informed by the large body of work in science and technology studies that is concerned with rhetoric and performance, especially actor-network theory; see esp., Callon 1986 and Latour 1987. (It is important to note, however, that I do not fully adopt the ontology of Latour and Callon's actor-network theory; my analysis quite self-consciously "sociologizes" actor-network theory in that I reserve a special place for human agency. For a discussion of sociological readings and misreadings of actor-network theory, see Lynch 1993, pp. 107–13.)

A concern with drama is also reflected in the work of Victor Turner (e.g., Turner 1974 and 1980); and in many works that use dramatic concepts to look at mass-mediated politics, including Gusfield 1981, Wagner-Pacifici 1986, Hilgartner and Bosk 1988, Edelman 1964 and 1988, and Gamson and Modigliani 1989.

18. On "information control," see esp. Goffman 1961b, ch. 2.

19. Goffman 1959; see also Wagner-Pacifici 1986.

20. Goffman 1959 and 1961b, esp. ch. 2.

21. For just a few examples, see Cambrosio and Keating 1995; Clarke and Fujimura 1992; Collins 1985; Fujimura 1996; Galison 1987; Kohler 1994; Knorr-Cetina 1981 and 1999; Latour 1987, 1988; Latour and Woolgar 1979; Lenoir 1997; Lynch 1985a; Lynch and Woolgar 1990; MacKenzie 1990; Pickering 1984 and 1995; Pinch 1986; Rheinberger 1997; Shapin and Schaffer 1985; Star 1989 and 1995; and Traweek 1998.

22. For a useful review of the large body of scholarship in science and technology studies that emphasizes rhetoric, discourse, and performance, see Ashmore, Myers, and Potter 1995. This area includes writings as diverse as Ashmore 1989; Bazerman 1988; Knorr-Cetina 1981; Gieryn 1999; Gilbert and Mulkay 1984; Law and Williams 1982; Latour 1987; Latour and Woolgar 1979; Lynch 1985a and 1985b; Mulkay 1985; Mulkay, Potter, and Yearley 1983; Myers 1990; and Shapin and Schaffer 1985.

23. Latour 1987, ch. 1.

24. Ibid.

25. See Latour and Woolgar 1979 on the concept of "inscription devices."

26. Jasanoff 1987.

27. On boundary work, see Gieryn 1983 and 1999.

28. Jasanoff 1990.

29. Shapin and Schaffer 1986. See also the discussion of Pasteur's laboratory as a theater of proof in Latour 1988.

30. T. M. Porter 1995. On "mechanical objectivity," see Daston and Galison 1992 and Daston 1992. See also Dear 1992 and T. M. Porter 1992.

31. The notion of "technologies of trust" is from Shapin and Schaffer 1985, ch. 2.

32. On region behavior and front- and backstage, see Goffman 1959, esp. ch. 3.

33. The story is possibly apocryphal.

34. Goffman 1959; see also id. 1961b, esp. ch. 2.

35. On teams, see Goffman 1959, esp. ch. 2. The phrase "dramaturgical cooperation" appears on p. 85.

36. This image of the self comes through especially clearly in Goffman 1959 and 1961b.

37. Ibid.; see also Waksler 1989.

38. Goffman 1959, p. 66.

39. On "identity norms," see Goffman 1961b, esp. pp. 126–30.

40. Goffman 1959, p. 19. See also Lynch and Bogen 1996, ch. 1, for an analysis of lying and displays of sincerity.

41. See Jasanoff 1990 and 1995; Wynne 1982; Douglas and Wildavsky 1982. The same is true of knowledge claims in other contexts, because scientists cannot appraise new knowledge claims without evaluating the individuals, laboratories, and communities that stand behind them; see, e.g., Collins 1985, Knorr-Cetina 1981, Latour and Woolgar 1979, Pinch 1981, and Shapin and Schaffer 1985.

42. Work on the theatricization of contemporary politics, such as Wagner-Pacifici 1986 and Lynch and Bogen 1996, is helpful here. See also Turner 1980.

43. Wynne 1992, p. 579.

44. As one indication of this lack of influence, one might note that Erving Goffman appears neither in the bibliography of the *Handbook of Science & Technology Studies* (Jasanoff et al. 1995) nor in the index of a recent reader on the field (Biagioli 1999). One recent work in science studies that makes extensive use of Goffman is Shapin 1994.

45. For a discussion of expert witnessing, see Lynch and Jasanoff 1998. See Goodwin 1994 for an ethnography of how expert witnesses project their professionally organized categories of visual objects and events into the courtroom; and see also Jasanoff 1998. For an analysis of the process of interrogation and the difficulty of converting testimony to history, see Lynch and Bogen 1996. For a discussion of the culture of adversary proceedings and the deconstruction of expert testimony, see Jasanoff 1995, esp. ch. 3.

46. See Lawrence and Shapin 1998 for a historical treatment of the theme of knowledge and the body.

47. On body idiom, see, e.g., Goffman 1963b. See also id. 1979, which examines the visual presentation of the body in a particular genre of document: print advertising.

48. To be sure, intimate conversations are sometimes overheard (and even tape-recorded), but the eavesdropper must capture a fleeting moment, not obtain access to a durable object.

49. The phrase "technologies of privacy" is meant to encompass a wide variety of devices, practices, and systems that are used to enclose information or limit the observational power of audiences. Examples might include walls, curtains, encryption algorithms, clothing, and locks.

50. As D. E. Smith 1974 points out, most of the factual documents that organizations routinely produce "are not made to be detachable from specific organizational contexts of interpretation."

51. On the shredding of documents and the fabrication of documents intended to create a false record, see Lynch and Bogen 1996.

52. On Watergate, see Schudson 1992; on the Iran-Contra affair, Lynch and Bogen 1996; on "Monicagate," Joan Didion, "Clinton Agonistes" (The Presidential Sex Scandal)," *New York Review of Books*, Oct. 22, 1998.

53. On public demonstrations, see Collins 1988; on the "theater of proof," see Latour 1988, esp. 85–90.

54. Lynch and Bogen 1996 beautifully analyzes the leakage, lying, and information containment in the context of the congressional investigation of the Iran-Contra affair.

55. See Lynch and Bogen 1996 for an analysis of the audiovisual field of the Iran-Contra hearings. See also Goodwin 1994 and Jasanoff 1998.

56. See, e.g., Collins 1985 and Pinch and Bijker 1984.

57. In addition to Americans, the NAS, NEA, and IOM also elect foreign associates.

58. Boffey 1975, p. 20. See also Cole and Cole 1973, p. 47; Boffey 1977; and Goldschmidt 1971.

59. See, e.g., National Academy of Sciences 1989, p. 8; and see also Press 1985a.

60. National Academy of Sciences 1994, p. 4.

61. In some cases, this is not possible and the Academy permits publication of majority and minority views, statements describing the pros and cons of alternative policies, and even dissenting statements by individual members of a panel.

62. See Bimber 1996 for a history of the OTA.

63. National Academy of Sciences, "The National Research Council," http://www.nas.edu/about/faq3.html, downloaded Jan. 18, 1999.

64. See, e.g., Alberts 1997e and National Academy of Sciences 1996. See also Boffey 1975, pp. 257–58.

65. See, e.g., Boffey 1975; D. S. Greenberg 1967a, 1967b, and 1967c; Barfield 1971; and Walsh 1971a and 1971b. See also Lawler 1997.

66. On the distrust of experts, see, e.g., Brickman et al. 1995; and see also Dupree 1957.

67. Boffey 1975.

68. Ibid., pp. 46–47.

69. Ibid., p. 55. He continues: "It would be unfair to suggest that a scientist's background automatically condemns him to reach a particular conclusion on an issue. Such an assumption would suggest that all human beings are slavishly programmed by their past experience, with no room for independent judgment and willingness to accept new facts and new viewpoints. Nevertheless, one can often predict how a scientist will lean on a particular issue simply by knowing his background" (ibid.).

70. Ibid., pp. 257–59. Boffey concluded by offering a number of proposals for reform, such as attempting to break out of *"its servant-master relationship to the government agencies and industrial interests which provide financial support,"* "soliciting participation of the activists it traditionally shuns," and "opening its advisory processes to outside scrutiny" (ibid., pp. 253–54; italics in original).

71. *Lombardo v. Handler* 1975; Jasanoff 1995, p. 98. As discussed in Chapter 2, the matter of confidentiality also came up in litigation surrounding one of the reports analyzed below, *Diet, Nutrition, and Cancer,* and the judge once again sided with the Academy.

72. Public Law 105-153, December 17, 1997. The new amendments to the FACA forbade government agencies to use Academy reports unless the NAS followed certain procedures, such as publishing the names of committee members (which the Academy was already doing) and releasing the names of the reviewers from outside the institution who reviewed reports (which the Academy was not doing). The FACA cases and amendments are discussed further in Chapter 2.

73. Lawler 1997. The Academy responds that it has taken measures to cut costs and increase its effectiveness (see, e.g., Alberts 1997b).

74. Lawler 1997.

75. Indeed, systematic study of the Academy is overdue; given its important public role, it has attracted surprisingly little analytic attention. Nearly a quarter century after its publication, Boffey 1975 remains the most recent book-length examination of the institution.

76. Jasanoff 1997, p. 228.

77. For analyses of other systems of science advice, see Jasanoff 1990 on advisory committees to federal regulatory agencies; Bimber 1996 and the special issue of *Technology Forecasting and Social Change* edited by Bruce Bimber and David Guston (Bimber and Guston 1997) on the OTA; Childress 1991, National Academy of Sciences 1995, and Rothman 1991, pp. 168–89, on bioethical advice; Perry 1987; and B. L. R. Smith 1992. See also, e.g., Bimber and Guston 1995, Ted Greenwood 1984, Golden 1995, and Primack and von Hippel 1974.

78. National Academy of Sciences 1980 and 1982.

79. In the case of the 1985 draft of the Tenth RDA, which was never published, much of the reaction was to the act of canceling the report, rather than to the report itself.

80. The four examples below are taken from statements collected in Council for Agricultural Science and Technology 1982.

81. Ibid., p. 66.

82. Ibid., p. 55.

83. Ibid., p. 50.

84. Ibid., p. 72.

85. Numerical estimates of this sort of thing are problematic. Nevertheless, it is worth noting that one well-placed Academy official, familiar with the institution's record in the 1980s, estimated that roughly 5 reports out of 2,000 inspired this level of controversy.

86. On face-to-face interaction, see, e.g., Garfinkel 1967 and Goffman 1959 and 1961a; on controversies, see Collins 1985 and Nelkin 1979, 1984, and 1992; and on accidents and errors, see Bosk 1979, Clarke 1989, Perrow 1984, Galison 1997, Gieryn and Figert 1990, Hilgartner 1992, Jasanoff 1994, Vaughan 1996, and Wynne 1982.

87. Because these questions intersect one another in multiple ways, they cannot be collapsed into a linear list, from A to Z, that one needs merely to answer in order. In other words, there is no single way to "untangle" this network of questions, no unique starting point, no single logical hierarchy. The choice of a starting point for examining an issue is, therefore, itself a decision with implications for the outcome of the inquiry.

88. Note, though, that they frequently disagreed about the extent of uncertainty and the level of consensus among experts.

89. On diet-disease controversies during this period, see, e.g., Broad 1979, Garrety 1997, Hilgartner and Nelkin 1987, Levine 1986, McNutt 1980, and Proctor 1995.

90. U.S. Department of Agriculture 1957.

91. U.S. Senate Select Committee on Nutrition and Human Needs 1975, p. v.

92. U.S. Senate Select Committee on Nutrition and Human Needs 1974, 1975, 1977a, 1977c, and 1977d. On the American Heart Association's recommendations, see id. 1961, 1965, and 1968. See also McNutt 1980.

93. See, e.g., de Vet and van Leeuwen 1986. Nutritional epidemiology is now an established subfield of epidemiology, the study of the distribution and causes of human disease. For an influential text, see Willett 1990.

94. See, e.g., Hegsted 1985.

95. See, e.g., Olson 1986; and see also National Academy of Sciences 1980.

96. Hilgartner and Nelkin 1987. Related controversies developed about the question of how much evidence was required to support claims in advertisements

that foods or food supplements, such as vitamin pills, may help prevent cancer and other diseases (ibid.).

97. See, e.g., Bullock 1982.

98. U.S. Senate Select Committee on Nutrition and Human Needs 1977b, 1977c, 1977d, and 1977f. See also Levine 1986.

99. U.S. Senate Committee on Agriculture, Nutrition, and Forestry, Subcommittee on Nutrition 1978, *Nutrition and Cancer Research*, and 1979, *Diet and Cancer Relationship*. For Upton's presentation, see *Diet and Cancer Relationship*, pp. 54–57.

100. U.S. Department of Agriculture and U.S. Department of Health and Human Services 1980 and 1985. See also Brody 1980b and Levine 1986.

101. National Academy of Sciences 1980, pp. 2–3.

102. Ibid., p. 4.

103. The report supported some dietary advice, such as that directed at maintaining proper weight by avoiding excessive caloric intakes. It was opposed to recommendations aimed at the public at large but not necessarily against advice offered to individuals by their own doctors.

104. Ibid., p. 14.

105. National Academy of Sciences 1982, pp. 14–16.

106. Measuring the effect of such a report obviously poses methodological challenges. There is little doubt, however, that *Diet, Nutrition, and Cancer* was an influential document, which, along with a widely cited review by Richard Doll and Richard Peto (1981), served to draw together the literature and frame discussion about the topic during the first half of the 1980s, a period in which attention to diet and cancer increased substantially. See Hilgartner 1990 for a discussion of the public presentation of Doll and Peto 1981. See U.S. Department of Health and Human Services 1983 for a discussion of how federal health agencies should respond to *Diet, Nutrition, and Cancer*. The National Cancer Institute (NCI), which had formally chartered a program on diet, nutrition, and cancer in 1975, devoted increasing attention to dietary prevention during the 1980s; see, e.g., U.S. National Cancer Institute 1978a, 1979b, 1982, 1984a, 1984b, 1985a, 1985b, 1986, and 1987. See also U.S. Department of Health and Human Services 1984 and Greenwald and Cullen 1985. NCI 1979 was the agency's first dietary advice aimed at cancer prevention. Its 1984 recommendations on diet and cancer cited the NAS report, as did the American Cancer Society's recommendations; see NCI 1984b and American Cancer Society 1984.

107. The Academy finally published a tenth edition in October 1989; see National Academy of Sciences 1989.

108. This trend encompassed not only the marketing of cereals and fruits as disease-preventing products (see Hilgartner and Nelkin 1987), but also the promotion of low-fat meats and dairy products. For example, cattle were reengineered to lower the fat content of beef; see, e.g., Sweeten et al. 1990. See also Burros 1986.

Chapter 2

1. National Academy of Sciences 1982.

2. One ambiguity surrounds the stability of an actor's public identity, which can be viewed, at one extreme, as a fixed feature of social structure, or at the other, as a fluid phenomenon that is continually (re)enacted in action. The precise location of a public identity is also problematic. From one viewpoint, public identity can be seen as a portable property of the actor, a possession that the actor deploys in encounters with audiences. From another, public identity can be viewed as something that exists in the perceptions and understandings of an actor's audiences. This conception, which emphasizes how identities are distributed throughout social space, might underline the variations in how people perceive an actor. Public identity can probably best be understood as situated neither in the actor nor the audience, but in the encounter between them. A particularly important dimension of social location concerns agency. An actor-focused vision of public identity would stress the impression that a particular actor fosters in public via both the intentional and unintentional aspects of self-presentation. Alternatively, public identity might be taken as referring to the assignment an audience makes when it defines the actor as belonging to a particular cultural category. As Goffman explicates (e.g., 1959 and 1961b), the agency of actors and audiences are intimately related: actors work to present themselves in a manner that will qualify them as members of desirable categories, drawing on their understandings of cultural stereotypes; simultaneously, audiences use stereotyped categories (along with prevailing cultural ideas about the nature of the different types and the means for recognizing them) to reduce the complexity of the social world.

3. These changes are among the most significant aspects of both individual biography and cultural change, as Shapin 1994 illuminates. Shapin examines the processes through which Robert Boyle (and those around him) constructed an identity that not only defined "Boyle" the man, but also became the founding exemplar of a new type of person: the "experimental philosopher"—a kind of man uniquely qualified to speak for nature.

4. See also Gusfield 1981, p. 87.

5. National Academy of Sciences 1994.

6. See the discussion in the section on "Persuasive Rhetoric" in Chapter 1 of this book. See also such works as Ashmore, Myers, and Potter 1995. This area includes work as diverse as Ashmore 1989, Bazerman 1988, Knorr-Cetina 1981, Gieryn 1999, Gilbert and Mulkay 1984, Law and Williams 1982, Latour 1987, Latour and Woolgar 1979, Lynch 1985a and 1985b, Mulkay 1985, Mulkay, Potter, and Yearley 1983, Myers 1990, and Shapin and Schaffer 1985.

7. As Knorr-Cetina 1981, p. 95, argues, part of the persuasive power of a scientific paper stems from the institutionalized definition of the scientific paper as a particular form of writing. Similarly, an advisory report draws persuasive force from the institutionalized notion of what such reports are.

8. See Latour and Bastide 1986, p. 60.

9. Ibid., pp. 59–66; Latour 1987, ch. 1.

10. The idea of using a dialogue between the report and a skeptic as means of presenting the report's argument was inspired by Latour and Bastide 1986. The technique of constructing dialogues, although relatively unusual in social science writing, has been used fairly frequently in recent social studies of science; see, e.g., Mulkay 1985 and Ashmore, Mulkay, and Pinch 1989. See also Ashmore, Myers, and Potter 1995.

11. National Academy of Sciences 1982, p. v.

12. Ibid., p. ii.

13. Ibid., p. v.

14. Ibid., p. ii.

15. Ibid., p. v.

16. Ibid.

17. Ibid., pp. v–vi.

18. Ibid., p. vii.

19. Ibid.

20. Ibid., p. vi.

21. Ibid.

22. Ibid., p. 31.

23. Ibid., pp. 43–44.

24. Ibid., p. 44.

25. Ibid.

26. Ibid., p. ii.

27. And if it did, as Latour points out, the argument would grow increasingly technical; see Latour 1987.

28. This parallels H. M. Collins's notion that the members of "core sets" should be understood as "delegates"; see Collins 1985, p. 148.

29. This stands in marked contrast to some mechanisms for producing science advice that designate relevant organizations, such as professional societies or trade associations, which supply individual representatives. The recent Task Force on Genetic Testing, established by the National Institutes of Health and Department of Energy Working Group on the Ethical, Legal, and Social Implications of genome research, followed this form; see Holtzman and Watson 1997.

30. National Academy of Sciences 1982, p. v.

31. Shapin 1994, pp. 305–6, 400–401.

32. In a curious way, these chains of associations also rebound back toward the universities, which in a sense end up also vouching for one another.

33. In using the number 1,738, I have chosen to trust rather than replicate the count of the references provided in U.S. General Accounting Office 1984, p. 18.

34. This network has the structural property of linking together many actors in a manner similar to the description of scientific texts in actor network theory; see Latour 1987. Rather than emphasizing the heterogeneity of the entities that constitute the network, however, I mean to emphasize the connection to reputational resources.

35. Gilbert and Mulkay 1984.

36. National Academy of Sciences 1996, p. 17.

37. Often there is ambiguity about what the committee is presenting as "the evidence" speaking for itself (based on empirical fact) and what it is presenting as "the committee" speaking (based on its own opinion reached through careful deliberation). As an example, consider the sentence: "Thus, in the judgment of the committee, evidence from both epidemiological and laboratory studies suggests that high protein intake *may* be associated with an increased risk of cancers at certain sites" (National Academy of Sciences 1982, p. 6). Depending on the weight one gives to the phrase "in the judgment of the committee," one can read this sentence either as (1) a straightforward example of the empiricist repertoire, or as (2) an example of expert opinion. Such ambiguities can be exploited—both in creating reports (e.g., to resolve debate among committee members) and in assertions (postpublication) about what a report "really" says.

38. Alberts 1994, p. 1.

39. Attached to Alberts's memorandum (ibid.) was a two-page "Statement on Consensus and Dissent: Guidance to NRC/IOM Staff, Approved by the Governing Board on Feb. 16, 1994."

40. The only portion of the report that is not explicitly presented as having been authored by the committee is the preface, signed by Clifford Grobstein, who is identified as chairman. The preface is written in a tone that clearly suggests even if it was not signed by the committee, it was written on behalf of the committee. The preface reports on the committee's actions and history. It contains no personal references to Grobstein himself (or to any other committee member). See National Academy of Sciences 1982, pp. v–viii.

41. On scientific controversies, see, e.g., Collins 1985, Martin and Richards 1995, Nelkin 1979, 1984, and 1992, Pinch 1986, and Richards 1991. For studies of the negotiations that took place around, and shaped, scientific papers, see, e.g., Law and Williams 1982 and Myers 1990; and see also Knorr-Cetina 1981, ch. 5.

42. National Academy of Sciences 1996, p. 14. See also Dam 1996, p. 21. Dam attributes the success of an NRC report on cryptography to the 23 days of meetings in which committee members—"none of whom could be considered a shrinking violet"—"talked out each and every issue at length."

43. According to the General Accounting Office, the idea for an analysis of diet and cancer originated in the NAS, which approached NCI with a formal proposal in February 1979, leading to discussions and eventually a contract. See U.S. General Accounting Office 1984, pp. 10–12.

44. A report on the report prepared by an analyst for the Congressional Research Service describes in general terms the process through which the committee was selected:

> Selection of persons to serve on ALS-NAS [Assembly of Life Sciences] study committees generally begins with a solicitation of names of possible candidates and/or disciplines to be represented. Such a solicitation is directed to members of the Academy in general, as

well as to the standing boards or committees of NAS with particular interest in the subject to be studied. (In this case, the Food and Nutrition Board and the Board of Toxicology and Environmental Health Hazards, which have overlapping jurisdictions in the topic were contacted.) In addition, professionals and scientific organizations outside the Academy are also approached for names. Once names have been submitted (500 were submitted for the DNC panel), the background of each individual is checked in terms of research published, the sources of research support and any public statements they have made which might indicate bias on the subject. The screening of individuals includes matching subject expertise to the topics which need to be addressed in the study. The list of first choices and alternative candidates are sent through several levels of review in the Assembly for approval. When the final list of candidates is approved, each individual is contacted to determine his or her willingness to participate. (D. V. Porter 1983, p. 5)

45. For example, one NRC document aimed at participants in the Academy's review process states that "[t]he numerical results of individual votes taken to reach . . . consensus, like other aspects of the deliberative process, should be omitted from the report" (National Academy of Sciences 1993, p. 7).

46. National Academy of Sciences 1996, p. 18.

47. Alberts 1997e.

48. National Academy of Sciences 1994, p. 15.

49. Ibid.

50. Ibid.

51. Ibid.

52. Ibid.

53. National Academy of Sciences 1996, pp. 18–19.

54. Ibid., p. 19.

55. Ibid., p. 20.

56. Ibid., pp. 19–20.

57. Ibid., pp. 21–22.

58. Ibid., p. 21.

59. National Academy of Sciences 1993, p. 3. Reviewers are instructed not to discuss reports with the press until after they are released and even then to "refrain from references to earlier drafts." See National Academy of Sciences 1979.

60. U.S. General Accounting Office 1984, pp. 7, 13, 21. The science writer Phillip M. Boffey was also denied access to internal Academy documents when researching his 1975 book *The Brain Bank of America*; see ibid. pp. x–xi.

61. Boffey 1975, pp. 257–58. On the central role of transparency and public witnessing in democratic politics, especially in the United States, see Yaron Ezrahi's contention in "Technology and the Civil Epistemology of Democracy" (1993) that the openness of science provides a model for the "civil epistemology" of democracy.

62. *Lombardo v. Handler* 1975. See also Jasanoff 1995, pp. 98–99.

63. Order Granting Motion to Limit Discovery Subpoena, In the Matter of General Nutrition, Inc., Federal Trade Commission Docket No. 9175, Mar. 19, 1985, pp. 1–2.

64. Ibid., p. 6.

65. Ibid, p. 5.

66. *Animal Legal Defense Fund, Inc. v. Shalala* 1997.

67. E. William Colglazier quoted in Wade 1997, p. A18. See also M. R. C. Greenwood 1997.

68. See, e.g., Wade 1997, M. R. C. Greenwood 1997, and Alberts 1997a, 1997c, 1997d, 1997e, and 1997f.

69. Federal Advisory Committee Act Amendments of 1997, Public Law 105-153, H.R. 2977, An Act to Amend the Federal Advisory Committee Act to Clarify Public Disclosure Requirements That Are Applicable to the National Academy of Sciences and the National Academy of Public Administration, Approved Dec. 17, 1997.

70. See Alberts 1998. See also U.S. General Accounting Office 1999.

71. Alberts 1998.

72. National Academy of Sciences 1994, p. 12.

73. Ibid., p. 3.

74. National Academy of Sciences 1996, p. 9.

75. National Academy of Sciences 1994, p. 14.

76. National Academy of Sciences 1996, p. 9.

77. National Academy of Sciences 1994, pp. 12–15.

78. Ibid., pp. 14–15.

79. National Academy of Sciences 1993, p. 6.

80. Although detailed social studies of the internal operation of the Academy are not available, it is well known that organizational self-descriptions typically conform incompletely to, and deviate systematically from, actual processes.

81. Shapin and Schaffer 1985.

82. On witnessing and "virtual witnessing," see ibid., pp. 55–79. See also Ezrahi 1990 and 1993; Jasanoff 1992.

83. National Academy of Sciences 1996, p. 1.

84. Ibid., p. 10.

85. Ibid., p. 15.

86. This rule that the committee is the "author of record" applies even to chapters or portions of a report that an individual committee member prepares. Authorship, the Academy stresses, is the collective responsibility of the committee: "Individual authorship generally is not credited; the report and all copyrights become the property of the National Academy of Sciences" (National Academy of Sciences 1996, p. 14).

87. The complexities, controversies, and paradoxes surrounding authorship have attracted considerable attention in recent decades in areas ranging from critical theory (e.g., Foucault 1977), to critical studies of law (e.g., Boyle 1996 and Rose 1988), to research on scientific publication, collaboration, and ownership (e.g., Biagioli 1998, LaFollette 1992, and Hilgartner and Brandt-Rauf 1994.)

88. Some staff members, in their less guarded moments, present themselves as

rather central characters. Prior to the initiation of projects, NRC study directors and other staff members interact with sponsors, sometimes negotiating about the direction and scope of projects that agencies propose and sometimes pitching their own ideas for projects in the hope of stimulating agency requests. Informally, staff comment that they adjust the composition of committees, balancing expertise, perspectives, and personalities and seeking to produce creative conflicts among members. They also describe using briefings strategically to present viewpoints that committees lack or to shift the dynamics of a deadlocked committee. They sometimes say that they ghostwrite reports. In short, the NRC staff often play an active and influential role in shaping the evolution of reports—although, clearly, they do so through interaction with committees.

89. As Wynne 1988 points out, rules follow evolving practices not the other way around.

90. It is likely that small "leaks," especially in informal conversation, often occur. But spectacular failures of stage management are rare.

91. Pear 1985a.

92. Regarding these disclosures, it is worth noting a moral asymmetry in the position of high Academy officials, on the one hand, and members of committees, reviewers, and Academy project managers, on the other. If members of the latter group disclose information about the negotiations surrounding a report without authorization, that action constitutes a blameworthy violation of Academy policy (in the moral order of the Academy). On the other hand, if a high Academy official, such as the NRC chairman, issues an official statement that discloses information about the negotiations, this action produces an authorized "statement," not a "leak," and is not blameworthy.

93. Published accounts of, and commentaries, on the RDA dispute can be found in Colburn 1985, Dosti 1985b, Edwards 1985, Guthrie 1985, Harper 1986, Kamin 1985b, Marshall 1985, Monmaney 1986, Olson 1985a, 1985b, Pear 1985a, 1985b, and 1985c, Press 1985a and 1985b, and Toufexis 1985. My summary of the dispute also draws on unpublished letters by some of the principals in the dispute.

94. Henry Kamin, chairman of the RDA committee, describes the process the committee used to prepare the report in Kamin 1985a.

95. Helen A. Guthrie, a member of the committee, describes its perspective on how RDAs should be set; see Guthrie 1985. For a defense of the committee's approach, see Harper 1986.

96. According to Frank Press, president of the Academy and NRC chairman, the "differences of opinion among committee members and reviewers extended to such issues as the appropriate data base for developing the RDAs, the adequate size of body stores for specific nutrients, and the advisability of modifying the definition of the RDAs. All these points of contention led to different conclusions about the allowance levels" (Press 1985a; see Appendix A, ll. 67–71).

97. In July 1985, when the negotiations about the report were nearing the endgame, the Food and Nutrition Board consisted of Kurt J. Isselbacher, chairman;

Richard J. Havel, vice-chairman; Hamish N. Munro, vice-chairman; William E. Connor; Peter Greenwald; M. R. C. Greenwood; Joan D. Gussow; James R. Kirk; Reynaldo Martorell; Walter Mertz; J. Michael McGinnis; Malden C. Nesheim; Ronald C. Shank; Robert H. Wasserman; and Myron Winick (cf. Table 3).

98. Quoted in Marshall 1985.

99. Quoted in ibid.

100. Dosti 1985a.

101. Marshall 1985.

102. The proposed footnote was attached to Frank Press to Henry Kamin, Aug. 15, 1985.

103. Press's first option, thus, would allow the report to give voice to two conflicting views on the disputed nutrients; at all other points, the report would speak with a unified voice.

104. Pear 1985a, p. 1.

105. Marshall 1985, p. 421.

106. Edwards 1985.

107. Press 1985a.

108. Pear 1985b, p. 1; Colburn 1985, p. 12.

109. National Academy of Sciences 1989. The preface begins:

> This tenth edition of the *Recommended Dietary Allowances* (RDAs) reflects the work of two panels of the Food and Nutrition Board. The first, the Committee on Dietary Allowances, was appointed in 1980 and by 1985 had prepared a draft of this edition that, after an outside review overseen by the Report Review Committee of the National Research Council (NRC), was postponed for further consideration [reference to Press 1985a]. The second panel, a subcommittee of the Food and Nutrition Board (FNB) itself, was appointed in 1987 to complete this, the tenth edition of the RDAs. (ibid. p. vii)

See also Burros 1989.

110. *Herbert v. National Academy of Sciences* 1991. Herbert was ultimately ordered to pay attorney's fees.

111. Lynch and Bogen 1996.

112. See ibid., esp. ch. 2, for an insightful analysis of this process in the context of the Iran-Contra hearings.

113. The "documentary evidence of history," Lynch and Bogen write "comes to us, as it were, already warm" (ibid., p. 65). In the Iran-Contra hearings, they contend, the parties engaged in a struggle over how history would be emplotted (e.g., by leaking, shredding, and fabricating documents):

> Specific testimonies and shards of documentary evidence were appropriated and put to use as elements within some developing story. . . . The proper image, then, is not of the solitary author sitting down with the stable record of relevant events, dates, places, and personages involved, and from this record, deducing a singular chronology of events; instead, the image is of a multiplicity of contending and ever-shifting factions, each working to capture the facts within a plot structure most favorable to their interests.

Even deeper, it is a record through which each faction tries to produce facts of particular kinds in anticipation of a later need to organize those facts in line with a specific mode of emplotment. (ibid., p. 78)

On emplotment, see White 1978, pp. 58–67.

114. See Bruno Latour's related discussion of how a "black box" is positioned between its "sociogram" and its "technogram" (Latour 1987, pp. 138–39).

115. National Academy of Sciences 1996, p. 18.

116. James B. Wyngaarden to Henry Kamin, Dec. 3, 1985.

117. Note that this sort of "consensus" means that the actors have agreed to the *words* of the text; they need not read or understand the text in precisely the same way.

Chapter 3

1. The metaphor of controversy has its limitations for understanding the place of scientific knowledge in politics, since it tends to split multidimensional struggles into stylized "sides" and to reify interest groups; see Wynne 1996 and Jasanoff 1996. At certain moments, however, the metaphor becomes one that actors "live by" — at least for a time; see Lakoff and Johnson 1980 for a discussion of how metaphors infiltrate and structure our experiences. Controversies thus can become venues with well-articulated, collectively understood, adversarial structures, not unlike trials and election campaigns. Diet and health in the early 1980s had crystallized into a debate with "sides" that participants experienced as intensely polarized.

2. On such operatives, see Hilgartner and Bosk 1988.

3. Again, this formulation does not imply that these critics are necessarily cynical about their performances. See the discussion in Chapter 1.

4. In addressing this topic, it is not my goal to focus on how particular individuals or organizations criticized the reports (since obviously there were variations), but rather to identify recurring lines of argument and overall patterns of attack.

5. See, e.g., Clark 1980.

6. Barnhill 1980. See also Semling 1980; "How Risky Is a Diet Rich in Fats?" *U.S. News & World Report*, June 16, 1980, p. 100; "The Heart-Breaking Cholesterol Issue," *Economist*, June 14, 1980, pp. 100–101; and "Diet and Heart Disease," *Consumer Reports*, May 1981, pp. 256–60.

7. See, e.g., Kotulak 1983. For examples of diet plans, see American Institute for Cancer Research 1984 and Cleveland and Pfeffer 1987.

8. As noted in Chapter 1, *Diet, Nutrition, and Cancer* was an influential document that served to draw together the literature and frame discussion about the topic during the first half of the 1980s, a period in which attention to diet and cancer increased substantially.

9. Cole 1988 reviews much of this coverage.

10. U.S. House Committee on Agriculture 1980; U.S. Senate Committee on

Appropriations 1980. On the Consumer Liaison Panel, see the former, pp. 55–62, and National Academy of Sciences, Food and Nutrition Board, Consumer Liaison Panel 1980.

11. U.S. Department of Health and Human Services 1983, U.S. Department of Agriculture 1983, D. V. Porter 1983, Council for Agricultural Science and Technology 1982, and R. Greenberg et al. 1983. To "determine the report's implications for its respective programs," the USDA and DHHS each prepared "internal Department reviews" of *Diet, Nutrition, and Cancer*, which, however, according to the agencies were "not designed to be comprehensive assessments" of the report (Mary Jarratt, assistant secretary for food and consumer services, U.S. Department of Agriculture, and Edward N. Brandt, Jr., M.D., assistant secretary for health, U.S. Department of Health and Human Services, to Representative Leon E. Panetta, chairman, Subcommittee on Domestic Marketing, Consumer Relations and Nutrition, Committee on Agriculture, U.S. House of Representatives, June 22, 1983). The DHHS task force on *Diet, Nutrition, and Cancer* was co-chaired by the director of the Bureau of Foods, Food and Drug Administration and the director of the Division of Resources, Centers and Community Activities, National Cancer Institute. The task force included representatives of the Office of Human Development Services, the Centers for Disease Control, the National Center for Health Statistics, and the Office of the Assistant Secretary for Health. The review consists of 23 single-spaced pages. The USDA report was prepared by a task force that included representatives from the Agricultural Marketing Service, Agricultural Research Service, Cooperative State Research Service, Economic Research Service, Extension Service, Food and Nutrition Service, Food Safety and Inspection Service, and the Human Nutrition Information Service. The USDA review consists of 70 double-spaced pages. In contrast to the USDA review, the DHHS review did not attack the report or its executive summary and news release; on the USDA review, see also "USDA Disputes NAS Findings on Diet and Cancer; Raps News Coverage," *Nutrition Action*, Sept. 1983, p. 5. Donna V. Porter prepared the Congressional Research Service analysis (26 double-spaced pages), which describes the history of the report, summarizes its recommendations, compares them with dietary advice from other bodies, and briefly discusses methods for identifying carcinogens in the diet. The Council for Agricultural Science and Technology (CAST), an association of 25 food and agricultural science societies, published an 80-page report. Under a contract from the American Meat Institute (AMI) and the National Live Stock and Meat Board, an epidemiological consulting firm, Epistat Associates, Inc., examined the epidemiologic evidence used to support the NAS interim recommendations relevant to consumption of meats, fats, and meat products; R. Greenberg et al. 1983.

12. U.S. General Accounting Office 1984. Prepared at the request of eleven members of Congress who were unhappy with *Diet, Nutrition, and Cancer* (National Academy of Sciences 1982), this analysis examined both that report and National Academy of Sciences 1980, *Toward Healthful Diets*, as well as the controversy about the relationship of diet and cancer and the Academy's process for preparing reports.

13. D. S. Greenberg 1980. See also D. S. Greenberg 1967a, 1967b, and 1967c, his series of critical articles in *Science* about the Academy.

14. D. S. Greenberg 1980.

15. Ibid.

16. Ibid.

17. Ibid. Greenberg identifies these figures, Alfred E. Harper and Robert E. Olson, as "paid consultants to the food industry." The conflict of interest charge is discussed later in this chapter.

18. National Academy of Sciences 1980, p. 3.

19. See, e.g., the editorial "A Confusing Diet of Fact," *New York Times*, June 3, 1980, p. 18.

20. Statement of Jeremiah Stamler, M.D., professor of cardiology and chairman of the Department of Community Health and Preventive Medicine, Northwestern University, in Chicago Heart Association 1980, pp. 3–4.

21. James S. Turner to Philip Handler, June 11, 1980, reprinted in U.S. Senate Committee on Appropriations, *Dietary Guidelines for Americans*, p. 112.

22. D. S. Greenberg 1980.

23. On ignoring epidemiology, see the testimony of D. Mark Hegsted, administrator, Human Nutrition Center, U.S. Department of Agriculture, in U.S. House Committee on Agriculture 1980, p. 12. Another argument charged that the committee did not interpret evidence consistently: Robert Levy, M.D., director of the National Heart, Lung, and Blood Institute, National Institutes of Health, testified that he was puzzled that the committee favored advising people to lower their salt intake but did not support telling them to lower their cholesterol consumption, even though similar kinds of evidence supported both recommendations (U.S. Senate Committee on Appropriations 1980, p. 222). See also the statements of Jeremiah Stamler and Richard B. Shekelle in Chicago Heart Association 1980; McGinnis 1980; and Center for Science in the Public Interest n.d.

24. Center for Science in the Public Interest n.d., p. 1.

25. Ibid., p. 2. Similar arguments were made by other critics; see, e.g., Chicago Heart Association 1980.

26. The phrase "brief report" is from McGinnis 1980.

27. D. S. Greenberg 1980.

28. See, e.g., Hegsted 1983, p. 472; U.S. House Committee on Agriculture 1980, pp. 18–19; D. S. Greenberg 1980.

29. James S. Turner to Philip Handler, June 11, 1980, reprinted in U.S. Senate Committee on Appropriations, *Dietary Guidelines for Americans*, p. 111.

30. Ibid.

31. See Cohn 1980.

32. Risser 1980.

33. "A Confusing Diet of Fact," *New York Times*, June 3, 1980, p. 18.

34. "A Few Kind Words for Cholesterol," *Time*, June 9, 1980, p. 51.

35. Broad 1980, p. 1355.

36. Samuel S. Epstein, letter to the editor, *New York Times*, June 28, 1980, p. 20.

37. Chicago Heart Association 1980, p. 12.

38. See, e.g., the testimony of Robert I. Levy, M.D., in U.S. House Committee on Agriculture 1980, esp. pp. 87–88.

39. D. S. Greenberg 1980.

40. See, e.g., the comment of a representative of the National Live Stock and Meat Board quoted in Clark 1980.

41. The chair of the Food and Nutrition Board, for example, wrote in a letter to the *New York Times*:

> It is a devastating commentary on the attitude toward freedom of scientific inquiry in this country when an assessment of nutrition information is condemned by a major newspaper because it does not conform with recommendations made by other groups. Impugning by innuendo the integrity of some Food and Nutrition Board members is an equally devastating commentary on attitudes toward freedom of inquiry and freedom of expression. (Alfred E. Harper, letter to the editor, *New York Times*, June 16, 1980, p. 22)

The letter contained references to Lysenkoism and the Nazi occupation of the Netherlands. For another example, see Victor Herbert, letter to the editor, *New York Times*, July 11, 1980, p. 24.

42. See, e.g., testimony of Robert E. Olson, in U.S. House Committee on Agriculture 1980, p. 113.

43. U.S. House Committee on Agriculture 1980, p. 214.

44. Ibid., p. 187. See also U.S. Senate Committee on Appropriations 1980, pp. 54–72.

45. Garment 1980.

46. Documents supporting this interpretation appear in U.S. House Committee on Agriculture 1980, pp. 258–311; see esp. Karen W. Seaton, secretary, Consumer Liaison Panel, to Dr. Ned D. Bayley, Office of the Secretary, USDA, Feb. 10, 1978 (ibid., p. 310); and Bayley to Seaton, Feb. 24, 1978 (ibid., p. 311). See also testimony of James S. Turner (ibid., pp. 55–62); testimony of Philip Handler (ibid., pp. 184–85); James S. Turner to Handler, June 11, 1980, in U.S. Senate Committee on Appropriations 1980, pp. 111; and testimony of Handler in ibid., pp. 82–83.

47. Testimony of Handler in U.S. House Committee on Agriculture 1980, pp. 185–88.

48. U.S. Department of Agriculture 1983, p. 11.

49. Ibid., pp. 6–7.

50. The USDA (ibid., p. 11) contended that if the missing areas of expertise had been included on the committee, two of the report's guidelines (nos. 1 and 3) would probably have been "differently worded." On meat industry groups, see American Meat Institute 1982 and C. Manly Molpus, quoted later in this chapter.

51. Olson 1982, p. 57.

52. Another line of attack on the committee was to suggest that the NRC staff

might be the real author of the report. Alfred E. Harper (of *Toward Healthful Diets*) argued that the General Accounting Office's investigation showed that *Diet, Nutrition, and Cancer* "was in large measure a staff report rather than a Committee report," because the "literature searches, preliminary analyses of research studies and preparation of background papers on scientific issues were done by staff." See Harper's comments published as an appendix to U.S. General Accounting Office 1984, p. 80.

53. Harper 1982, p. 17.

54. See Harper's comments in U.S. General Accounting Office 1984, p. 79.

55. On the uses of claims about the extent of uncertainty in different contexts, see, e.g., Pinch 1981, Campbell 1985, and Yearley 1991. See S. L. Star 1989, ch. 3, for a discussion of various types of uncertainty that emerge in scientific work.

56. McMillan is quoted in "USDA's McMillan Cautions against 'Precipitous Response' to NAS Report," *Food Chemical News*, June 28, 1982, pp. 24–25. He stated that the USDA would establish an "expert committee" to review the report (ibid., p. 24).

57. American Meat Institute 1982. The AMI went on to quote *Toward Healthful Diets* and a 1981 NAS report on dietary sources of nitrites and N-nitroso compounds.

58. C. Manly Molpus et al. 1982. The organizations were the American Meat Institute, the Poultry and Egg Institute of America, the United Egg Producers, the National Turkey Federation, the National Milk Producers Federation, the National Cattlemen's Association, the National Broiler Council, the National Live Stock and Meat Board, and the National Pork Producers Council. The letter was released to the media; see, e.g., Kendall 1982 and Neiman 1982.

59. National Meat Association 1982. The news release argued:

> Today, this committee [i.e., the Committee on Diet, Nutrition, and Cancer] suggests there is evidence that most common cancers are influenced by diet and recommends, among other things, that Americans eat less foods high in saturated and unsaturated fats. Only two years ago, the National Research Council's Food and Nutrition Board, that too made up of eminent scientists from around the nation, issued a conflicting opinion [i.e., National Academy of Sciences 1980], and advised against recommending changes in the basic diet.

60. Council for Agricultural Science and Technology 1982, pp. ii, iv. Most of these experts were natural scientists or food technologists, but agricultural economists and other social scientists were also asked to consider the report's social impact.

61. See Shapin and Schaffer 1985, ch. 2, for a discussion of "literary technology." As a reflexive note, I want to point out that Chapter 1 draws on the CAST report to introduce the reader of this book to the debate over diet and health, using quotations from four of CAST's commentators.

62. Council for Agricultural Science and Technology 1982, pp. 5–7. Other critics used similar strategies to partition the scientific community and place *Diet,*

Nutrition, and Cancer in a field of controversy, although the category systems differed slightly. For example, one food scientist, Owen Fennema, drew an analogy to judges and legal scholars, partitioning the scientific community into "strict constructionists" and "broad constructionists" (ibid., p. 20). See also R. Greenberg et al. 1983, pp. 14–17, which uses the categories "activist" versus "conservative."

63. Council for Agricultural Science and Technology 1982, p. 5.
64. Ibid.
65. Ibid., pp. 5–7.
66. The recommenders, CAST wrote:

> note that the occurrence of cancer is greatly influenced by the environment and that diet is apparently the major environmental factor of importance. These scientists admit that it may be a long time before we have ironclad evidence to document the connections, but they nonetheless are of the opinion that the evidence we now have is strong enough, and the consequences of failure to act are so important, that we should proceed at once to try to alter people's diets in an attempt to reduce the incidence of cancer. (ibid., p. 5)

In contrast, the hesitant recommenders:

> acknowledge that certain epidemiologic associations observed in humans as well as the results of certain experiments with animals may be strongly suggestive, but they say the data are "soft" and do not represent scientifically acceptable evidence of causation. In the words of Philip Handler, the late President of the National Academy of Sciences, they argue that "the necessity of scientific rigor is even greater when scientific evidence is being offered as the basis for formulation of public policy than when it is simply expected to find its way into the marketplace of accepted scientific understanding." (ibid., p. 6)

67. Ibid., p. 3. Critics (e.g., CAST, AMI, USDA, and others, as we shall see) also charged that media coverage of the report misrepresented its content.
68. U.S. Department of Agriculture 1983, p. 10.
69. Ibid. Elsewhere in the review, the USDA said: "The problems presented by the summary and press release do not, however, negate the general excellence of a report encyclopedic in its scope and admirably rigorous in its method" (ibid., p. 1).
70. Council for Agricultural Science and Technology 1982, p. 3. The GAO disputed these charges, arguing that "the executive summary's statements about committee conclusions almost exactly repeat the language found in other sections of the report" (U.S. General Accounting Office 1984, p. 20).
71. The agency concentrated its objections on guidelines nos. 1 (reduce fat consumption to 30 percent of calories) and 3 (minimize consumption of salt-cured and smoked foods). Guidelines 1 and 3 were the only ones that suggested *reductions* in the consumption of foods. These guidelines, thus, conflicted with the USDA's traditional promotional orientation toward agriculture and the food industry. The USDA did not comment on guideline no. 6, which suggested minimizing consumption of alcohol, because, it said, the agency is not "directly involved in this area" (U.S. Department of Agriculture 1983, p. 2). Disagreeing "with the Committee's assump-

tion that sustained fat intakes can readily be reduced to 30 percent of calories" (guideline no. 1), the USDA argued that this goal was incompatible with the types of food consumed in the United States and suggested 35 percent instead (U.S. Department of Agriculture 1983, pp. 13, 27).

72. Ibid., p. 4.

73. The statement of J. P. Fontenot, a professor of animal science at the Virginia Polytechnic Institute, provides another example:

> The report is very detailed and quite comprehensive. The Committee that prepared the publication was composed of competent scientists from different disciplines and locations. The committee members are to be commended for an exhaustive coverage of the subject. . . . It appears that the Committee has done a good job of searching and summarizing the literature . . . and pointing out the many voids which prevent firm conclusions. It is unfortunate that the Committee felt compelled to formulate "interim dietary guidelines." The evidence cited in the report seemed to be too fragmentary and inconclusive to recommend such guidelines. (Council for Agricultural Science and Technology 1982, p. 27)

74. Ibid., p. 61.

75. U.S. Department of Agriculture 1983, p. 1.

76. See, e.g., Council for Agricultural Science and Technology 1982, p. 3; a section of the overview of the CAST report was titled: "Discrepancies between the News Release and the Report."

77. See "AMI Asks NAS to Correct Misconceptions Based on 1982 Report," *Food Chemical News*, Jan. 20, 1986, pp. 15–17. Accompanying Molpus's letter to the NAS was a "commentary" by Robert G. Cassens of the Department of Meat and Animal Science at the University of Wisconsin, who charged that the suggestion in the news release that people minimize consumption of bacon, ham, bologna, and hot dogs "represents an inexcusable distortion of a rather narrow set of facts" (ibid., p. 16). Cassens went on to say that the credibility of science was being damaged, not by the report, but by the news release (ibid., p. 17).

78. The Academy's arguments that the executive summary was part of the report appear inter alia in U.S. General Accounting Office 1984, p. 20. In addition to the chair of the Diet, Nutrition, and Cancer committee, the executive director of the NAS Assembly of Life Sciences reviewed the news release (ibid., pp. 26–27).

79. On the use of the notion of "popularization" in boundary work, see Hilgartner 1990.

80. To be sure, there were a few cases of relatively comprehensive efforts to rewrite the report narrative. For example, Robert E. Olson's commentary on *Diet, Nutrition, and Cancer*, which appeared in the CAST report, attacked most of the elements of the basic narrative of Academy reports, as well as criticizing the executive summary, news release, and guidelines (Council for Agricultural Science and Technology 1982, pp. 55–61). Olson wrote the longest critique of any of the contributors to the CAST report.

81. In Bruno Latour's terms, the cancer report was backed by a robust, heterogeneous network; see Latour 1987.

82. The quotation is from D. S. Greenberg 1980.

83. Handler testimony, U.S. House Committee on Agriculture 1980, p. 188.

84. Indeed, Handler seems almost to reach this conclusion himself when he writes, in his prepared testimony, that in "hindsight" he might have added an epidemiologist or "ardent proponent of cholesterol avoidance" to the committee (ibid., p. 187).

85. R. Greenberg et al. 1983, p. 6. The contract specified that Epistat should review the epidemiologic literature pertaining to dietary fat, meat, and processed meats. Among other tasks, Epistat was to identify studies not cited in the NAS report that could have been cited or that had been published after the committee prepared the report (ibid., p. 5).

86. The AMI continued, however, to complain about the news release. The Epistat report was completed in 1983; C. Manly Molpus (quoted above) asked for "written acknowledgement" that the news release was "erroneous" in 1986.

87. Dennis T. Gordon, quoted in Council for Agricultural Science and Technology 1982, p. 29.

88. Ibid., p. 30.

89. I want to stress that I am making this assertion at the aggregate level: it refers to groups, not individuals. To a lesser degree, the same comment applies to groups of organizations as opposed to individual ones.

90. This notion of "public identity" assumes a world based less on the intimate knowledge of others than on a knowledge of social categories, and trust less in individuals than in institutions and procedures. I do not mean to suggest that more personalized trust relations are unimportant. See Shapin 1994, pp. 409–17, for an interesting argument about the continuing importance of interpersonal trust in warranting knowledge even in these depersonalized times.

91. The institutional affiliations of the scientists who criticized *Diet, Nutrition, and Cancer* in the CAST report provide an example. Although some critics were affiliated with "core" "health-oriented" areas, such as departments of biochemistry, medicine, and nutrition, "applied" "food-oriented" areas, such as animal science, food science, food technology, meat science, and poultry science, were more heavily represented.

92. These differences are integrated into cultural classifications and structured relations that place "core" science above "applied" science, and "medicine" above "agriculture." These hierarchies in science resemble in some ways the "taste cultures" that Bourdieu 1984 analyzes with respect to culture and art. They also have practical consequences in shaping who is likely to be able to assert claims to professional "jurisdiction" over a domain more strongly; on jurisdictional contests, see Abbott 1988.

93. The public identities of the "friends" of these reports also influenced their reception. For example, when meat and dairy producers lauded *Toward Healthful*

Diets at the same time that health groups attacked it, this reinforced the framing of the dispute along a "health science vs. food industry interests" axis.

94. For example, in a *New York Times* article that reported that Harper considered *Diet, Nutrition, and Cancer*'s recommendations "misleading," he was identified as "professor of nutrition and biochemistry at the University of Wisconsin and chairman of the Academy's Food and Nutrition Board. . . . In addition to his academic work, Dr. Harper says, he derives about 10 percent of his income from 'industry consultantships,' mainly for Pillsbury, producer of many bakery and other products, and Kraft, the nation's largest purveyor of cheese products." See Burros 1982.

95. A strong argument, for example, can be made that expertise in food science and technology may have critical contributions to make to analysis of diet and health, as the USDA and others pointed out.

96. See, e.g., Gans 1979 and Gamson and Modigliani 1989.

Chapter 4

1. On emplotment, see White 1978, ch. 2. See also Burke 1989, Gusfield 1981, Lynch and Bogen 1996, Turner 1974, and Wagner-Pacifici 1986.

2. See Lynch and Bogen 1996.

3. See, e.g., Burke 1989, Gusfield 1981, Lynch and Bogen 1996, Turner 1974, Wagner-Pacifici 1986, and White 1978.

4. The RDA committee and the panel that wrote *Toward Healthful Diets* (National Academy of Sciences 1980) also shared two important members, Henry Kamin and Victor Herbert (see Table 3).

5. The available documents do not make it possible to determine exactly when the decision not to release the report was made, other than to say that it occurred sometime between late August and the official announcement on October 7. To compound the limits of available records, there is some evidence that the committee and the Academy may have disagreed about when this occurred.

6. Helen A. Guthrie, a member of the committee, wrote another interesting account, which describes the committee's approach to the RDAs and emphasizes its efforts to produce a sound report; see Guthrie 1985.

7. Press 1985a.

8. Kamin 1985b; Marshall 1985; Olson 1985a.

9. Press 1985b.

10. For example, critics of a decision to cancel *any* report might be expected to attribute its cancellation to illegitimate political pressures; however, in this case, the advance news coverage — which quoted representatives of Washington-based advocacy groups and highlighted points of disagreement between the report and recent government advice — might easily be read in such a way as to make this line of argument appear plausible.

11. A similar approach of repackaging verbatim quotations to create a play was also employed by the journalist Richard Norton-Taylor in his play *Half the*

Picture, which draws on excerpts from the public hearings of the Scott inquiry, an investigation of a scandal concerning the sale of military technology to Iraq; see Norton-Taylor and Lloyd 1995. Plays or playlike dialogs have also appeared in several works in social studies of science, including Ashmore, Mulkay, and Pinch 1989.

12. See T. M. Porter 1995 on how quantification can help stabilize social action.

13. It is also striking how the chairman emplots the breach (a failure to reach agreement on the text of the report) as an event that simply arose; responsibility for it is not clearly and dramatically localized. On social dramas, see Turner 1980, which depicts them as "processual units" within groups that share values and interests. Such dramas have four discernible stages: they progress from an initial normative "breach," through a period of "crisis," a phase of "redress," and finally either a "reintegration" (if the redress is successful) or a "continuation of schism" (ibid., p. 149). See also Turner 1974 and Wagner-Pacifici 1986.

14. Kamin 1985b. See also Marshall 1985, Monmaney 1986, and Pear 1985b and 1985c.

15. Kamin 1985b, l. 6.

16. Ibid., l. 18.

17. Ibid., ll. 69–71.

18. Ibid., ll. 6–9.

19. Ibid., ll. 29–33.

20. Ibid., l. 2.

21. Ibid., ll. 4–5.

22. Ibid., l. 6.

23. Ibid., ll. 6, 66–70.

24. Ibid., ll. 7–8.

25. Ibid., ll. 8–11.

26. Ibid., ll. 15–17. Marshall 1985 describes how Lemov wrote the Academy concerned about the implications of the report for nutritionally vulnerable populations.

27. Kamin 1985b, ll.12–15.

28. Ibid., ll. 54, 37–39.

29. Ibid., l. 12.

30. Ibid., ll. 36–43.

31. Ibid., l. 18–24.

32. Ibid., ll. 23–26. Kamin goes on to quote Peterkin as saying: "RDA changes, since the development of the school lunch meal pattern in the 1940's, the poverty formula in the 1960's, and the food stamp standard in the early 1970's have *not* affected the dollar-related aspects of these standards" (ll. 26–28).

33. Kamin 1985b, ll. 33–36.

34. Ibid. ll. 54–59. Note that Kamin, along with Victor Herbert, who also served on the RDA committee, is listed among the authors of *Toward Healthful Diets* (see Table 3).

35. Kamin 1985b, ll. 78–79.

36. Ibid., ll. 55–57.

37. Ibid., ll. 61–67. Note how Kamin's use of "thus far" and his claim that the committee remained open to serious discourse on the issues suggest that he was unwilling to rule out the possibility of reopening negotiations with the Academy.

38. Ibid., ll. 75–79.

39. I have not included in the list above several characters who represent bystanders to the central moral struggle. These include "previous RDA committees," which are not involved in the dispute, and in any case no longer exist, because they have disbanded, and "James Wyngaarden," director of the NIH, who appears in Kamin's account only as the recipient of a letter from Kamin.

40. Even scientific reports end up surrounded. According to Kamin 1985b, ll. 39–42, "the publicity-based mythology that surrounds it" distorted the meaning of *Diet, Nutrition, and Cancer.*

41. Olson 1985a.

42. Ibid. In the letter, he suggests that "a possible conflict of interest" might exist for "persons who are members of the Food and Nutrition Board and at the same time represent federal agencies such as the National Cancer Institute," which are actively engaged in nutrition education programs, including some that involve participating in controversial food industry advertising that promotes products, such as bran cereals, as anticancer foods.

43. Ibid.

44. In comparing the characters in the two dramas, I am looking at these texts as separate semiotic worlds that can be compared. It is also possible to attempt to translate between them. Hegsted, who was one of the reviewers of the report, provides an example. Kamin refers to Hegsted by name but does not mention his role as a reviewer. The chairman's letter refers to the reviewers but does not mention their names. One might therefore claim that Kamin "refers" to a reviewer and the chairman "refers" to Hegsted. This sort of reformulation, however, does violence to the ontologies that inform each account and fundamentally deforms their dramatic structure.

45. Ibid. Olson's mention of the reviewers occurs during a discussion of arguments made by Hegsted that Olson considers to be absurd: "With this type of argument, it is not difficult to see why the Academy and its reviewers reached a standoff with the committee." His goal seems to be to use the example of Hegsted to discredit the reviewers in general.

46. Chairman Press's characters seem incapable of taking brutal action, such as "suppressing a report that cost the National Institutes of Health $600,000" (Olson 1985a). The chairman's characters are more suited to finding, after appropriate consultation, that they "have concluded that the National Research Council will be unable to issue" a report "at this time" (Press 1985b, ll. 1–3).

47. Arguably, Wyngaarden and Press both appear more as occupants of official posts — the director of the NIH, the chairman of the NRC — than as individuals.

48. See T. M. Porter 1995 on procedures versus persons.

49. Following a pattern that Jasanoff 1987 has identified in other contexts, the committee and the NAS defined the boundary separating "science" from "policy" in ways that not only conflicted but also had implications for who should participate in decision making.

50. Press 1985b.

51. Press 1985a.

52. Press 1985b.

53. Ibid.

54. Ibid.

55. Ibid.

56. Ibid.

57. Ibid.

58. Ibid. What Press frames as "peer review," Kamin and Olson see as "suppression," showing how the concept of "peer review" can be used as boundary work (see Jasanoff 1987, 1990, and 1995). Press's definition of the issue — as a scientific one to be resolved through peer review — legitimates the NAS's decision to stop publication. Kamin, by treating it as a nonscientific act of suppression, is also engaging in boundary work, but he puts the decision to cancel on the other side of the line. On criticisms of peer review, see also Chubin and Hackett 1990.

59. Press's reply did not, of course, put an end to the debate about the cancellation. Indeed, in less visible forums than the letter pages of *Science*, such as personal correspondence, members of the committee replied to Press's reply, charging that he was unfairly attacking their scientific integrity. Kamin and his supporters also unsuccessfully campaigned for a reconsideration of the decision to cancel the report.

60. Discursive containment is a specific type of the kinds of strategies, discussed in Lynch and Bogen 1996, that protagonists use to shape the story line of history, emplotting events in a narrative favorable to their interests. Discursive containment offers a strategy for recapturing events that have (at least partially) escaped the performer's prior information-management efforts.

Chapter 5

1. The title of an editorial ("Raiders of the Last Bastion?"), published in *Science* in the midst of the struggle over whether NRC committees would be subject to the (unamended) Federal Advisory Committee Act, captures this apocalyptic view; see M. R. C. Greenwood 1997.

Abbott, Andrew. 1988. *The System of the Professions: An Essay on the Division of Expert Labor.* Chicago: University of Chicago Press.

"Academy Critic Shoots Wildly but Hits Sore Spot." 1971. *Nature* 229 (Jan. 15): 151–52.

Alberts, Bruce. 1994. "Consensus and Dissent in NRC Reports." National Research Council memorandum, Mar. 1.

———. 1997a. "Statement from Bruce Alberts, President, National Academy of Sciences, and Chair, National Research Council Regarding January 10, 1997 U.S. Court of Appeals Ruling." Jan. 30.

———. 1997b. Letter to the editor. *Science* 277 (Aug. 1): 625.

———. 1997c. "Statement Regarding Ruling to Deny Rehearing in U.S. Court of Appeals." May 6.

———. 1997d. "Statement Regarding Supreme Court Decision to Deny Certiorari in ADLF v. Shalala." Nov. 4.

———. 1997e. "Oversight of the Federal Advisory Committee Act." Statement before the Subcommittee on Government Management, Information, and Technology, Committee on Government Reform and Oversight, U.S. House of Representatives. Nov. 5.

———. 1997f. "Statement Regarding Passage of Bill to Exempt the National Academy of Sciences from FACA." Nov. 13.

———. 1998. "Statement before the Subcommittee on Government Information and Management, Committee of Government Reform and Oversight, U.S. House of Representatives." July 14.

American Cancer Society. 1984. *Nutrition and Cancer: Cause and Prevention: An American Cancer Society Special Report.* Pamphlet 84-50M-No. 3389-PE. New York: American Cancer Society.

———. 1985. *Eating to Live: What Food May Help You Reduce Your Cancer Risk?* Pamphlet 85-(30MM) No. 2099-LE. New York: American Cancer Society.

American Heart Association. 1961. "Dietary Fat and Its Relation to Heart Attacks and Strokes: Report by the Central Committee for Medical and Community Program." *Circulation* 23 (Jan.): 133–36.

———. 1965. *Diet and Heart Disease: Report of the Committee on Nutrition.* New York: American Heart Association.

———. 1968. *Diet and Heart Disease: Report of the Committee on Nutrition.* New York: American Heart Association.

———. 1978. "Diet and Coronary Heart Disease" (statement of the AHA Nutrition Committee). *Circulation* 58: 762A–766A.

———. 1982. "Rationale of the Diet-Heart Statement of the American Heart Association: Report of the AHA Nutrition Committee." *Arteriosclerosis* 4 (Mar.–Apr.): 177–91.

American Institute for Cancer Research. 1984. *Planning Meals That Lower Cancer Risk: A Reference Guide.* Washington, D.C.: American Institute for Cancer Research.

American Meat Institute. 1982. "The American Meat Institute Challenges NAS Study on Diet and Cancer." News Release, June 16.

American Medical Association, Council on Scientific Affairs. 1979. "American Medical Association Concepts of Nutrition and Health." *Journal of the American Medical Association* 242 (Nov. 23): 2335–38.

Animal Legal Defense Fund, Inc. v. Shalala. 1997. WL 7050 (D.C. Cir.).

Ashmore, Malcolm. 1989. *The Reflexive Thesis: Wrighting Sociology of Scientific Knowledge.* Chicago: University of Chicago Press.

Ashmore, Malcolm, Greg Myers, and Jonathan Potter. 1995. "Discourse, Rhetoric, Reflexivity: Seven Days in the Library." In *Handbook of Science and Technology Studies,* ed. S. Jasanoff et al., pp. 321–42. Newbury Park, Calif.: Sage.

Ashmore, Malcolm, Michael Mulkay, and Trevor Pinch. 1989. *Health and Efficiency: A Sociology of Health Economics.* Milton Keynes, Eng.: Open University Press.

Austin, James E., and John A. Quelch. 1979. "US National Dietary Goals: Food Industry Threat or Opportunity." *Food Policy,* May, pp. 115–28.

Barfield, Claude E. 1971. "National Academy of Sciences Tackles Sensitive Policy Questions." *National Journal,* Jan. 16, pp. 101–12.

Barnes, Barry. 1977. *Interests and the Growth of Knowledge.* London: Routledge.

Barnes, Barry, and David Edge. 1982. *Science in Context: Readings in the Sociology of Science.* Cambridge, Mass.: MIT Press.

Barnhill, William. 1980. "The Cholesterol Controversy." *Family Health,* Sept., p. 12.

Bazerman, Charles. 1988. *Shaping Written Knowledge: The Genre and Activity of the Experimental Article in Science.* Madison: University of Wisconsin Press.

Beck, Ulrich. 1992. *Risk Society: Towards a New Modernity.* Newbury Park, Calif.: Sage.

Best, Joel. 1990. *Threatened Children: Rhetoric and Concern about Child-Victims.* Chicago: University of Chicago Press.

Biagioli, Mario. 1998. "The Instability of Authorship: Credit and Responsibility in Contemporary Biomedicine." *FASEB Journal* 12: 3–16.

———, ed. 1999. *The Science Studies Reader.* New York: Routledge.

Bijker, Wiebe E., Trevor Pinch, and Thomas P. Hughes, eds. 1987. *The Social Construction of Technological Systems*. Cambridge, Mass.: MIT Press.

Bimber, Bruce. 1996. *The Politics of Expertise in Congress: The Rise and Fall of the Office of Technology Assessment*. Albany: State University of New York Press.

Bimber, Bruce, and David Guston. 1995. "Politics by the Same Means: Government and Science in the United States." In *Handbook of Science and Technology Studies*, ed. S. Jasanoff, pp. 554–71. Newbury Park, Calif.: Sage.

———. 1997. "Introduction: The End of OTA and the Future of Technology Assessment." *Technological Forecasting and Social Change* 54: 125–13.

Boffey, Philip M. 1975. *The Brain Bank of America: An Inquiry into the Politics of Science*. Introduction by Ralph Nader. New York: McGraw-Hill.

———. 1977. "National Academy of Sciences: How the Elite Choose Their Peers." *Science* 196 (May 13): 738–42.

———. 1982. "Cancer Experts Lean Toward Vigilance, but Less Alarm on Environment." *New York Times*, Mar. 2, p. C1.

———. 1984. "After Years of Cancer Alarms, Progress amid the Mistakes." *New York Times*, Mar. 20, p. C1.

Bosk, Charles L. 1979. *Forgive and Remember: Managing Medical Failure*. Chicago: University of Chicago Press.

Bourdieu, Pierre. 1984. *Distinction: A Social Critique of the Judgement of Taste*. Translated by Richard Nice. Cambridge, Mass.: Harvard University Press.

Boyle, James. 1996. *Shamans, Software, and Spleens: Law and Construction of the Information Society*. Cambridge, Mass.: Harvard University Press.

Brickman, Ronald, Sheila Jasanoff, and Thomas Ilgen. 1985. *Controlling Chemicals: The Politics of Regulation in Europe and the United States*. Ithaca, N.Y.: Cornell University Press.

Broad, William J. 1979. "NIH Deals Gingerly with Diet-Disease Link." *Science* 204 (June 15): 1175–78.

———. 1980. "Academy Says Curb on Cholesterol Not Needed." *Science* 208 (June 20): 1354–55.

Brody, Jane. 1980a. "Experts Assail Report Declaring Curb on Cholesterol Isn't Needed." *New York Times*, June 1, p. 1.

———. 1980b. "U.S. Acts to Reshape Diets of Americans." *New York Times*, Feb. 5, p. A1.

Bullock, J. Bruce. 1982. "Impact on American Agriculture if American Consumers Were to Implement the Dietary Guidelines Proposed in the Report on *Diet, Nutrition, and Cancer*." In Council for Agricultural Science and Technology, *Diet, Nutrition, and Cancer: A Critique*," 12–14. Special Report No. 13. Ames, Iowa: Council for Agricultural Science and Technology.

Burke, Kenneth. 1989. *On Symbols and Society*. Edited by Joseph R. Gusfield. Chicago: University of Chicago Press.

Burros, Marian. 1982. "Prudent Diet and Cancer Risk." *New York Times*, June 23, C1.

————. 1986. "Meat Is Getting Trimmer for a Comeback Fight." *New York Times*, Oct. 8, C1.

————. 1989. "Panel Changes Dietary Standards for Calcium." *New York Times*, Oct. 24, C10.

Butrum, Ritva R., Elaine Lanza, and Carolyn K. Clifford. Undated. "The Diet and Cancer Branch, NCI: Current Projects and Future Research Directions." National Cancer Institute, Division of Cancer Prevention and Control, Diet and Cancer Branch. Photocopy.

Cairns, John. 1978. *Cancer: Science and Society*. San Francisco: W. H. Freeman.

Callon, Michel. 1986. "Some Elements of a Sociology of Translation: Domestication of the Scallops and the Fishermen of St. Brieuc Bay." In *Power, Action, and Belief: A New Sociology of Knowledge?* ed. John Law, pp. 186–229. New York: Routledge & Kegan Paul.

Callon, Michel, John Law, and Arie Rip, eds. 1986. *Mapping the Dynamics of Science and Technology: Sociology of Science in the Real World*. London: Macmillan.

Cambrosio, Alberto, and Peter Keating. 1995. *Exquisite Specificity: The Monoclonal Antibodies Revolution*. New York: Oxford University Press.

Campbell, Brian L. 1985. "Uncertainty as Symbolic Action in Disputes among Experts." *Social Studies of Science* 15: 429–53.

Center for Science in the Public Interest. 1985. "Groups Demand End to Secrecy of Fast Food Contents." News Release, June 24.

————. N.d. "Comments on 'Toward Healthful Diets.' " Photocopy.

Chicago Heart Association. 1980. Edited transcript of press conference, May 30.

Childress, James F. 1991. "Deliberations of the Human Fetal Tissue Transplantation Research Panel." In *Biomedical Politics*, ed. Kathi E. Hanna, pp. 215–48. Washington, D.C.: National Academy Press.

Chubin, Daryl E., and Edward J. Hackett. 1990. *Peerless Science: Peer Review and U.S. Science Policy*. Albany, N.Y.: State University of New York Press.

Clark, Matt. 1980. "How Bad Is Cholesterol?" *Newsweek*, June 9, p. 111.

Clarke, Adele, and Joan H. Fujimura, eds. 1992. *The Right Tools for the Job: At Work in the Twentieth-Century Life Sciences*. Princeton, N.J.: Princeton University Press.

Clarke, Lee. 1989. *Acceptable Risk? Making Decisions in a Toxic Environment*. Berkeley and Los Angeles: University of California Press.

Cleveland, Linda E., and Andrea B. Pfeffer. 1987. "Planning Diets to Meet the National Research Council's Guidelines for Reducing Cancer Risk." *Journal of the American Dietetic Association* 87, 2: 162–68.

Cohn, Victor. 1980. "Two on Food Panel Are Advisers." *Washington Post*, May 31, p. A1.

————. 1982. "Reshaping the Nation's Diet; Drastic Changes Urged to Avoid Cancer." *Washington Post*, June 17, p. 1.

Colburn, Don. 1985. "The RDA: A Fuzzy Guide to What You Need." *Washington Post*, Oct. 16, p. 12.

Cole, Jonathan R. 1988. "Dietary Cholesterol and Heart Disease: The Construction of a Scientific 'Fact.' " In *Surveying Social Life: Papers in Honor of Herbert H. Hyman*, ed. Hubert J. O'Gorman, pp. 437–66. Middletown, Conn.: Wesleyan University Press.

Cole, Jonathan R., and Stephen Cole. 1973. *Social Stratification in Science*. Chicago: University of Chicago Press.

Collingridge, David, and Colin Reeve. 1986. *Science Speaks to Power: The Role of Experts in Policy Making*. New York: St. Martin's Press.

Collins, H. M. 1985. *Changing Order: Replication and Induction in Scientific Practice*. Beverly Hills, Calif.: Sage.

———. 1988. "Public Experiments and Displays of Virtuosity: The Core-Set Revisited." *Social Studies of Science* 18: 725–48.

"A Confusing Diet of Fact." 1980. *New York Times*, June 3, p. 18.

Council for Agricultural Science and Technology. 1982. *Diet, Nutrition, and Cancer: A Critique*. Special Report No. 13. Ames, Iowa: Council for Agricultural Science and Technology.

Daemmrich, Arthur. 1998. "The Evidence Does Not Speak for Itself: Expert Witnesses and the Organization of DNA-Typing Companies." *Social Studies of Science* 28: 741–72.

Dam, Kenneth W. 1996. *The Role of Private Groups in Public Policy: Cryptography and the National Research Council*. Occasional Paper Number 38. Chicago: University of Chicago Law School.

Daston, Lorraine. 1992. "Objectivity and the Escape from Perspective." *Social Studies of Science* 22: 597–618.

Daston, Lorraine, and Peter Galison. 1992. "The Image of Objectivity." *Representations* 40: 81–128.

de Vet, Henrica Cornelia Wilhelmina, and Flora Elizabeth van Leeuwen. 1986. "Dietary Guidelines for Cancer Prevention: The Etiology of a Confused Debate." *Nutrition and Cancer* 8: 223–29.

Dear, Peter. 1992. "From Truth to Disinterestedness in the Seventeenth Century." *Social Studies of Science* 22: 619–31.

Dickson, David. 1984. *The New Politics of Science*. New York: Pantheon Books.

Doering, Otto C. 1982. "Potential Impact of the *Diet, Nutrition, and Cancer* Report on the U.S. Agricultural Industry." In Council for Agricultural Science and Technology, *Diet, Nutrition, and Cancer: A Critique*, 18–19. Special Report No. 13. Ames, Iowa: Council for Agricultural Science and Technology.

Doll, Richard, and Richard Peto. 1981. "The Causes of Cancer: Quantitative Estimates of Avoidable Risks of Cancer in the United States Today." *Journal of the National Cancer Institute* 66, 6: 1192–308.

Dosti, Rose. 1985a. " RDA Changes Expected; Nutrient Allowances to Be Altered." *Los Angeles Times*, July 18, pt. 8, p. 22.

———. 1985b. "Requirements for Vitamins A and C Disputed; Revised Recommended Dietary Allowance Figures Won't Be Released." *Los Angeles Times,* Oct. 31, pt. 8, p. 33.

Douglas, Mary, and Aaron Wildavsky. 1982. *Risk and Culture: An Essay on the Selection of Technical and Environmental Dangers.* Berkeley and Los Angeles: University of California Press.

Downey, Gary T. 1988. "Structure and Practice in the Cultural Identities of Scientists: Negotiating Nuclear Waste in New Mexico." *Anthropological Quarterly,* Jan. 1988, pp. 26–38.

Dupree, A. Hunter. 1957. *Science in the Federal Government: A History of Policies and Activities to 1940.* Cambridge, Mass.: Harvard University Press, Belknap Press.

Edelman, Murray. 1964. *The Symbolic Uses of Politics.* Urbana: University of Illinois Press.

———. 1988. *Constructing the Political Spectacle.* Chicago: University of Chicago Press.

Edwards, Diane D. 1985. "Diet Allowances to Slim Down? Draft Report Proposes Reduction of Recommended Dietary Allowances." *Science News,* Sept. 28, p. 109.

Epstein, Steven. 1996. *Impure Science: AIDS, Activism, and the Politics of Knowledge.* Berkeley and Los Angeles: University of California Press.

———. 1997. "Activism, Drug Regulation, and the Politics of Therapeutic Evaluation in the AIDS Era: A Case Study of ddC and the 'Surrogate Markers' Debate." *Social Studies of Science* 27: 691–726.

Exon, J. James, Charles E. Grassley, Roger W. Jepsen, and John Melcher. 1982. Letter to Charles A. Bowsher, Sept. 30. In U.S. General Accounting Office, *National Academy of Sciences' Reports on Diet and Health — Are They Credible and Consistent?* pp. 51–55. GAO/RCED-84-109. Aug. 21, 1984.

Ezrahi, Yaron. 1980. "Science and the Problem of Authority in Democracy." In *Science and Social Structure,* ed. T. F. Gieryn, pp. 43–60. Transactions of the New York Academy of Sciences, 2d ser., 39.

———. 1990. *The Descent of Icarus: Science and the Transformation of Contemporary Democracy.* Cambridge, Mass.: Harvard University Press.

———. 1993. "Technology and the Civil Epistemology of Democracy." *Inquiry* 35: 363–76.

Ferris, John. 1982. "Economic Impact of the Interim Dietary Guidelines from the Report of the Committee on *Diet, Nutrition, and Cancer,* National Academy of Sciences." In Council for Agricultural Science and Technology, *Diet, Nutrition, and Cancer: A Critique,* pp. 20–26. Special Report No. 13. Ames, Iowa: Council for Agricultural Science and Technology.

Foucault, Michel. 1977. "What Is an Author?" In id., *Language, Counter-Memory, Practice: Select Essays and Interviews,* edited by Donald F. Bouchard, translated by Donald F. Bouchard and Sherry Simon, pp. 113–38. Ithaca, N.Y.: Cornell University Press.

Fujimura, Joan H. 1996. *Crafting Science: A Sociohistory of the Quest for the Genetics of Cancer.* Cambridge, Mass.: Harvard University Press.

Galison, Peter. 1987. *How Experiments End.* Chicago: University of Chicago Press.

———. 1997. "Accidents of History." Paper presented at conference on "Knowledge and Its Discontents," Cornell University, May 1997.

Gamson, William A., and André Modigliani. 1989. "Media Discourse and Public Opinion on Nuclear Power: A Constructionist Approach." *American Journal of Sociology* 95: 1–37.

Gans, Herbert J. 1979. *Deciding What's News: A Study of CBS Evening News, NBC Nightly News, Newsweek, and Time.* New York: Pantheon Books.

Garfinkel, Harold. 1967. *Studies in Ethnomethodology.* Englewood Cliffs, N.J.: Prentice-Hall.

Garment, Suzanne. 1980. "Science Academy's Cholesterol Report Spatters in Capitol." *Wall Street Journal,* June 27, 1980, p. 24.

Garrety, Karin. 1997. "Social Worlds, Actor-Networks and Controversy: The Case of Cholesterol, Dietary Fat, and Heart Disease." *Social Studies of Science* 27: 727–73.

Gieryn, Thomas F. 1983. "Boundary-Work and the Demarcation of Science from Non-Science: Strains and Interests in the Professional Ideologies of Scientists." *American Sociological Review* 48, 6: 781–95.

———. 1995. "Boundaries of Science." In *Handbook of Science and Technology Studies,* ed. S. Jasanoff et al., pp. 393–443. Newbury Park, Calif.: Sage.

———. 1999. *Cultural Boundaries of Science: Credibility on the Line.* Chicago: University of Chicago Press.

Gieryn, Thomas F., and Anne E. Figert. 1990. "Ingredients for a Theory of Science in Society: O-Rings, C-Clamp, Richard Feynman, and the Press." In *Theories of Science in Society,* ed. Susan E. Cozzens and Thomas F. Gieryn, pp. 67–97. Bloomington: Indiana University Press.

Gieryn, Thomas F., George M. Bevins, and Stephen C. Zehr. 1985. "The Professionalization of American Scientists." *American Sociological Review* 50, 3: 392–409.

Gilbert, G. Nigel. 1977. "Referencing as Persuasion." *Social Studies of Science* 7: 113–22.

Gilbert, G. Nigel, and Michael Mulkay. 1982. "Warranting Scientific Belief." *Social Studies of Science* 12: 383–408.

———. 1984. *Opening Pandora's Box: A Sociological Analysis of Scientists' Discourse.* Cambridge, Eng.: Cambridge University Press.

Goffman, Erving. 1959. *The Presentation of Self in Everyday Life.* Garden City, N.Y.: Doubleday, Anchor Books..

———. 1961a. *Encounters: Two Studies in the Sociology of Interaction.* Indianapolis: Bobbs-Merrill.

———. 1961b. *Stigma: Notes on the Management of Spoiled Identity.* Englewood Cliffs, N.J.: Prentice-Hall.

———. 1963a. *Asylums: Essays on the Social Situation of Mental Patients and Other Inmates.* Garden City, N.Y.: Doubleday, Anchor Books.

———. 1963b. *Behavior in Public Places: Notes on the Social Organization of Gatherings.* New York: Free Press.

———. 1974. *Frame Analysis: An Essay on the Organization of Experience.* New York: Harper & Row.

———. 1979. *Gender Advertisements.* Cambridge, Mass.: Harvard University Press.

Golden, William T. 1995. *Science and Technology Advice to the President, Congress, and Judiciary.* New Brunswick, N.J.: Transaction.

Goldschmidt, Walter. 1971. "Equinoxial Rites of the National Research Council." *Science* 174 (Oct. 29): 474–76.

Goodwin, Charles. 1994. "Professional Vision." *American Anthropologist* 96: 606–33.

Greenberg, Daniel S. 1967a. "The National Academy of Sciences: Profile of an Institution (I)." *Science* 156 (Apr. 14): 222–23, 226–28.

———. 1967b. "The National Academy of Sciences: Profile of an Institution (II)." *Science* 156 (Apr. 21): 360–64.

———. 1967c. "The National Academy of Sciences: Profile of an Institution (III)." *Science* 156 (Apr. 28): 488–93.

———. 1980. "How a Health Report Gets Written." *Maine Times,* June 27, 1980, p. 11.

Greenberg, Robert, Charles Hennekens, Theodore Colton, Bernard Rosner, and Susan Vogt. 1983. "Review of Diet, Nutrition, and Cancer — Investigation of the Epidemiologic Evidence Used to Support the National Academy of Sciences Recommendations Relevant to the Consumption of Meat." Report prepared by Epistat Associates. Photocopy.

Greenhouse, Steven. 1986. "Can the Cow Make a Comeback?" *New York Times,* Sept. 28, sec. 3, p. 1.

Greenwald, Peter, and Joseph W. Cullen. 1985. "The New Emphasis in Cancer Control." *Journal of the National Cancer Institute* 74, 3: 543–51.

Greenwood, M. R. C. 1997. "Raiders of the Last Bastion?" *Science* 227 (July 11): 163.

Greenwood, Ted. 1984. *Knowledge and Discretion in Government Regulation.* New York: Praeger.

Gusfield, Joseph R. 1981. *The Culture of Public Problems: Drinking-Driving and the Symbolic Order.* Chicago: University of Chicago Press.

———. 1989. "Introduction" to Kenneth Burke, *On Symbols and Society.* Chicago: University of Chicago Press.

Guthrie, Helen A. 1985. "The 1985 Recommended Dietary Allowance Committee: An Overview." *Journal of the American Dietetic Association* 85, 12 (Dec.): 1646–49.

Halfon, Saul. 1998. "Collecting, Testing and Convincing: Forensic DNA Experts in the Courts." *Social Studies of Science* 28: 801–28.

Haraway, Donna. 1989. *Primate Visions: Gender, Race, and Nature in the World of Modern Science.* New York: Routledge.

Harper, Alfred E. 1982. "Firm Recommendations, Infirm Basis." *Nutrition Today,* July–Aug., pp. 16–17.

———. 1986. "Recommended Dietary Allowances in Perspective." *Food & Nutrition News,* Mar.–Apr., pp. 7–10.

Hegsted, D. M. 1983. "Diet, Nutrition, and Cancer." *Preventive Medicine* 12: 470–74.

———. 1985. "Nutrition: The Changing Scene." *Nutrition Reviews* 43, 12: 357–67.

Herbert, Victor. 1981. "Nutrition Cultism." *Western Journal of Medicine* 135: 252–56.

———. 1986. Letter to the editor. *Science* 232 (Apr. 4): 11.

Herbert, Victor, and Stephen Barrett. 1985. *Vitamins and "Health" Foods: The Great American Hustle.* Philadelphia: George F. Stickley Co.

Herbert v. National Academy of Sciences. 1991. *Herbert v. National Academy of Sciences,* 1991 U.S. Dist. LEXIS 7074; *Herbert v. National Academy of Sciences,* 297 U.S. App. D.C. 406; *United States ex rel., Herbert v. National Academy of Sciences,* 1992 U.S. Dist. LEXIS 14063.

Hilgartner, Stephen. 1990. "The Dominant View of Popularization." *Social Studies of Science* 20: 519–39.

———. 1992. "The Social Construction of Risk Objects." In *Organizations, Uncertainties, and Risks,* ed. James F. Short, Jr., and Lee Clarke, pp. 39–53. Boulder, Colo.: Westview Press.

Hilgartner, Stephen, and Charles L. Bosk. 1988. "The Rise and Fall of Social Problems: A Public Arenas Model." *American Journal of Sociology* 94, 1: 53–78.

Hilgartner, Stephen, and Sherry I. Brandt-Rauf. 1994. "Data Access, Ownership, and Control: Toward Empirical Studies of Access Practices." *Knowledge: Creation, Diffusion, Utilization* 15: 355–72.

Hilgartner, Stephen, and Dorothy Nelkin. 1987. "Communication Controversies over Dietary Risks." *Science, Technology, and Human Values* 12, 3–4; 41–7.

Holtzman, Neil A., and Michael S. Watson, eds. 1997. *Promoting Safe and Effective Genetic Testing in the United States: Final Report of the Task Force on Genetic Testing.* Baltimore: Task Force on Genetic Testing.

Hughes, Thomas P. 1986. "The Seamless Web: Technology, Science, Etcetera, Etcetera." *Social Studies of Science* 16: 281–92.

In the Matter of General Nutrition, Inc. 1986. Initial Decision, U.S. Federal Trade Commission, Montgomery K. Hyun, administrative law judge, Feb. 24, 1986, Docket No. 9175.

Jasanoff, Sheila S. 1987. "Contested Boundaries in Policy-Relevant Science." *Social Studies of Science* 17: 195–230.

———. 1990. *The Fifth Branch: Science Advisors as Policymakers*. Cambridge, Mass.: Harvard University Press.

———. 1992. "Science, Politics, and the Renegotiation of Expertise at EPA." *OSIRIS*, 2d ser., 7: 195–217.

———, ed. 1994. *Learning from Disaster: Risk Management after Bhopal*. Philadelphia: University of Pennsylvania Press.

———. 1995. *Science at the Bar: Law, Science, and Technology in America*. Cambridge, Mass.: Harvard University Press.

———. 1996. "Beyond Epistemology: Relativism and Engagement in the Politics of Science." *Social Studies of Science* 26: 393–418.

———. 1997. "Civilization and Madness: The Great BSE Scare of 1996." *Public Understanding of Science* 6: 221–32.

———. 1998. "The Eye of Everyman: Witnessing DNA in the Simpson Trial." *Social Studies of Science* 28: 687–712.

Jasanoff, Sheila, Gerald E. Markle, James C. Petersen, and Trevor Pinch, eds. 1995. *Handbook of Science and Technology Studies*. Thousand Oaks, Calif.: Sage.

Kamin, Henry. 1985a. "Status of the 10th Edition of the Recommended Dietary Allowances — Prospects for the Future." *American Journal of Clinical Nutrition* 41 (Jan.): 165–70.

———. 1985b. Letter to the editor. *Science* 230 (Dec. 20): 1324, 1326.

Keller, Evelyn Fox. 1995. "The Origin, History, and Politics of the Subject Called 'Gender and Science': A First Person Account." In *Handbook of Science and Technology Studies*, edited by Sheila Jasanoff, Gerald E. Markle, James C. Petersen, and Trevor Pinch. Thousand Oaks, Calif.: Sage.

Kendall, Don. 1982. "Meat Industry Skeptical of Report on Cancer-Diet Link." Associated Press, June 20.

Knorr-Cetina, Karin D. 1981. *The Manufacture of Knowledge: An Essay on the Constructivist and Contextual Nature of Science*. New York: Pergamon.

———. 1983. "The Ethnographic Study of Scientific Work: Toward a Constructivist Interpretation of Science." In *Science Observed: Perspectives on the Social Study of Science*, ed. Karin D. Knorr-Cetina and Michael Mulkay, pp. 115–40. Beverly Hills, Calif.: Sage.

———. 1999. *Epistemic Cultures: How the Sciences Make Knowledge*. Cambridge, Mass.: Harvard University Press.

Kohler, Robert E. 1994. *Lords of the Fly: Drosophila Genetics and the Experimental Life*. Chicago: University of Chicago Press.

Kotulak, Robert. 1983. "Food for Thought on Cancer Cause, Cure." *Chicago Tribune*, Aug. 10, p. 1.

LaFollette, Marcel C. 1992. *Stealing into Print: Fraud, Plagiarism, and Misconduct in Scientific Publishing*. Berkeley and Los Angeles: University of California Press.

Lakoff, George, and Mark Johnson. 1980. *Metaphors We Live By*. Chicago: University of Chicago Press.

Latour, Bruno. 1987. *Science in Action: How to Follow Scientists and Engineers Through Society*. Cambridge, Mass.: Harvard University Press.

———. 1988. *The Pasteurization of France*. Translated by Alan Sheridan and John Law. Cambridge, Mass.: Harvard University Press.

———. 1993. *We Have Never Been Modern*. Translated by Catherine Porter. Cambridge, Mass.: Harvard University Press.

Latour, Bruno, and Françoise Bastide. 1986. "Writing Science — Fact and Fiction." In *Mapping the Dynamics of Science and Technology: Sociology of Science in the Real World*, ed. Michel Callon, John Law, and Arie Rip, pp. 51–66. Basingstoke, Hants.: Macmillan.

Latour, Bruno, and Steve Woolgar. 1979. *Laboratory Life: The Social Construction of Scientific Facts*. Introduction by Jonas Salk. Beverly Hills, Calif.: Sage.

Law, John, and R. J. Williams. 1982. "Putting Facts Together: A Study of Scientific Persuasion." *Social Studies of Science* 12: 535–58.

Lawler, Andrew. 1997. "Is the NRC Ready for Reform?" *Science* 276 (May 9): 900–904.

Lawrence, Christopher, and Steven Shapin, eds. 1998. *Science Incarnate: Historical Embodiments of Natural Knowledge*. Chicago: University of Chicago Press.

Leary, Warren E. 1985. "Academy of Sciences Says It Won't Release Nutrition Findings." Associated Press, 7 Oct.

Lenoir, Timothy. 1997. *Instituting Science: The Cultural Production of Scientific Disciplines*. Stanford: Stanford University Press.

Levine, Janet M. 1986. "Hearts and Minds: The Politics of Diet and Heart Disease." In *Consuming Fears: The Politics of Product Risks*, ed. Harvey M. Sapolsky, 40–79. New York: Basic Books.

Lombardo v. Handler. 1975. 397 F. Suppl. 792 (D.D.C. 1975). Aff'd 546 F.2d 1043 (D.C. Cir. 1976). Cert. denied, 431 U.S. 932 (1977).

Lynch, Michael. 1985a. *Art and Artifact in Laboratory Science: A Study of Shop Work and Shop Talk in a Research Laboratory*. Boston: Routledge & Kegan Paul.

———. 1985b. "Discipline and the Material Form of Images: An Analysis of Scientific Visibility." *Social Studies of Science* 15: 37–66.

———. 1993. *Scientific Practice and Ordinary Action: Ethnomethodology and Social Studies of Science*. New York: Cambridge University Press.

———. 1998. "The Discursive Production of Uncertainty: The O. J. Simpson 'Dream Team' and Sociology of Knowledge Machine." *Social Studies of Science* 28: 829–68.

Lynch, Michael, and David Bogen. 1996. *The Spectacle of History: Speech, Text, and Memory at the Iran-Contra Hearings*. Durham, N.C.: Duke University Press.

Lynch, Michael, and Sheila Jasanoff, eds. 1998. *Contested Identities: Science, Law, and Forensic Practice*. Special issue, *Social Studies of Science* 28 (Oct.).

Lynch, Michael, and Steve Woolgar, eds. 1990. *Representation in Scientific Practice*. Cambridge, Mass.: MIT Press.

Mackenzie, Donald. 1990. *Inventing Accuracy: A Historical Sociology of Nuclear Missile Guidance*. Cambridge, Mass.: MIT Press.

Marshall, Eliot. 1985. "The Academy Kills a Nutrition Report." *Science* 230 (Oct. 25): 420–21.

———. 1986. "Diet Advice, with a Grain of Salt and a Large Helping of Pepper." *Science* 231 (Feb. 7): 537–39.

Martin, Brian, and Evelleen Richards. 1995. "Scientific Knowledge, Controversy, and Public Decision Making." In *Handbook of Science and Technology Studies*, edited by Sheila Jasanoff, Gerald E. Markle, James C. Petersen, and Trevor Pinch, pp. 506–26. Thousand Oaks, Calif.: Sage.

McGinnis, J. Michael, M.D. [deputy assistant secretary, U.S. Department of Health and Human Services]. 1980. "Statement on NAS/NRC Food and Nutrition Board Report, 'Toward Healthful Diets.' " May 30. Photocopy.

McNutt, Kristen. 1980. "Dietary Advice to the Public: 1957–1980." *Nutrition Reviews* 38, 10: 353–60.

Mendeloff, Albert I. 1983. "Appraisal of 'Diet, Nutrition, and Cancer.' " *American Journal of Clinical Nutrition* 37 (Mar.): 495–98.

Molpus, C. Manly, Lee Campbell, Al Pope, G. L. Walts, Patrick B. Healy, W. T. Berry Jr., George B. Watts, John Huston, and Orville Sweet. 1982. Letter to Frank Press, June 16.

Monmaney, Terence. 1986. "Vitamins: Much Ado about Milligrams." *Science '86*, Jan.–Feb., pp. 10–11.

Mueller, Allan G. 1982. "The NAS Report Diet, Nutrition, and Cancer: Implications for Agriculture." In Council for Agricultural Science and Technology, *Diet, Nutrition, and Cancer: A Critique*, 51–53. Special Report No. 13. Ames, Iowa: Council for Agricultural Science and Technology.

Mulkay, Michael. 1985. *The Word and the World: Explorations in the Form of Sociological Analysis*. London: George Allen & Unwin.

———. 1995. "Galileo and Embryos: Religion and Science in Parliamentary Debate over Research on Human Embryos." *Social Studies of Science* 25: 499–532.

Mulkay, Michael, Jonathan Potter, and Steven Yearley. 1983. "Why an Analysis of Scientific Discourse Is Needed." In *Science Observed: Perspectives on the Social Study of Science*, ed. Karin D. Knorr-Cetina and Michael Mulkay, pp. 171–203. Beverly Hills, Calif.: Sage.

Mulkay, Michael, Trevor Pinch, and Malcolm Ashmore. 1987. "Colonizing the Mind: Dilemmas in the Application of Social Science." *Social Studies of Science* 17: 231–56.

Myers, Greg. 1990. *Writing Biology: Texts and the Social Construction of Scientific Knowledge*. Madison: University of Wisconsin Press.

National Academy of Sciences. 1979. "Guidelines for Review of Reports." Memorandum, June 15.

———. 1980. *Toward Healthful Diets*. Food and Nutrition Board, Division of Biological Sciences, Assembly of Life Sciences, National Research Council. Washington, D.C.: National Academy of Sciences.

———. 1982. *Diet, Nutrition, and Cancer.* Report of Committee on Diet, Nutrition, and Cancer, Assembly of Life Sciences, National Research Council. Washington, D.C.: National Academy Press.

———. 1983. *Diet, Nutrition, and Cancer: Directions for Research.* Report of Committee on Diet, Nutrition, and Cancer, Assembly of Life Sciences, National Research Council. Washington, D.C.: National Academy Press.

———. 1989a. *Diet and Health: Implications for Reducing Chronic Disease Risk.* Report of the Committee on Diet and Health, Food and Nutrition Board, Commission on Life Sciences, National Research Council. Washington, D.C.: National Academy Press.

———. 1989b. *Recommended Dietary Allowances.* 10th ed. Food and Nutrition Board, Division of Biological Sciences, Assembly of Life Sciences, National Research Council. Washington, D.C.: National Academy Press.

———. 1993. *Report Review: Guidelines for Committees and Staff.* Brochure. Prepared by the Report Review Committee, National Research Council. Oct. 1993.

———. 1994. *A Unique National Resource.* Brochure. Prepared by the Office of News and Public Information, National Academy of Sciences, National Academy of Engineering, Institute of Medicine, National Research Council, Washington, D.C.

———. 1995. *Society's Choices: Social and Ethical Decision Making in Biomedicine.* Report of the Committee on the Social and Ethical Impacts of Developments in Biomedicine, Institute of Medicine. Washington, D.C.: National Academy Press.

———. 1996. *Getting to Know the Committee Process.* Brochure. Prepared by the Office of News and Public Information, National Research Council, Institute of Medicine, Washington, D.C.

National Academy of Sciences. Food and Nutrition Board. Consumer Liaison Panel. 1980. "News Release: Consumer Nutrition Panel Breaks Ties in Protest over National Academy of Sciences Report." Photocopy. June 11.

National Meat Association. 1982. "Statement in Response to the National Research Council's Recommendations." News release, June 16.

Neiman, Janet. 1982. "Food Groups Cry Foul over Cancer Link Data." *Advertising Age,* June 21.

Nelkin, Dorothy, ed. 1979. *Controversy: Politics of Technical Decisions.* Beverly Hills, Calif.: Sage.

———. 1984. *Controversy: Politics of Technical Decisions.* 2d ed. Beverly Hills, Calif.: Sage.

———. 1992. *Controversy: Politics of Technical Decisions.* 3d. ed. Newbury Park, Calif.: Sage.

Noble, David. 1984. *Forces of Production: A Social History of Industrial Automation.* New York: Knopf.

Norton-Taylor, Richard, with Mark Lloyd. 1995. *Truth Is a Difficult Concept: Inside the Scott Inquiry.* London: Fourth Estate.

Novak, Joseph D., and D. Bob Gowin. 1984. *Learning How to Learn*. New York: Cambridge University Press.

Olson, Robert E. 1982. "*Diet, Nutrition, and Cancer*: A Critical Review." In Council for Agricultural Science and Technology, *Diet, Nutrition, and Cancer: A Critique*, 55–61. Special Report No. 13. Ames, Iowa: Council for Agricultural Science and Technology.

———. 1985a. Letter to the editor. *Science* 230 (Dec. 20): 1326.

———. 1985b. Letter to the editor. *New York Times*, Oct. 26, p. 26.

———. 1986. "Mass Intervention vs Screening Selective Intervention for the Prevention of Coronary Heart Disease." *Journal of the American Medical Association* 255: 2204–7.

Palmer, Sushma, and Kulbir Bakshi. 1983. "Public Health Considerations in Reducing Cancer Risk: Interim Dietary Guidelines." *Seminars in Oncology* 10 (Sept.): 342–47.

Pariza, Michael W. 1984. "A Perspective on Diet, Nutrition, and Cancer." *Cancer* 251, 11: 1455–58.

———. 1986. "Analyzing Current Recommendations on Diet, Nutrition and Cancer." *Food and Nutrition News*, Jan.–Feb., pp. 1–4.

Pear, Robert. 1985a. "Lower Nutrient Levels Proposed in Draft Report on American Diet." *New York Times*, Sept. 23, p. A1.

———. 1985b. "Impasse Delays Proposal to Cut Diet Guidelines." *New York Times*, Oct. 8, p. A1.

———. 1985c. "For Scientists, the Impasse on Vitamins Is a Bitter Pill." *New York Times*, Oct. 13, p. 22E.

Perrow, Charles. 1984. *Normal Accidents: Living with High-Risk Technologies*. New York: Basic Books.

Perry, Seymour. 1987. "The NIH Consensus Development Program: A Decade Later." *New England Journal of Medicine* 317, 8: 485–88.

Pickering, Andrew. 1984. *Constructing Quarks: A Sociological History of Particle Physics*. Chicago: University of Chicago Press.

———. 1995. *The Mangle of Practice: Time, Agency, and Science*. Chicago: University of Chicago Press.

Pinch, Trevor J. 1981. "The Sun Set: The Presentation of Certainty in Scientific Life." *Social Studies of Science* 11: 131–58.

———. 1986. *Confronting Nature: The Sociology of Solar-Neutrino Detection*. Dordrecht: Reidel.

Pinch, Trevor J., and Wiebe Bijker. 1984. "The Social Construction of Facts and Artifacts, or, How the Sociology of Science and the Sociology of Technology Might Benefit Each Other." *Social Studies of Science* 14: 399–441.

Porter, Donna V. 1983. "Diet, Nutrition and Cancer: An Analysis of the National Academy of Sciences Report." Congressional Research Service. Photocopy.

Porter, Theodore M. 1992. "Quantification and the Accounting Ideal in Science." *Social Studies of Science* 22: 633–51.

———. 1995. *Trust in Numbers: The Pursuit of Objectivity in Science and Public Life*. Princeton: Princeton University Press.

Press, Frank. 1985a. Frank Press, chairman of the National Research Council, to Dr. James B. Wyngaarden, director, National Institutes of Health, Oct. 7, 1985. Reprinted as "Postponement of the 10th edition of the RDAs." *Journal of the American Dietetic Association* 85, 12: 1644–45.

———. 1985b. Letter to the editor. *Science* 230 (Dec. 20): 1326, 1410.

———. 1985c. Letter to the editor. *New York Times*, Nov. 9, p. 26.

Primack, Joel, and Frank von Hippel. 1974. *Advice and Dissent: Scientists in the Political Arena*. New York: Basic Books.

Proctor, Robert N. 1995. *Cancer Wars: How Politics Shapes What We Know and Don't Know about Cancer*. New York: Basic Books.

"Review of Dietary Goals of the United States." 1977. *The Lancet*, Apr. 23. Reprinted in U.S. Senate Select Committee on Nutrition and Human Needs 1977e.

Rheinberger, Hans-Jörg. 1997. *Toward a History of Epistemic Things: Synthesizing Proteins in the Test Tube*. Stanford: Stanford University Press.

Richards, Evelleen. 1988. "The Politics of Therapeutic Evaluation: The Vitamin C and Cancer Controversy." *Social Studies of Science* 18, 4: 653–701.

———. 1991. *Vitamin C and Cancer: Medicine or Politics?* London: Macmillan.

Rip, Arie. 1982. "The Development of Restrictedness in the Sciences." In *Scientific Establishments and Hierarchies*, ed. Norbert Elias, Herminio Martins, and Richard Whitley, 219–38. Sociology of the Sciences Yearbook. Boston: Reidel.

———. 1986. "Controversies as Informal Technology Assessment." *Knowledge: Creation, Diffusion, Utilization* 8, 2: 349–71.

Risser, James. 1980. "Food Firms Helped Fund Diet Report." *Des Moines Register*, May 30, p. 1.

Rose, Mark. 1988. "The Author as Proprietor: *Donaldson v. Becket* and the Genealogy of Modern Authorship." *Representations* 23: 51–85.

Rothman, David J. 1991. *Strangers at the Bedside: How Law and Bioethics Changed Medical Decision Making*. New York: Basic Books.

Schudson, Michael. 1992. *Watergate in American Memory: How We Remember, Forget, and Reconstruct the Past*. New York: Basic Books.

Sclove, Richard E. 1995. *Democracy and Technology*. New York: Guilford Press.

Scott, Pam, Evelleen Richards, and Brian Martin. 1990. "Captives of Controversy: The Myth of the Neutral Social Researcher in Contemporary Science Controversies." *Science, Technology, and Human Values* 15: 474–94.

Seligmann, Jean. 1984. "America's Nutrition Revolution." *Newsweek*, Nov. 19, pp. 111–18.

Semling, Harold V., Jr. 1980. "Nutrition Board Report Sparks Controversy." *Food Processing*, Aug., p. 8.

Shapin, Steven. 1994. *A Social History of Truth: Science and Civility in Seventeenth-Century England*. Chicago: University of Chicago Press.

———. 1995. "Cordelia's Love: Credibility and the Social Studies of Science." *Perspectives on Science* 3, 3: 255–75.

Shapin, Steven, and Simon Schaffer. 1985. *Leviathan and the Air Pump: Hobbes, Boyle, and the Experimental Life*. Princeton, N.J.: Princeton University Press.

Smith, Bruce L. R. 1992. *The Advisers: Scientists in the Policy Process*. Washington, D.C.: Brookings Institution.

Smith, Dorothy E. 1974. "The Social Construction of Documentary Reality." *Sociological Inquiry* 44: 257–68.

Star, Susan Leigh. 1989. *Regions of the Mind: Brain Research and the Quest for Scientific Certainty*. Stanford: Stanford University Press.

———, ed. 1995. *Ecologies of Knowledge: Work and Politics in Science and Technology*. Albany, N.Y.: State University of New York Press.

Star, Susan Leigh, and James R. Griesemer. 1989. "Institutional Ecology, 'Translation,' and Boundary Objects." *Social Studies of Science* 19: 387–420.

Starr, Paul. 1982. *The Social Transformation of American Medicine*. New York: Basic Books.

Sweeten, Mary Kinney, H. Russell Cross, Gary C. Smith, Jeffrey W. Savell, and Stephen B. Smith. 1990. "Lean Beef: Impetus for Lipid Modifications." *Journal of the American Dietetic Association* 90: 87–92.

Toufexis, Anastasia. 1985. "Advice on Eating Right: Two New Reports Stir Confusion about a Healthy Diet." *Time*, Oct. 7, p. 61.

Traweek, Sharon. 1988. *Beamtimes and Lifetimes: The World of High Energy Physicists*. Cambridge, Mass.: Harvard University Press.

Turner, Victor. 1974. *Dramas, Fields, and Metaphors: Symbolic Action in Human Society*. Ithaca, N.Y.: Cornell University Press.

———. 1980. "Social Dramas and Stories about Them." *Critical Inquiry*, Autumn, pp. 141–68.

"USDA Disputes NAS Findings on Diet and Cancer; Raps News Coverage." 1983. *Nutrition Action*, Sept., p. 5.

U.S. Congress. House. Committee on Agriculture. Subcommittee on Domestic Marketing, Consumer Relations, and Nutrition. 1980. *National Academy of Sciences Report on Healthful Diets*. Hearings held June 18 and 19, 1980, 96th Cong., 2d sess. Serial No. 96-JJJ.

U.S. Congress. Senate. Committee on Agriculture, Nutrition, and Forestry, Subcommittee on Nutrition. 1978. *Nutrition and Cancer Research*. Hearings held June 12 and 13, 1978. 95th Cong., 2d sess.

———. 1979. *Diet and Cancer Relationship*. Hearing held Oct. 2, 1979. 96th Cong., 1st sess.

U.S. Congress. Senate. Committee on Appropriations. Subcommittee on Agriculture, Rural Development, and Related Agencies. *Dietary Guidelines for Americans*. Hearing held July 16, 1980. 96th Congress, 2d sess.

U.S. Congress. Senate. Committee on Labor and Public Welfare. Subcommittee on

Health. 1974. *National Cancer Act of 1974.* Hearing held Jan. 30, 1974. 93rd Cong., 2d sess.

U.S. Congress. Senate. Select Committee on Nutrition and Human Needs. 1974. *National Nutrition Policy Study — 1974, Part 6 — Nutrition and Health.* Hearing held June 21, 1974. 93d Congress, 2d sess.

———. 1975. *Nutrition and Health.* 94th Cong., 1st sess., Dec. 1975.

———. 1976. *Diet Related to Killer Diseases.* Vol. 1. Hearings held July 27 and 28, 1976. 94th Cong., 2d sess.

———. 1977a. *Diet and Killer Diseases with Press Reaction and Additional Information.* 95th Cong., 1st sess., Jan. 1977.

———. 1977b. *Dietary Goals for the United States.* 95th Cong., 1st sess., Feb. 1977.

———. 1977c. *Diet Related to Killer Diseases, III: Response to Dietary Goals of the United States: Re Meat.* Hearing held Mar. 24, 1977. 95th Cong., 1st sess.

———. 1977d. *Diet Related to Killer Diseases, VI: Response to Dietary Goals of the United States: Re Eggs.* Hearing held July 26, 1977. 95th Cong., 1st sess.

———. 1977e. *Dietary Goals for the United States — Supplemental Views,* 95th Cong., 1st sess., Nov. 1977.

———. 1977f. *Dietary Goals for the United States.* 2d ed. 95th Cong., 1st. sess., Dec. 1977.

U.S. Department of Agriculture. 1957. *Essentials of an Adequate Diet. Agricultural Research Service, Home Economics Research Report No. 3.* Washington, D.C.: Government Printing Office.

———. 1983. "Response to the Report 'Diet, Nutrition, and Cancer,' of the Committee on Diet, Nutrition, and Cancer, Assembly of Life Sciences, National Research Council, 1982." Photocopy.

U.S. Department of Agriculture and Department of Health and Human Services. 1980. *Nutrition and Your Health: Dietary Guidelines for Americans.* Home and Garden Bulletin No. 232. Washington, D.C.: Government Printing Office.

———. 1985. *Nutrition and Your Health: Dietary Guidelines for Americans, Second Edition.* Home and Garden Bulletin No. 232. Washington, D.C.: Government Printing Office.

U.S. Department of Health and Human Services. Public Health Service. Office of the Assistant Secretary for Health. 1988. *The Surgeon General's Report on Nutrition and Health.* DHHS Publication No. 88-50210. Washington D.C.: Government Printing Office.

U.S. Department of Health, Education and Welfare. Public Health Service. Office of the Assistant Secretary for Health and Surgeon General. 1979. *Healthy People: The Surgeon General's Report on Health Promotion and Disease Prevention.* Rockville, Md.: Washington, D.C.: Government Printing Office.

U.S. Department of Health and Human Services. 1983. "Report of the DHHS Task Force on Diet, Nutrition, and Cancer." May 25. Photocopy.

———. 1984. "HHS News." U.S., Department of Health and Human Services,

Public Health Service, National Cancer Institute. News Release, Mar. 6. Photocopy.

U.S. General Accounting Office. 1978. *Recommended Dietary Allowances: More Research and Better Food Guides Needed.* CED-78-169. Washington, D.C.: GAO.

———. 1984. *National Academy of Sciences' Reports on Diet and Health — Are They Credible and Consistent?* GAO/RCED-84-109. Washington, D.C.: GAO.

———. 1998. *Federal Research: The National Academy of Sciences and the Federal Advisory Committee Act.* GAO/RCED-99-17. Washington, D.C.: GAO.

"U.S. Institute Latest to Stress Connection Between Diet and Cancer." 1984. *Nutrition Action*, May, p. 3.

U.S. National Cancer Institute. 1979a. *Diet, Nutrition and Cancer Program Status Report, September 1978.* Bethesda, Md.: Department of Health, Education, and Welfare, Public Health Service, National Institutes of Health, National Cancer Institute. NIH Publication No. 79-1992.

———. 1979b. "Statement on Diet, Nutrition, and Cancer." Presented by NCI Director Arthur C. Upton at Diet and Cancer Relationship Hearings, U.S. Congress, Senate Committee on Agriculture, Nutrition, and Forestry, Subcommittee on Nutrition, October 2.

———. 1982. *Diet, Nutrition and Cancer Program Status Report, October 1981.* Bethesda, Md.: Department of Health and Human Services, Public Health Service, National Institutes of Health, National Cancer Institute. NIH Publication No. 82-1992.

———. 1984a. "Dietary Fiber and Lower Colon Cancer Risk." National Cancer Institute, Division of Cancer Prevention and Control. Photocopy.

———. 1984b. *Diet, Nutrition & Cancer Prevention: A Guide to Food Choices.* Bethesda, Md.: Department of Health and Human Services, Public Health Service, National Institutes of Health. NIH Publication No. 85-2711.

———. 1985a. *Division of Cancer Prevention and Control: Annual Report 1984.* Bethesda, Md.: Department of Health and Human Services, Public Health Service, National Institutes of Health, National Cancer Institute, Division of Cancer Prevention and Control.

———. 1985b. *National Cancer Program: 1983–1984 Director's Report and Annual Plan FY 1986–1990.* Bethesda, Md.: Department of Health and Human Services, Public Health Service, National Institutes of Health. NIH Publication No. 86–2765.

———. 1986. *Cancer Control Objectives for the Nation: 1985–2000.* Bethesda, Md.: Department of Health and Human Services, Public Health Service, National Institutes of Health. NCI Monographs, 1986, No. 2. NIH Publication No. 86-2880.

———. 1987. *Diet, Nutrition & Cancer Prevention: A Guide to Food Choices.* Bethesda, Md.: Department of Health and Human Services, Public Health Service, National Institutes of Health. NIH Publication No. 87-2878.

U.S. National Institutes of Health. 1985. "Consensus Conference: Lowering Blood Cholesterol to Prevent Heart Disease." *Journal of the American Medical Association* 253 (Apr. 12): 2080–86.

Vaughan, Diane. 1996. *The Challenger Launch Decision: Risky Technology, Culture, and Deviance at NASA*. Chicago: University of Chicago Press.

Wade, Nicholas. 1997. "Academy of Sciences, Fighting to Keep Its Panels Closed, Is Rebuffed by Supreme Court." *New York Times*, 4 Nov., p. A18.

Wagner-Pacifici, Robin Erica. 1986. *The Moro Morality Play: Terrorism as Social Drama*. Chicago: University of Chicago Press.

Waksler, F. Chaput. 1989. "Erving Goffman's Sociology: An Introductory Essay." *Human Studies* 12, 1–2: 1–18.

Walsh, John. 1971a. "National Research Council: And How It Got That Way." *Science* 172 (Apr. 16): 242–46.

———. 1971b. "National Research Council (II): Answering the Right Questions?" *Science* 172 (Apr. 23): 353–57.

Weber, Max. 1978. *Economy and Society*. Edited by Guenther Roth and Claus Wittich. Berkeley and Los Angeles: University of California Press.

White, Hayden. 1978. *Tropics of Discourse: Essays in Cultural Criticism*. Baltimore: Johns Hopkins University Press. Reprinted 1985.

Willett, Walter. 1990. *Nutritional Epidemiology*. New York: Oxford University Press.

Winner, Langdon. 1980. "Do Artifacts Have Politics?" *Daedalus* 109, 1: 121–36.

———. 1986. *The Whale and the Reactor: A Search for Limits in an Age of High Technology*. Chicago: University of Chicago Press.

"Wolf Resigns as Dietary Guideline Review Nears Completion." 1985. *Food Chemical News*, Apr. 8, p. 7.

Wynder, Ernst, and Gio B. Gori. 1977. "Contribution of the Environment to Cancer Incidence: An Epidemiologic Exercise." *Journal of the National Cancer Institute* 58: 825–32.

Wynne, Brian. 1982. *Rationality and Ritual: The Windscale Inquiry and Nuclear Decisions in Britain*. Chalfont St. Giles, Bucks.: British Society for the History of Science.

———. 1988. "Unruly Technology: Practical Rules, Impractical Discourses and Public Understanding." *Social Studies of Science* 18: 147–67.

———. 1992. "Representing Policy Constructions and Interests in SSK." *Social Studies of Science* 22: 575–80.

———. 1996. "SSK's Identity Parade: Signing Up, Off-and-On." *Social Studies of Science* 26: 357–91.

Yearley, Steven. 1991. *The Green Case: A Sociology of Environmental Issues, Arguments, and Politics*. New York: Routledge.

INDEX

In this index an "f" after a number indicates a separate reference on the next page, and an "ff" indicates separate references on the next two pages. A continuous discussion over two or more pages is indicated by a span of page numbers, e.g., "57–59." *Passim* is used for a cluster of references in close but not consecutive sequence.

Abbott, Andrew, 180n92
Academy, see National Academy of Sciences
Actor-network theory, 160n17, 167n34
Advice, science, *see* Science advice
Advisory bodies, 4–15 *passim*, 23, 26–27, 146
Agency, human, 124, 160n17, 161n44, 166n2
Agricultural interests, *see* Meat, dairy, and egg industries
Alberts, Bruce, 60
American Cancer Society, 35, 165n106
American Heart Association, 31, 34–35, 109
American Meat Institute (AMI), 99–103 *passim*, 108f, 174n11, 179n77, 180n86
Audiences, 7–20 *passim*, 58, 66, 68, 86, 112, 145, 150; participation of, 4, 9, 83, 147.
Authority, cultural, 5, 159n10. *See also* Credibility; Expertise
Authorized voices, 83–85, 147
Authorship, 52, 69, 82–84, 170n86, 170n87, 170n88; distributed, 84, 88; reconcentration of, 88–89, 176n52

Backstage, 11–12, 18, 83–85, 146–47, 148f; leaks and, 17–18, 71f, 81–82, 94–95, 107; enclosure of, 19–20, 54–60; official descriptions of, 60–70 *passim*, 128; unauthorized accounts of, 70–83 *passim*; emplotment of, 114, 135–41 *passim*, 144.

See also Confidentiality; Stage management
Berliner, Robert J., 39, 50
Boffey, Philip M., 24f, 58, 163n69, 163n70, 163n75, 169n60
Bogen, David, 80, 162n50, 172n113, 184n60
Boundary work, 10, 100–103 *passim*, 109, 178n66, 179n79, 184n49, 184n58
Bourdieu, Pierre, 180n92
Boyle, Robert, 10, 66, 166n3
Brain Bank of America, The, 58
Broad, William, 92
Brody, Jane, 92

Cairns, John, 39, 46
Callon, Michel, 160n17
Cardiology, 89f, 96, 109
Cassens, Robert G., 179n77
CAST, *see* Council for Agricultural Science and Technology
Center for Science in the Public Interest, 92, 108
Character, 7f, 13, 113–48. *See also* Public identity; Self-presentation
Characters, 68–70, 91–93, 98; in Academy announcement, 127–28, 135–39, 183n44, 183n46, 183n47; in Kamin letter, 130–39, 183n44. *See also* Advisory bodies; Critics; Committees; Melodrama; Public identity; Self-presentation
Chicago Heart Association, 90, 92, 108

Writing Science

Helmut Müller-Sievers, *Self-Generation: Biology, Philosophy, and Literature Around 1800*

Karen Newman, *Fetal Positions: Individualism, Science, Visuality*

Peter Galison and David J. Stump, eds., *The Disunity of Science: Boundaries, Contexts, and Power*

Niklas Luhmann, *Social Systems*

Hans Ulrich Gumbrecht and K. Ludwig Pfeiffer, eds., *Materialities of Communication*

Managing the
Diabetic Foot

T0258397

Contents

Acknowledgements

I would like to express my gratitude for the excellent assistance of Rachael Winter in the production of this third edition.

We are grateful to Mr Hisham Rashid, Consultant Vascular Surgeon, and Mr Venu Kavarthapu, Consultant Orthopaedic Surgeon, for their excellent surgical leadership in the Diabetic Foot Service.

We are grateful to colleagues past and present, who include: Simon Fraser, Huw Walters, Mary Blundell, Cathy Eaton, Mark Greenhill, Susie Spencer, Maureen McColgan-Bates, Mel Doxford, Sally Wilson, Adora Hatrapal, E Maelor Thomas, Mick Morris, John Philpott-Howard, Jim Wade, Andrew Hay, Robert Lewis, Anne-Marie Ryan, Irina Mantey, Robert Hills, Rachel Ben-Salem, Muriel Buxton-Thomas, Mazin Al-Janabi, Dawn Hurley, Stephanie Amiel, Stephen Thomas, Daniela Pitei, Paul Baskerville, Anthony Giddings, Irving Benjamin, Mark Myerson, Paul Sidhu, Joydeep Sinha, Patricia Wallace, Gillian Cavell, Lesley Boys, Magdi Hanna, Sue Peat, Colin Roberts, David Goss, Colin Deane, Sue Snowdon, Ana Grenfell, Tim Cundy, Pat Ascott, Lindis Richards, Kate Spicer, Debbie Broome, Liz Hampton, Timothy Jemmott, Michelle Buckley, Rosalind Phelan, Maggie Boase, Maria Back, Julie Lambert, Avril Witherington, Daniel Rajan, Ghulam Mufti, Karen Fairbairn, Ian Eltringham, Nina Petrova, Lindy Begg, Barbara Wall, Mark O'Brien, Sacha Andrews, Barry Pike, Jane Preece, Briony Sloper, Christian Pankhurst, Jim Beaumont, Matthew McShane, Tim Cooney, Lin Pan, Cheryl Clark, Marcello Perez, Nicholas Cooley, Paul Bains, Patricia Yerbury, Charlotte Biggs, Anna Korzon Burakowska, David Ross, Jason Wilkins, David Evans, Dean Huang, Carol Gayle, David Hopkins, Rifat Malik, Pratik Choudhary, Keith Jones, Bob Edmondson, Enid Joseph, Karen Reid, David Williams, Doris Agyemang-Duah, Jennifer Tremlett, Om Lahoti, Mark Phillips, Sarah Phillips, Dom Valenti, Hani Slim, Indira Maharaj, Surabhi Taori, Paula Gardiner, Ian Alejandro, Barbara Chirara, Victoria Morris, Hany Zayed,

Igor Kubelka, Daksheka Jayaratnam, Thoraya Ammar, Nicola Mulholland, Gill Vivian, Riddhika Chakravartty, Naveen Cavale, Wegin Tang, Natalya Hedger, Sophie Whitelaw, Joanne Casey, Leye Stephen, Jody Lucas, Vesna Vincent, Olla Shitta-Bey, Leila Howe, Marcus Simmgen, Rajan Patel, Chris Manu, Paul Donohoe, Sui Phin Kon, David Elias, Lisa Meakin, Ben Whitelaw, James Dent, Ben Freedman, Victoria Rose, Esther Dontoh and two great stalwarts of the Foot Clinic, Peter Watkins and the late David Pyke.

The Podiatry Managers and Community Podiatrists from Lambeth, Southwark and Lewisham have also contributed greatly to the work of the Foot Clinic at King's over many years. We are also grateful to Lee Sanders, who was our co-author in writing *A Practical Manual of Diabetic Foot Care*.

We are particularly grateful for the advice of the members of the Dermatology Department, Anthony du Vivier, Daniel Creamer, Claire Fuller, Elisabeth Higgins, Sarah MacFarlane, Rachel Morris-Jones, Sarah Walsh and Saqib Bashir. We give special thanks to Yvonne Bartlett, Alex Dionysiou, David Langdon, Lucy Wallace, Margaret Delaney and Moira Lovell from the Department of Medical Photography.

I would like to thank Audrey Edmonds for her support and patience.

We are particularly grateful to Jennifer Seward, Senior Development Editor, Rebecca Huxley, Senior Production Editor, and Oliver Walter, Senior Editor Wiley-Blackwell for their patience and help.

This is a practical hands-on manual uninterrupted by references. At the end of the book we have given a further reading list.

Preface

It was C.S. Lewis who said 'I wrote the books I should have liked to read if I could have got them.' and this was rather our approach when we first developed *Managing the Diabetic Foot*. Back in 2000, our aim was to fill what we perceived as a need for a very practical handbook. We wanted a book that could be used within the clinic as a basis for rapid and effective clinical decisions; a book incorporating a very simple and practical method of classifying and staging the diabetic foot that could be used as a framework for care, even by health-care practitioners who did not necessarily have a lot of previous experience in managing the diabetic foot. We wanted a book that would be useful for all members of the diabetic foot multidisciplinary team, a book that would help individual members of the team to appreciate the differing roles of other members, and above all, a book to emphasize the need for a multidisciplinary team approach in this most challenging field of health care; a book that could save the lives and limbs of diabetic foot patients.

These principles live on in this third updated edition of *Managing the Diabetic Foot*. Since the second edition in 2005, we have refined our classification of the diabetic foot, subdividing the ischaemic foot into the neuroischaemic foot, the critically ischaemic foot, acutely ischaemic foot and the renal ischaemic foot. We have developed our simple staging system, to emphasize that there is a rapid progress to necrosis in the natural history of the diabetic foot and this amounts to what we call a 'diabetic foot attack', which demands immediate treatment just like a heart or brain attack.

Over the years we have been increasingly alarmed by the devastating impact of neuropathy on our patients and have developed the concept of the need to practise neuropathic medicine. When classical signs of disease are absent or minimal and yet the pathology advances quickly, practitioners need to be aware of this and act like good detectives to recognize the early and subtle signs of disease and react quickly. When it is not possible to rely on the nervous system to reflect accurately what is going on inside the body, we have to use modern imaging more readily. This edition has illustrated the use of single-photon emission computer tomography and conventional computed tomography (SPECT/ CT) in the diagnosis of Charcot foot, grey-scale ultrasound and magnetic resonance imaging (MRI) in the diagnosis of infection and CT angiography and magnetic resonance angiography in delineating disease of the peripheral arterial system.

We describe major advances in the management of the diabetic foot since 2005. Reconstruction of the unstable Charcot hindfoot by internal stabilization has saved legs from certain amputation. Revascularization of the ischaemic foot has recently been achieved by very distal angioplasty and bypasses to the plantar arteries of the foot as well as by hybrid techniques involving both angioplasty and bypass in the same leg. Wound healing has also progressed with the increasing usage of negative pressure wound therapy and soft tissue reconstruction techniques including skin grafts and flaps. There has been increasing use of intravenous antibiotic therapy in the patients' homes utilizing peripherally inserted central catheter lines.

We stress the importance of the foot protection team in the community as well as the multidisciplinary foot care team based in the diabetic foot clinic, to which patients should have ready and open access when they are in trouble. We have come to learn that such is the vulnerability of the diabetic foot patient that the clinic door must always be open to give rapid treatment to a patient having a 'diabetic foot attack'.

My co-author Ali Foster sadly died at the initial stages of this third edition. However, Ali had been greatly involved in the planning of this edition and I hope her thoughts and experience of her beloved diabetic foot patients live on in this completed edition.

In tribute to Ali Foster at the International Symposium on the Diabetic Foot in 2011, I stated that she was a great source of inspiration to us all. Ali transformed diabetic podiatry and planted seeds of friendship throughout the world. Indeed, these have lived on and will never die. Ali was a great teacher and keen to share her experience and expertise with all health-care professionals. To honour this, the authors' royalties from this book will be devoted to the Ali Foster Travel fund to support the visit of young foot practitioners to centres of excellence of their choice.

I sincerely hope (as also did Ali) that this third edition will be of assistance to all heath-care professionals throughout the world who so nobly strive to look after diabetic patients with foot problems. May it help to improve their outcome and prevent amputations, an aspiration to which Ali was so unselfishly devoted.

Michael E Edmonds
Alethea VM Foster (died January 2011)
London 2013

Abbreviations

ABPI	ankle brachial pressure index
ACCORD	Action to Control Cardiovascular Risk in Diabetes
AFO	ankle–foot orthosis
b.d.	twice daily
BCM	bilayered cellular matrix
CAPD	continuous ambulatory peritoneal dialysis
CARDS	Collaborative-AtoRvastatin Diabetes Study
CAV/VVHD	continuous arteriovenous/venovenous haemodialysis
cm	centimetre
CROW	Charcot restraint orthotic walker
CRP	C-reactive protein
CT	computed tomography
CTA	computed tomography angiography
DCCT	Diabetes Control and Complications Trial
DSA	digital subtraction angiography
ECG	electrocardiogram
ECM	extracellular matrix
EDIC	Epidemiology of Diabetes Interventions and Complications
eGFR	estimated Glomerular Filtration Rate
ESBLs	extended-spectrum beta lactamases
EVA	ethylene-vinyl acetate
g	grams
GFR	Glomerular Filtration Rate
h	hour
HD	intermittent haemodialysis
HDF	haemodiafiltration
HDL	high-density lipoprotein
Hg	mercury

HOPE	Heart Outcomes Prevention Evaluation
HPS	Heart Protection Study
Hz	hertz
IM	intramuscular
IV	intravenous
L	litre
LDL	low-density lipoprotein
min	minutes
mL	millilitre
mm	millimetre
mol	mole
mmol	millimole
MRA	magnetic resonance angiography
MRI	magnetic resonance imaging
MRSA	methicillin-resistant *Staphylococcus aureus*
NPWT	negative pressure wound therapy
o.d.	once daily
po	orally
PTA	percutaneous transluminal angioplasty
PNA	partial nail avulsion
PRAFO	pressure relief ankle foot orthosis
q.d.s.	four times daily
s	seconds
SPECT	single-photon emission computed tomography
t.d.s.	three times daily
TENS	transcutaneous electrical nerve stimulation
UKPDS	United Kingdom Prospective Diabetes Study
V	volts

1

Introduction

NEW APPROACH TO THE DIABETIC FOOT

Diabetes has reached epidemic proportions, and with it has come a growing number of complex diabetic foot problems. This book is written to help practitioners tackle these problems. It attempts to give enough simple practical information to enable practitioners to understand the natural history of the diabetic foot, rapidly diagnose its problems and confidently undertake appropriate interventions in a timely manner.

Three great pathologies come together in the diabetic foot: neuropathy, ischaemia and infection. Their combined impact results in a swift progression to tissue necrosis, which is the fundamental hallmark of the natural history of the diabetic foot. Progress towards necrosis can be so rapid and devastating that it has come to be regarded as a 'diabetic foot attack', similar to the heart and brain attacks of the coronary and cerebrovascular systems. A 'diabetic foot attack' can quickly reach the point of no return, with overwhelming necrosis. Thus, it is vital to diagnose it early and provide rapid and intensive treatment. Furthermore, it is important to achieve early recognition of the at-risk foot so as to institute prompt measures to prevent the onset of the 'diabetic foot attack'. Although there have been many advances in the management of the diabetic foot, it nevertheless remains a major global public health problem. All over the world, health-care systems have failed the diabetic foot patient and a major amputation occurs every 20 s. However, amputations are not inevitable.

In this book we describe a system of multidisciplinary care that has been shown to reduce the number of amputations. It is easily

Managing the Diabetic Foot, Third Edition. Michael E Edmonds and Alethea VM Foster.
© 2014 John Wiley & Sons, Ltd. Published 2014 by John Wiley & Sons, Ltd.

reproducible and has been developed as a successful model of care throughout the world. This system is always being improved and refined, and this book describes the modern version of our diabetic foot management.

One important facet of this approach is the realization that neuropathy revolutionizes the practice of medicine and surgery. Classical symptoms and signs of disease are often absent because their expression depends on an intact peripheral nervous system. Thus, in traditional medical practice, a patient has a symptom, complains of this to their practitioner, who then makes a diagnosis. However, this approach may not work in the patient who has neuropathy. Instead, there must be a meticulous assessment of the patient to elicit subtle symptoms and signs that are clues to disease. Furthermore, an intact nervous system usually reflects symptomatically a 'picture' of what is going on inside the body, but in the presence of neuropathy this picture is absent and prompt use of imaging is required. Also, particular attention must be paid to inflammatory markers. Overall, it is important to practise what we call 'neuropathic medicine'. All practitioners looking after diabetic feet should understand this and adapt their practice of working with diabetic foot patients.

MODERN MANAGEMENT OF THE DIABETIC FOOT

This consists of four simple steps: assessment, classification, staging and intervention.

Assessment

A simple assessment of the diabetic foot is described to classify and stage the foot, looking for eight clinical features (Table 1.1). This assessment should take no longer than 5 min.

Table 1.1 **Eight clinical features in the assessment of the foot.**
Neuropathy
Ischaemia
Deformity
Callus
Swelling
Skin breakdown
Infection
Necrosis

Classification

The diabetic foot can be classified into two groups:

1 Neuropathic foot with palpable pulses

2 Ischaemic foot without pulses and a varying degree of neuropathy.

The neuropathic foot may be further divided into two clinical scenarios:

1 Foot with neuropathic ulceration

2 Charcot foot, which may be secondarily complicated by ulceration.

The ischaemic foot may be divided into four clinical scenarios:

1 Neuroischaemic foot characterized by both ischaemia and neuropathy and complicated by ulcer

2 Critically ischaemic foot

3 Acutely ischaemic foot

4 Renal ischaemic foot characterized by digital necrosis.

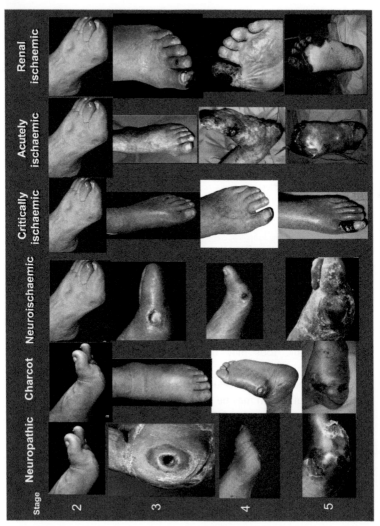

Fig. 1.1 The natural history and staging of the neuropathic and ischaemic foot.

Staging

Each of these six clinical scenarios (two neuropathic and four ischaemic) have specific stages in their natural history, and these stages have been described in a simple staging system (Fig. 1.1). This system covers the whole spectrum of diabetic foot disease and describes six stages in the natural history of each of the six clinical scenarios and emphasizes the relentless progression to the end stage necrosis. The stages are briefly summarized in Table 1.2 and will be described in detail in subsequent chapters devoted to each stage.

Intervention

A simple management plan is described for each stage, outlining six aspects of patient treatment within a multidisciplinary framework (Table 1.3).

ASSESSING THE DIABETIC FOOT

The initial approach to the diabetic foot starts with a simple assessment to enable the practitioner to make a basic classification and staging.

Table 1.2 **Staging the diabetic foot.**

Stage	Clinical condition
1	Normal
2	High risk
3	Ulcerated
4	Infected
5	Necrotic
6	Unsalvageable

Table 1.3 **Six aspects of patient treatment, within a multidisciplinary framework.**

Wound control
Microbiological control
Mechanical control
Vascular control
Metabolic control
Educational control

There is a specific search for eight factors, as shown in Table 1.1. Many of these features can be detected by an examination that includes:
- Simple inspection
- Palpation
- Sensory testing.

A complicated examination is not necessary. This chapter describes the search for these individual features and then presents an integrated examination. It is often helpful to detect abnormalities by comparing one foot with the other.

Shoe inspection should be included in the foot assessment and this is described in Chapter 2.

Neuropathy

Peripheral neuropathy is the most common complication of diabetes, affecting 50% of all diabetic patients. Although neuropathy may present with tingling and a feeling of numbness, it is asymptomatic in the majority of patients and neuropathy will only be detected by clinical examination. An important indication of neuropathy will be a patient who fails to complain of pain, even when significant foot lesions are present. Neuropathic patients are at increased risk of injury while walking because of impaired sensation and motor function. Neuropathy also damages proprioception and falls are common.

The presentation of peripheral neuropathy is determined by the impairment of sensory, motor and autonomic nerves. Simple inspection will usually reveal signs of motor and autonomic neuropathy of the feet, but sensory neuropathy must be detected by screening or by a simple sensory examination.

The diabetic patient with peripheral neuropathy affecting the feet and legs may also have systemic symptoms resulting from autonomic neuropathy of the heart, gut and bladder. We have seen cases of sudden death in young, apparently robust neuropathic patients. Also, there may be poor neurological control of ventilation, leading to sleep apnoea and susceptibility to pulmonary infections. Other neuropathic complications include postural hypotension and hypoglycaemic episodes without any warnings.

The peripheral nervous system is an early warning system. It detects external insults to the body and internal faults within and is programmed to direct appropriate protective responses to maintain the homeostatic integrity of the body. Diabetic patients with neuropathy have impaired homeostatic balance with diminished response to changes in the external and internal environment, and as a result they are very vulnerable and prone to disease. The signs and symptoms of disease in the foot and also in the rest of the body may be minimal and in some cases absent, reflecting 'silent disease'. Damage to the nerve supply of the heart can lead to silent ischaemia and silent myocardial infarction. Nevertheless, the pathology proceeds rapidly. There is a limited window of opportunity, and the end stage of tissue death in the foot and elsewhere is quickly reached.

Motor neuropathy
The classical sign of a motor neuropathy is a high medial longitudinal arch, leading to prominent metatarsal heads and pressure points over the plantar forefoot (Fig. 1.2). In severe cases, pressure points also develop over the apices and dorsal interphalangeal joints of associated claw toes. However, claw toe is a common deformity and may not always

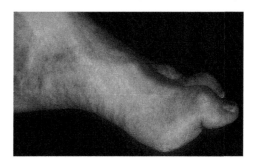

Fig. 1.2 Neuropathic foot showing motor neuropathy with high medial longitudinal arch, leading to prominent metatarsal heads and pressure points over the plantar forefoot.

be related to a motor neuropathy and atrophy of small muscles. It may be caused by wearing unsuitable shoes, trauma or may be congenital.

Complicated assessment of motor power in the foot or leg is not usually necessary, but it is advisable to test dorsiflexion of the foot to detect a foot drop secondary to a common peroneal nerve palsy. This is usually unilateral and will affect the patient's gait.

Autonomic neuropathy

The classical signs of peripheral autonomic neuropathy are:
- Dry skin which can lead to fissuring (Fig. 1.3)
- Distended veins over the dorsum of the foot and ankle (Fig. 1.4).

The dry skin is secondary to decreased sweating. The sweating loss normally occurs in a stocking distribution, which can extend up to the knee. The distended veins are secondary to arteriovenous shunting associated with autonomic neuropathy.

Autonomic neuropathy can be tested using a Neuropad® to assess the moisture status of the foot. This is an adhesive pad containing a cobalt II salt. It is placed on the first metatarsal and in the presence of sweat

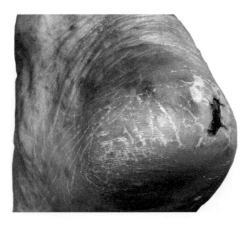

Fig. 1.3 Dry skin and fissuring of the heel with superficial necrosis in a neuroischaemic foot.

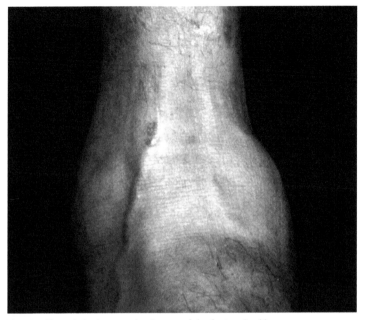

Fig. 1.4 Distended veins over the dorsum of the foot and ankle.

the pad will undergo a blue to pink colour change. Failure to change colour indicates autonomic neuropathy.

Sensory neuropathy

Sensory neuropathy can be simply detected by monofilaments (Fig. 1.5) or neurothesiometry (Fig. 1.6).

The advantage of the assessment with monofilaments or neurothesiometry is that it detects patients who have lost protective pain sensation and who are, therefore, susceptible to foot ulceration.

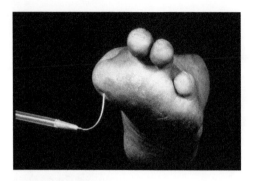

Fig. 1.5 Nylon monofilament buckles at a force of 10 g when applied perpendicularly to the foot. If the patient cannot feel this pressure then protective sensation has been lost.

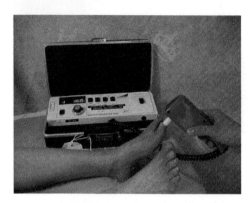

Fig. 1.6 A neurothesiometer is a device that delivers a vibratory stimulus which increases as the voltage is raised.

A simple technique for detecting neuropathy is to use a nylon mono-filament, which, when applied perpendicular to the foot, buckles at a given force of 10 g. The filament should be applied at the plantar aspects of the first toe, the first, third and fifth metatarsal heads, the plantar surface of the heel and the dorsum of the foot. The filament should not be applied at any site until callus has been removed. If the patient cannot feel the filament at a tested area, then significant neuropathy is present and protective pain sensation is lost. After using a monofilament on 10 consecutive patients, there should be a recovery time of 24h before further usage.

The degree of neuropathy can be further quantified by the neurothesiometer. When applied to the foot, this device delivers a vibratory stimulus, which increases as the voltage is raised. The vibration threshold increases with age, but, for practical purposes, any patient unable to feel a vibratory stimulus of 25V is at risk of ulceration.

If monofilaments or a neurothesiometer are not available, then a simple clinical examination detecting sensation to light touch using a cotton wisp and to vibration using a 128Hz tuning fork will suffice, comparing a proximal site with a distal site to confirm a symmetrical stocking-like distribution of the neuropathy.

Recently, the 'Touch the toes' test, also known as the Ipswich touch test, has been developed. This involves lightly touching the tips of the first and fifth toes on the right foot, then the first and fifth toes on the left foot and finally the third toes of the right and left foot. If the touch is not felt at two or more toes then the patient has significant neuropathy.

Also recently, Vibratip™, a simple, disposable, pocket-sized device that uses a button battery-driven vibrator motor to deliver a uniform source of vibration to the skin has been used to assess vibration in diabetic patients.

Touch and vibration are carried by large myelinated nerve fibres, but some patients have a small-fibre neuropathy with impaired pain and temperature perception but with intact touch and vibration. They are prone to ulceration and thermal traumas but test normally with filaments and the neurothesiometer and a clinical assessment of light touch and vibration is normal. As yet, there is no inexpensive method of detecting and quantifying small-fibre neuropathy. However, a simple assessment of cold sensation can be made by placing a cold tuning fork on the patient's foot and leg.

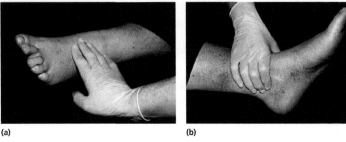

(a)   **(b)**

Fig. 1.7 Palpation of (a) the dorsalis pedis pulse on the dorsum of the foot and (b) the posterior tibial pulse at the ankle.

Ischaemia

Classical symptoms of ischaemia, namely claudication and rest pain, are often absent because of concomitant neuropathy. The most important manoeuvre to detect ischaemia is the palpation of foot pulses:

- The dorsalis pedis pulse is lateral to the extensor hallucis longus tendon on the dorsum of the foot (Fig. 1.7a)
- The posterior tibial pulse is below and behind the medial malleolus (Fig. 1.7b)
- If either of these foot pulses can be felt then it is highly unlikely that there is significant ischaemia.

A small, hand-held Doppler can be used to confirm the presence of pulses and to assess the vascular supply. Used together with a sphygmomanometer, the brachial systolic pressure and ankle systolic pressure can be measured, and the ankle brachial pressure index (ABPI), which is the ratio of ankle systolic pressure to brachial systolic pressure, can be calculated. In normal subjects, the ABPI is usually >1, but in the presence of ischaemia it is <1. Thus, absence of pulses and an ABPI of <1 confirms ischaemia. Conversely, the presence of pulses and an ABPI of >1 rules out ischaemia. This has important implications for management, namely that macrovascular disease is not an important factor and further vascular investigations are not necessary.

Many diabetic patients have medial arterial calcification, giving an artificially elevated systolic pressure, even in the presence of ischaemia. It is thus difficult to assess the diabetic foot when the pulses are not palpable but ABPI is >1. There are two explanations:

- The examiner may have missed the pulses, particularly in an oedematous foot, and should go back to palpate the foot after the arteries have been located by Doppler ultrasound
- If the pulses remain impalpable, then ischaemia probably exists in the presence of medial wall calcification. It is then necessary to use other methods to assess flow in the arteries of the foot, such as examining the pattern of the Doppler arterial waveform or measuring transcutaneous oxygen tension or toe systolic pressures (see Chapter 4).

Despite the difficulties of interpreting ankle systolic pressures in the presence of medial calcification, an ABPI of 0.5 or less indicates severe ischaemia whether the patient is calcified or not.

Deformity

It is important to recognize deformity in the diabetic foot. Deformity often leads to bony prominences, which are associated with high mechanical pressures on the overlying skin. This results in ulceration, particularly in the absence of protective pain sensation and when shoes are unsuitable. Ideally, the deformity should be recognized early and accommodated in properly fitting shoes before ulceration occurs.

Common deformities include:

- Claw toes
- Pes cavus
- Hallux rigidus
- Hallux valgus
- Hammer toe
- Mallet toe

- Fibro-fatty padding depletion
- Charcot foot
- Deformities related to previous trauma and surgery
- Nail deformities.

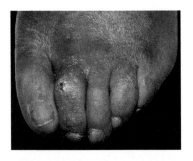

Fig. 1.8 Clawed second toe with early skin breakdown.

Claw toes

Claw toes (Fig. 1.8) have fixed flexion deformities at the interphalangeal joints and are associated with callus and ulceration of the apices and dorsal aspects of the interphalangeal joints. Although claw toes may be associated with neuropathy, they are often unrelated, especially when the clawing is unilateral and associated with trauma or surgery of the forefoot. Claw toes may result from acute rupture of the plantar fascia.

Pes cavus

Normally the dorsum of the foot is domed due to the medial longitudinal arch which extends between the first metatarsal head and the calcaneus. When it is abnormally high, the deformity is called pes cavus and the abnormal distribution of pressure leads to high mechanical pressure over the metatarsal heads (Fig. 1.2).

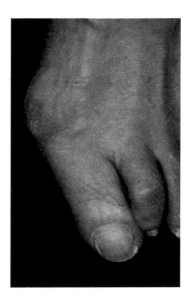

Fig. 1.9 Hallux valgus with erythema at first metatarso-phalangeal joint from tight shoe.

Hallux rigidus

This leads to limited joint mobility of the first metatarso-phalangeal joint with loss of dorsiflexion and results in excessive pressure on the plantar surface of the first toe, causing callus formation.

Hallux valgus

Hallux valgus is a deformity of the first metatarso-phalangeal joint with lateral deviation of the hallux and a medial prominence on the margin of the foot. This site is particularly vulnerable in the neuroischae-mic foot and frequently breaks down under pressure from a tight shoe (Fig. 1.9).

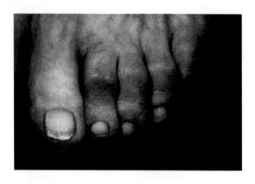

Fig. 1.10 Hammer toes (second, third and fourth toes) with hyperflexion of the proximal interphalangeal joints and hyperextension of the distal interphalangeal joints.

Hammer toe
Hammer toe is a flexion deformity of the proximal interphalangeal joint of a lesser toe with hyperextension of the distal interphalangeal joint (Fig. 1.10). The toe is at risk of dorsal ulceration.

Mallet toe
This deformity is a flexion contracture at the distal interphalangeal joint.

Fibro-fatty padding depletion
The plantar soft-tissue overlying the metatarsal heads is frequently pushed forward or destroyed by previous ulceration or infection. Also, motor neuropathy leads to anterior fat pad displacement and increased focal plantar pressures.

Charcot foot
Bone and joint damage in the metatarso-tarsal region is the commonest site of involvement and leads to two classical deformities:
• Rocker bottom deformity (Fig. 1.11), in which there is displacement and subluxation of the tarsus downwards
• Medial convexity, which results from dislocation of the talo-navicular or tarso-metatarsal joint.

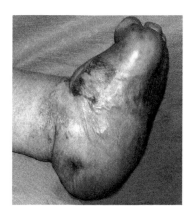

Fig. 1.11 Charcot foot showing rocker bottom deformity.

Both are often associated with a bony prominence which is very prone to ulceration. If these deformities are not diagnosed early and accommodated in properly fitting footwear, ulceration at vulnerable pressure points often develops (Fig. 1.12).

Deformities related to previous trauma and surgery

Deformities of the hip and fractures of the tibia or fibula lead to leg-shortening and hence abnormal gait, which predisposes to foot ulceration. Ray amputations remove the toe together with part of the metatarsal. They are usually very successful but disturb the biomechanics of the foot, leading to high pressure under the adjacent metatarsal heads. Removal of the fifth ray may lead to varus deformity of the foot if the fifth metatarsal base and its muscle attachments are not preserved. After amputation of a toe, deformities are often seen in adjoining toes (Fig. 1.13).

Nail deformities

It is important to inspect the nails closely as these may become the site of ulceration. Thickened nails are common in the population at large and may lead to ulceration.

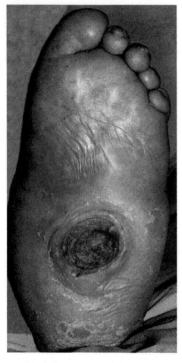

Fig. 1.12 Ulceration over bony prominence on the plantar surface of a rocker bottom deformity.

Ingrowing toe nail (onychocryptosis) arises when the nail plate is excessively wide and thin, or develops a convex deformity, putting pressure on the tissues at the nail edge. Callus builds up in response to pressure and inflammation. Eventually, usually after incorrect nail cutting or trauma, the nail penetrates the flesh (see Fig. 2.5a and b).

Callus

This is a thickened area of epidermis which develops at sites of pressure, shear and friction. It should not be allowed to become excessive, as callus is a common forerunner of ulceration in the presence of neuropathy.

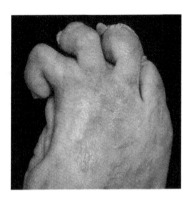

Fig. 1.13 Deformity of toe adjacent to amputated first toe.

Swelling

Swelling of the tissues of the foot is a major factor predisposing to ulceration, and often exacerbates a tight fit inside poorly fitting shoes. It also impedes healing of established ulcers. Swelling may be bilateral or unilateral.

Bilateral swelling

This is usually secondary to:

- Cardiac failure
- Hypoalbuminaemia
- Renal failure
- Venous insufficiency (sometimes unilateral)
- Inferior vena caval obstruction
- Lymphoedema (Fig. 1.14)
- Diabetic neuropathy, when it is related to increased arterial blood flow and arteriovenous shunting and is known as neuropathic oedema.

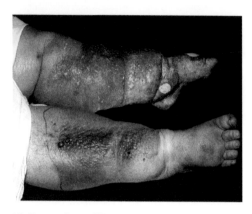

Fig. 1.14 Bilateral lymphoedema with cellulitis of both legs.

Unilateral swelling

This is usually associated with local pathology in the foot or leg. Causes are:

- Infection, when it is usually associated with erythema and a break in the skin (Fig. 1.15a and b)
- Charcot foot (a unilateral hot, red, swollen foot is often the first sign, and the swelling can extend to the knee)
- Gout, which may also present as a hot, red, swollen foot
- Trauma, sprain or fracture
- Deep vein thrombosis
- Venous insufficiency
- Lymphoedema, caused by lymphatic obstruction secondary to malignancy
- Venous obstruction by a pelvic mass, malignancy or ovarian cyst
- Localized collection of blood or pus which may present as a fluctuant swelling.

Skin breakdown

An active search should be made for breaks in the skin over the entire surface of the foot and ankle, not forgetting the areas between the toes

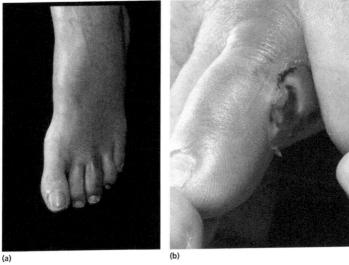

(a)   **(b)**

Fig. 1.15 (a) Erythema and swelling of the third toe spreading up the foot. (b) Interdigital ulcer as a source of sepsis with cellulitis and blue discolouration adjacent to ulcer.

and at the back of the heel. Toes should be gently held apart for inspection (Fig. 1.15b). If jerked apart, this can split the skin. The classical sign of tissue breakdown is the foot ulcer. However, fissures (Fig. 1.3) and bullae/blisters (see Fig. 4.5) also represent breakdown of the skin.

Some lesions will be obvious; others will make their presence known by their complications, such as:
- Discharge or exudate
- Colour changes under callus or nail plate
- Pain or discomfort
- Swelling
- Warmth
- Erythema.

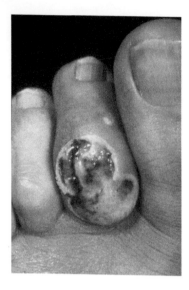

Fig. 1.16 Ulceration, cellulitis and purulent discharge from toe.

Infection

When skin breakdown develops, it may act as a portal of entry for infection (see Chapter 5). A close inspection for signs of infection should be made. These signs include purulent discharge from the lesion and erythema, swelling and warmth of the toe or foot (Fig. 1.16).

In the presence of neuropathy, the signs of infection may be subtle and include increased friability of granulation tissue, wound odour, wound breakdown and delayed healing.

Necrosis

Finally, lesions of skin breakdown may progress to underlying necrosis (Fig. 1.17). This can be identified by the presence of black or brown devitalized tissue (see Chapter 6).

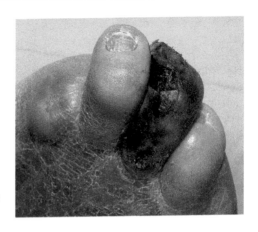

Fig. 1.17 Wet necrosis of fourth toe.

Integrated examination

In practice, the examination of the foot should be divided into three main parts: inspection, palpation and neurological assessment.

Inspection

The foot should be fully inspected, including dorsum, sole, back of the heel and interdigital areas with a full assessment of:
- Colour (as an indicator of ischaemia)
- Deformity
- Swelling
- Callus
- Skin breakdown
- Infection
- Necrosis.

Palpation

Pulses should be palpated and skin temperature compared between both feet with the back of the examining hand. The measurement of skin temperature is particularly helpful in the management of the Charcot foot, when a digital skin thermometer is useful (see Chapter 4).

Neurological assessment

Peripheral neuropathy can be detected by using the monofilament, neurothesiometer, Vibratip™ or by performing a simple sensory examination or 'Touch the toe' test.

After completing this basic examination, it will now be possible to classify the diabetic foot and to make the appropriate staging in its natural history.

CLASSIFYING THE DIABETIC FOOT

For practical purposes, the diabetic foot can be divided into two main entities: the neuropathic foot with palpable pulses and the ischaemic foot without palpable pulses. It is essential to differentiate between the neuropathic and the ischaemic foot as their management will differ.

Infection is the most frequent complication of ulceration in both the neuropathic and ischaemic foot. It is important to diagnose it early and intervene rapidly. It is responsible for considerable tissue necrosis in the diabetic foot and is the main reason for major amputation.

The neuropathic foot

- This is a warm, well-perfused foot with bounding pulses due to arteriovenous shunting and distended dorsal veins
- Sweating is diminished, the skin may be dry and prone to fissuring, and any callus tends to be hard and dry
- Toes may be clawed and the foot arch raised
- Ulceration can develop on the sole of the foot, associated with neglected callus and high plantar pressures
- Despite the good circulation, necrosis can develop secondary to severe infection

- The neuropathic foot may have an abnormal response to minor traumatic injuries, and this can lead to bone and joint problems (the Charcot foot)
- When patients are followed for many years, the neuropathic foot may develop ischaemia and become a neuroischaemic foot.

The ischaemic foot

This is a cool, pulseless foot with reduced perfusion. It may also be complicated by swelling, often secondary to cardiac failure or renal failure. If it becomes infected, the ischaemic foot may feel deceptively warm.

The various subdivisions of the ischaemic foot will have characteristic appearances.

Neuroischaemic foot

The most frequent presentation is that of ulceration. Ischaemic ulcers are commonly seen on the margins of the foot, including the tips of the toes and the areas around the back of the heel (Fig. 1.18). They

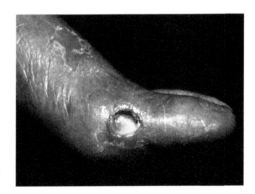

Fig. 1.18 Neuroischaemic foot ulcer.

are usually caused by minor trauma or by wearing unsuitable shoes. Even if neuropathy is present and plantar pressures are high, plantar ulceration is rare, probably because the foot does not develop heavy plantar callus, which requires good blood flow. Intermittent claudication and rest pain may be absent because of neuropathy and the distal distribution of the arterial disease to the leg.

Critically ischaemic foot
This presents as a pink, often painful foot with pallor on elevating the foot and rubor on dependency. The colour of the critically ischaemic foot can be a deceptively healthy pink or red, caused by dilatation of capillaries in an attempt to improve perfusion (Fig. 1.19).

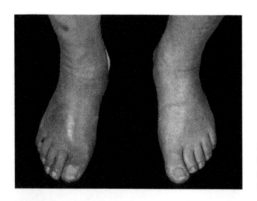

Fig. 1.19 Critically ischaemic right foot showing rubor on dependency.

Acutely ischaemic foot
This presents initially with sudden pallor and the foot becomes mottled (Fig. 1.20).

Renal ischaemic foot
A classical feature of this foot is the digital necrosis (Fig. 1.21).

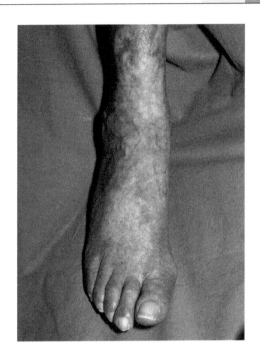

Fig. 1.20 Acutely ischaemic foot showing mottling of the skin.

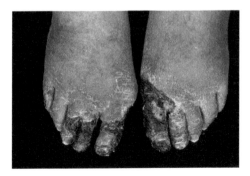

Fig. 1.21 Digital necrosis in renal ischaemic feet.

STAGING OF THE DIABETIC FOOT

The natural history of the diabetic foot can be divided into six stages, as shown in Table 1.2. The most frequently encountered types of diabetic foot are the neuropathic foot with ulceration and the neuroischaemic foot with ulceration. Their natural history is portrayed in Fig. 1.22. This represents pictorially the progression from Stage 2 to Stage 5 for each type of foot.

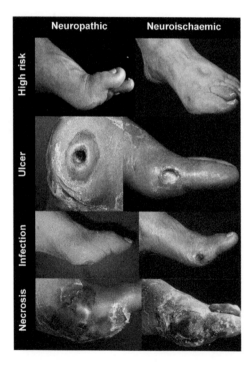

Fig. 1.22 Composite picture to show the natural history of the neuropathic and neuroischaemic foot as it passes from high risk through ulceration, infection and necrosis.

- *Stage 1*   The foot is not at risk. The patient does not have the risk factors of neuropathy, ischaemia, deformity, callus or swelling. Thus, the patient is not vulnerable to foot ulcers.
- *Stage 2*   The patient has developed one or more of the risk factors for ulceration and the foot may be divided into the neuropathic foot and the neuroischaemic foot.
- *Stage 3*   The neuropathic and neuroischaemic foot has developed a skin breakdown. This is usually an ulcer, but because some minor injuries, such as blisters, splits or grazes, have a propensity to become ulcers, they are included in Stage 3. Ulceration is usually on the plantar surface in the neuropathic foot and usually on the margin in the ischaemic foot.
- *Stage 4*   The ulcer has developed infection with the presence of cellulitis, which can complicate both the neuropathic and the neuroischaemic foot.
- *Stage 5*   Necrosis has supervened. In the neuropathic foot, infection is usually the cause; in the neuroischaemic foot, infection is still the most common reason for tissue destruction, although ischaemia contributes.
- *Stage 6*   The foot cannot be saved and will need a major amputation.

The staging system was developed primarily for the two main scenarios of the neuropathic and neuroischaemic foot, stressing the development of the ulcer as a pivotal stage in the natural history of the diabetic foot and the rapid progression through infection to necrosis (Fig. 1.22).

However, staging can be helpful for the four less common scenarios, namely the Charcot foot, the critically ischaemic foot, the acutely ischaemic foot and the renal ischaemic foot. The natural history of these feet, together with that of the neuropathic and neuroischaemic foot, has been described at the beginning of this chapter in Fig. 1.1.

The overwhelming feature of the natural history of all these scenarios of the diabetic foot is the rapid progression to necrosis, which clinically

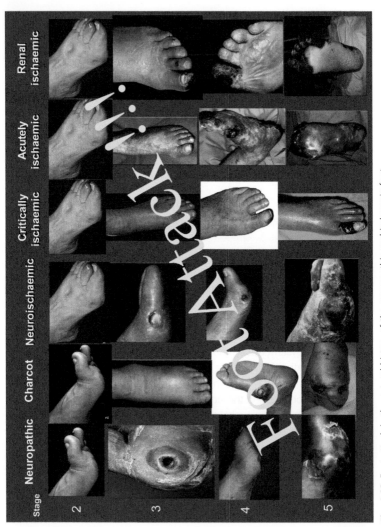

Fig. 1.23 Foot attack in the natural history of the neuropathic and ischaemic foot.

can be described as a 'diabetic foot attack' with similarities to the heart attack and brain attack (Fig. 1.23). Essentially, there are two drivers of the 'diabetic foot attack' which leads to necrosis: infection and ischaemia. Infection results in a septic vasculitis and is a prominent feature both of the neuropathic foot and the neuroischaemic foot. It can also complicate ulcers associated with the Charcot foot. In the remaining scenarios, the driver is ischaemia producing the clinical syndromes of critical ischaemia, acute ischaemia and the renal ischaemic foot.

INTERVENTION

At each stage of the diabetic foot it is necessary to intervene early and take control of the foot to prevent further progression. Management will be considered under the headings shown in Table 1.3. This book describes full details of practical management for each stage in the appropriate chapter with one colour-coded chapter for each of the six stages. The book contains sufficient, easily accessible information to enable the practitioner to make rapid, effective decisions which will prevent deterioration and progression to necrosis and amputation.

Multidisciplinary foot management

In the modern management of the diabetic foot, two teams have established importance: the multidisciplinary foot care team and the foot protection team.

The multidisciplinary foot care team

Successful management of the diabetic foot needs the expertise of a multidisciplinary foot care team which provides integrated care focused in a diabetic foot clinic. Members of the team comprise podiatrist, nurse, orthotist, microbiologist, physician, radiologist and surgeon, including vascular surgeon, orthopaedic surgeon and plastic surgeon. Some roles may overlap, depending on local expertise. The multidisciplinary foot care team should be available to assess outpatients with active foot disease, not only in routine appointments but also as emergencies. Patients in Stages 3–5 are best seen within a multidisciplinary foot service. Day-to-day multidisciplinary treatment is carried out by podiatrist, nurse, orthotist and physician in the diabetic foot clinic. Further management is achieved by holding regular joint multidisciplinary clinics with vascular and orthopaedic surgeons in the diabetic foot clinic. Through these specialist clinics, it is possible to organise a 'fast-track' service in a 'one-stop' visit, comprising clinical assessment, same-day investigations and urgent treatment.

In the joint clinic with the vascular surgeon, the need for angiography can be rapidly agreed upon and either angioplasty or bypass surgery can then be promptly carried out. Ischaemic patients are followed up postoperatively to provide continuity of care for wounds and amputation sites. Follow up includes routine preventive foot care, regular updating of education to detect problems early, rapid and aggressive care of ulcers, regular arterial and graft surveillance and the provision of statins and aspirin for secondary prevention of arterial disease.

In the joint clinic with the orthopaedic surgeon, patients with Charcot osteoarthopathy and patients needing complex deformity corrections and limb reconstructions can also be seen. In the joint clinic with the plastic surgeon, patients with tissue destruction and non-healing wounds are seen and considered for skin grafts and free flaps.

The diabetic foot clinic should offer rapid access, early diagnosis and prompt help for patients with urgent foot problems, providing podiatric, nursing, surgical and medical treatment. The use of modern imaging is important in diagnosis, and the foot clinic can facilitate urgent visits to radiology, nuclear medicine, ultrasound departments and the vascular laboratory. The clinic can facilitate urgent measurement of inflammatory parameters, such as serum C-reactive protein (CRP). Each team member should be available quickly for emergency appointments, which can be run concurrently with routine clinics so that patients with new ulcers, pain or discolouration can be seen the same day. This includes patients in whom overwhelming infection or ischaemia is 'attacking' the foot and leading to significant necrosis in a 'diabetic foot attack'. Such patients need rapid treatment and admission to hospital through the emergency service provided by the diabetic foot clinic.

When diabetic patients with severe foot problems have been admitted to hospital, they should be looked after by the multidisciplinary team. Some patients may be under the primary care of the vascular, orthopaedic or plastic surgeons and others under the care of the diabetologist. However, there should be joint ward rounds and multidisciplinary team meetings. This has been facilitated at King's College Hospital by the creation of the post of diabetic foot practitioner, who, as an experienced podiatrist, coordinates all aspects of inpatient care, including wound, microbiology, mechanical, vascular, metabolic and educational aspects, as shown in Table 1.3.

Overall, the diabetic foot clinic has taken the role of an 'operations' centre or a 'command' centre for the prevention of amputation in vulnerable diabetic neuropathic and ischaemic patients that are susceptible to trauma, ulceration, infection and necrosis.

The foot protection team

In contrast to patients with ulceration in Stages 3–5, patients in Stage 2 without ulcers, but at an increased risk of developing lower limb complications, should be treated by the foot protection team. Typically, members of this team include podiatrists, orthotists and other foot care specialists who are based in primary care. The important aspect of management is screening for patients at risk of ulceration and then providing follow-up care and education for those patients. However, there should be very rapid referral pathways between the foot protection team and the multidisciplinary foot care team if a patient develops ulceration.

2

Managing Stage 1: the normal foot

PRESENTATION AND DIAGNOSIS

The foot has none of the risk factors for foot ulcers, namely neuropathy, ischaemia, deformity, callus or swelling, and the diagnosis of Stage 1 is made by excluding these risk factors.

These patients have a low risk of ulceration with normal foot pulses, normal vibration and sensation to the 10 g monofilament, no history of foot ulceration and no significant foot deformity. However, despite this, patients can still suffer traumatic injuries, but the presence of intact nerves should make patients aware of this and they should be educated to take appropriate action.

Techniques for the assessment of risk factors and screening are described in the Chapter 1, and they should be carried out when the patient presents for annual review.

MANAGEMENT

Patients at low risk of diabetic foot disease are managed preventatively through annual screening, regular foot inspections/examinations and education supervised by the foot protection team. The aim of management is to keep the foot at Stage 1.

The following components of multidisciplinary management are important:

- Mechanical control
- Metabolic control
- Educational control.

This stage does not have any skin breakdown or ischaemia. Therefore, wound, microbiological and vascular control are not relevant.

Managing the Diabetic Foot, Third Edition. Michael E Edmonds and Alethea VM Foster.
© 2014 John Wiley & Sons, Ltd. Published 2014 by John Wiley & Sons, Ltd.

Mechanical control

Mechanical control is based upon wearing the correct footwear to prevent the foot from developing unnecessary deformity. It also involves the diagnosis and treatment of common problems affecting the biomechanics of the foot.

Correct footwear

If shoes are the wrong size or style, they can permanently damage the feet and lead to deformity, callus and ulceration.

All people at Stage 1 will be wearing their own shoes. Therefore, advice about footwear purchase is necessary and patients should be told the principles of good footwear (Table 2.1, Fig. 2.1 and Fig. 2.2). If pos-

Table 2.1 **Good shoe guide.**
The toe box should be sufficiently long, broad and deep to accommodate the toes without pressing on them, with a clear space between the apices of the toes and the toe box so that the toes are not too cramped to function
Shoes should fasten with adjustable lace, strap or Velcro high on the foot. (When the lace is fastened, the foot is firmly held inside the shoe, thus reducing the frictional forces when the patient walks and preventing the foot from sliding forwards and jamming the toes against the toe box.) Shoes should be foot shaped
The heel of the shoe should be under 5 cm high to avoid weight being thrown forward on to metatarsal heads (Fig. 2.1 and Fig. 2.3)
The inner lining of the shoe should be smooth
Shoes should be purchased in the afternoon because feet swell a little during the day
Stockings or socks should always be worn with shoes to avoid blisters. Socks with prominent seams should be worn inside out, and socks with holes should be replaced.

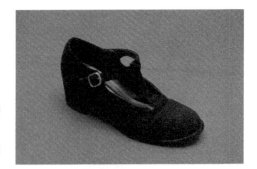

Fig. 2.1 A good woman's shoe with low heel, generous toe box and restraining strap fastening high on the foot.

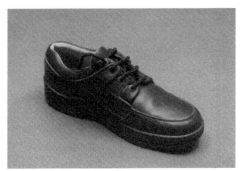

Fig. 2.2 A good 'high-street' man's shoe. The shoe is the shape of the foot.

sible, shoes should be purchased on approval and checked by a health-care professional. Trainer styles are useful. Shoes should be part of the foot assessment, and features of a bad shoe are shown in Fig. 2.3.

Minor foot problems

In achieving mechanical control, it is important to diagnose common foot problems which are not peculiar to diabetes but are very common in the population at large. Most people in Stage 1 will be able to cut their own nails (Table 2.2). However, specific nail and other minor foot problems will need treatment. Minor foot problems can become major problems unless they are diagnosed early and treated.

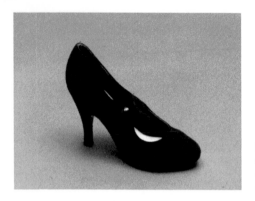

Fig. 2.3 A bad woman's shoe. Heel is too high and toe box is cramped and it has no fastening.

Table 2.2 **Patients who can safely cut their own toe nails.**
Pain-free normal nails with no pathology
Can see feet clearly
Can reach feet
Have been taught correct nail cutting techniques

Onychogryphosis

This is thickening of the nail with deformity (Fig. 2.4). The cause is a previous insult to the nail bed and it is necessary to file down the nail regularly otherwise it may grow at an angle and penetrate adjoining tissue.

Onychocryptosis

This is an ingrowing toe nail, often due to poor toe nail cutting technique or trauma. A splinter of nail, left behind by incomplete cutting or attempts to remove the corners of the nail, penetrates the nail sulcus (the groove of flesh at the side of the nail plate).

The offending splinter of nail (Fig. 2.5a) should be removed (Fig. 2.5b) and the ragged edge of the nail filed smooth. Unless the splinter of nail

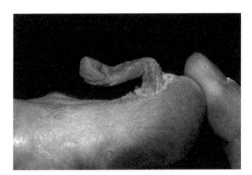

Fig. 2.4 Onychogryphosis – monster nail.

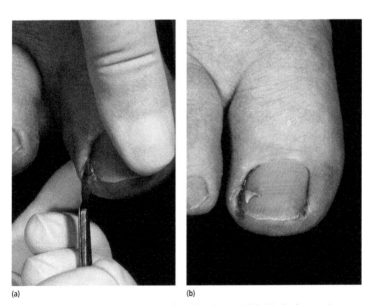

(a)   (b)

Fig. 2.5 Onychocryptosis. (a) A spike of nail has been 'left behind' after cutting. (b) The offending spike has been removed and lies on the nail plate.

is removed, the flesh will be penetrated and infection supervenes. The lesion will not heal and paronychia may develop.

If the problem does not resolve, partial nail avulsion under local anaesthetic and phenolysation of the nail matrix may be necessary although it can take several weeks to heal. It is safe to carry this out in a Stage 1 diabetic patient who, by definition, has good peripheral circulation.

Onychomycosis

Fungal infection can cause whitish or yellowish discolouration of the nail plate, which frequently becomes thickened and crumbly (Fig. 2.6).

The majority of infections are caused by dermatophytes or yeasts. Eradication is difficult. Unless the condition is spreading, painful or cosmetically unacceptable, palliative care is best. The bulk of the nail should be reduced at regular intervals. Active treatment involves topical or systemic agents. Topical agents include amorolfine nail lacquer. Terbinafine is the oral agent of choice. Onychomycosis predisposes to bacterial foot infection.

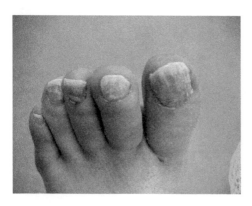

Fig. 2.6 Onychomycosis. Discoloured, friable nails.

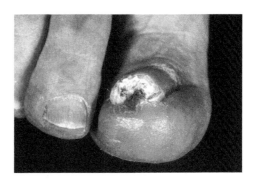

Fig. 2.7 Involuted first toe nail.

Involuted toe nails
These have an excessive lateral curvature and trap epithelial cells which accumulate in the sulcus and become painful (Fig. 2.7). The sulcus should be gently cleared with a Black's file (a small file specially designed to fit into the sulcus). Removal of the edge of the nail is also helpful.

Subungual haematoma
This follows trauma to the nail. Blood collects under the nail plate causing a red, purple or black discolouration. This may be painful. A large collection of blood can loosen the entire nail plate. The haematoma can be drained by making a small hole in the nail plate with a scalpel or with a podiatrist's nail drill. If the nail plate is loose, it is best to cut it back before it catches on the hose and causes further trauma.

Tinea pedis
This can present in several ways: moist, cracked areas with whitish macerated skin between the toes (Fig. 2.8), a dry, scaly hyperkeratotic area or a vesicular itchy rash are all presentations.

Canesten spray (clotrimazole 1% in 30% isopropyl alcohol) or cream may be prescribed, which should be continued for 2 weeks

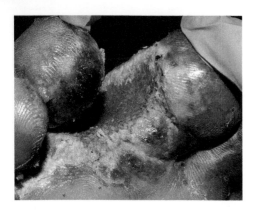

Fig. 2.8 Interdigital fungal infection.

after resolution of symptoms to avoid relapse. For other parts of the foot, Canesten cream can be applied. Whitfield's ointment is useful. Tinactin (tolnaftate) and Mycil (chlorphenesin) can be bought over the counter in powder or cream formulations.

Verrucae

Verrucae (warts) may occur on the sole of the foot (Fig. 2.9). They should be treated, if painful or spreading, by cryotherapy with liquid nitrogen. Most will resolve without treatment within 2 years.

Corns

These are areas where, in response to pressure or friction, the stratum corneum is thicker than in adjoining areas and has a deeper nucleus (Fig. 2.10). Corns between the toes are soft and white.

Corns should be removed and abnormal mechanical forces reduced with good footwear.

Bullae/blisters

Bullae are superficial fluid-filled sacs which develop when the skin is traumatized. The usual causes are inadequate footwear or failing to

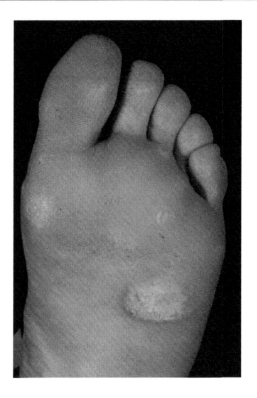

Fig. 2.9 Verrucae on plantar aspect of the foot.

wear socks. If the feet and shoes and socks are wet, then blistering is more likely to develop.

If the bulla is small and flaccid, it can be cleaned and covered with a sterile dressing. If large and tense, it should be lanced with a scalpel to release the contents before dressing. Aspiration with a syringe is less useful, because the hole may seal and the bulla may become tense again.

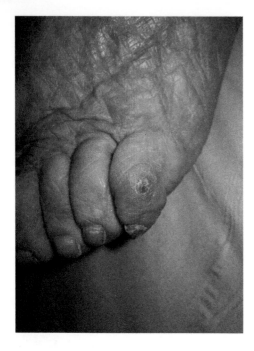

Fig. 2.10 Corn on lateral surface of fifth toe.

Chilblains

These are localized inflammatory lesions, provoked by cold. They present as dusky red swellings in the acute stage and, in the chronic stage, as purple lesions on the toes. They are best prevented by making sure that the feet are protected from the cold (Fig. 2.11).

Traumas

Patients without neuropathy or vascular disease can still be subjected to traumas. Superficial cuts and grazes may be cleaned with an antiseptic

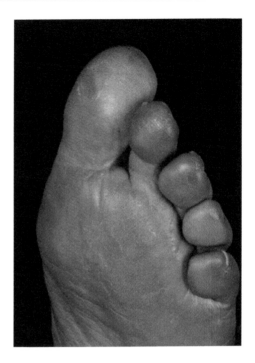

Fig. 2.11 Chilblains of second, third and fifth toes.

and covered with a sterile dressing. All diabetic patients should keep a first-aid box at home which is equipped with sterile dressings, tape and antiseptic cream to treat accidental injuries.

Any foot problem, no matter how apparently trivial, which is not healing well within 48 h should be treated as Stage 3. The main risk to Stage 1 patients is the rapid development of infection complicating a skin breakdown. This should lead to considerable pain and an early request for help. If this does not happen, patients in Stage 1 can quickly be overwhelmed by infection.

Dry skin and fissures

It is essential for people with diabetes to keep the skin clean and free from scales, hyperkeratosis and cracks. This can be achieved with regular washing, application of emollient to dry skin, and podiatric debridement of hyperkeratosis. Clearing the edges of fissures to achieve closure is important. Many ulcers can be prevented if care is taken to treat dry skin early.

Metabolic control

Hyperglycaemia, hypertension, hyperlipidaemia and smoking are the great quartet of factors that predispose the patient to neuropathy and ischaemia. Thus, good control of blood glucose, blood pressure, blood cholesterol and triglycerides and refraining from smoking are extremely important at Stage 1 to preserve neurological and cardiovascular function. Poorly controlled patients may be more prone to develop infection.

The results of the Diabetes Control and Complications Trial (DCCT) for type 1 diabetes and the UK Prospective Diabetes Study (UKPDS) for type 2 diabetes indicated the value of good blood glucose control in preventing microvascular complications. A reduction in glycated haemoglobin to less than 7% (53 mmol/mol) may also lower the risk of myocardial infarction and cardiovascular death. Furthermore the 'legacy' effect of tight control at an early stage of diabetes has a long-lasting influence on the reduction of both microvascular and macrovascular complications, as shown by the Epidemiology of Diabetes Interventions and Complications (EDIC) Study.

However, in type 2 diabetes, there is some concern that too tight control by bringing glycated haemoglobin to less than 6.5% (48 mmol/mol) is associated with increased mortality, as was demonstrated in the Action to Control Cardiovascular Risk in Diabetes (ACCORD) trial (2010). It included mostly patients who were middle-aged and older who had a long duration of diabetes and a high risk of cardiovascular disease.

For patients having more than 10 years of diabetes, the benefit of tight control in reducing macrovascular and microvascular complications may thus be limited.

High blood pressure is a major risk factor for cardiovascular disease and microvascular complications, and the target should be below 140/80 mmHg. In patients with microalbuminuria, the target should be below 130/80 mmHg. Angiotensin-converting enzyme inhibitors or angiotensin-II receptor blockers are the first-line therapy for hypertensive patients with microalbuminuria.

Blood lipid control involves lowering low-density lipoprotein (LDL) cholesterol, raising high-density lipoprotein (HDL) cholesterol and lowering triglycerides. Achieving this reduces macrovascular disease and mortality in patients with type 2 diabetes. LDL cholesterol is the main target for type 2 diabetes, aiming for levels below 2 mmol/L. Patients should reduce saturated fat and cholesterol intake, and achieve weight loss and increased physical activity levels. When life-style changes are not successful, statins are the first-line therapy for hypercholesterolaemia. The Collaborative-AtoRvastatin Diabetes Study (CARDS) has shown the benefit of cholesterol lowering with statins in patients without existing cardiovascular disease. CARDS demonstrated that atorvastatin, compared with placebo, resulted in a significant 37% reduction in the combined primary endpoint of major cardiovascular events in patients with type 2 diabetes but with no previous history of cardiovascular disease.

Fibrates can be used to reduce very high levels of triglycerides above 5 mmol/L, but fibrates are not used commonly in primary prevention to decrease triglycerides and increase HDL cholesterol.

Smoking is a very high risk factor for peripheral vascular disease. Clear unequivocal advice should be given to stop smoking. Enrolment in a smokers' clinic programme may help.

All patients with any degree of cardiovascular risk should take daily aspirin. However, aspirin is not recommended for the primary prevention of vascular events in people with diabetes.

Hypoglycaemia is a common complication of diabetic treatment. Capillary blood glucose measurement should be available wherever diabetic foot patients are treated, as well as first-aid treatment. Warning signs of hypoglycaemia include trembling, paraesthesiae around the mouth, shakiness, anxiety, hunger and sweating, confusion, altered behaviour, slurred speech, irritability, drowsiness and, in severe cases, fits and loss of consciousness. If hypoglycaemia is suspected, the capillary blood glucose should be measured. A reading below 3.5 mmol/L confirms hypoglycaemia. If the patient is not drowsy and can swallow, then 130 mL Lucozade or 200 mL fresh orange juice should be given. On recovery, a slice of bread or two digestive biscuits should be taken. If the patient cannot swallow, Glucogel (formerly Hypostop) can be applied around the gums or glucagon given 1 mg subcutaneously or intramuscularly. If very drowsy, 75 mL of 20% glucose or 150 mL of 10% glucose can be administered intravenously. Hypoglycaemia secondary to sulphonylurea therapy can be prolonged, and patients will need intravenous glucose therapy. Advice on hypoglycaemia prevention should be given.

Educational control

It is easy to teach people the theory of foot care, but it is extremely difficult to change behaviour. Throughout this book, simple educational material is provided for adaptation and presentation to individual patients and groups (who may include relatives) or to provide topics for workshops or worksheets. Written words need verbal reinforcement and vice versa. Education should be adapted so as to make it relevant for patients of varying ages, backgrounds and cultures. Patients should never be made to feel that they are back in the classroom with an unsympathetic teacher. Patient educators are useful. Frequent educational updating is necessary. Stage 1 patients should be taught about neuropathy and peripheral vascular disease and reassured that good control can delay or prevent complications. They should be taught to expect foot inspection as part of their diabetes annual review.

Patient information

Shoes
- Buy well-fitting shoes which fasten with lace or strap
- Look for a foot-shaped shoe
- Shoe heels should be under 5 cm high
- Have your feet measured
- Avoid slippers and slip-ons.

Foot care
- Wash feet every day and check for problems
- Regular skin care is very important. Apply cream to dry skin. Regular washing should help to prevent skin scales from accumulating
- If problems develop (hard skin, scaly skin, splits, blisters, warts, athletes foot or injuries), seek help from a doctor or podiatrist. Never try to treat the problem yourself, except for simple first aid. Avoid proprietary remedies.

First aid
- Keep a first-aid box at home containing sterile dressings, tape, bandages and antiseptic cream
- If the foot is injured, clean the wound under the tap. Apply antiseptic cream and a bandage or a dressing.

Nails
- Cut nails after a bath or shower when they are softer
- Do not try to cut the whole nail in one piece
- Do not cut nails too short or leave them poking beyond the end of the toe
- Never cut out the corner of the nail or dig down the sides
- If nails are painful or difficult to cut, then see a podiatrist.

Daily foot check
- Check feet for danger signs of swelling, colour change, pain or breaks in the skin and seek immediate help if these occur
- Seek advice for minor wounds which do not heal.

(Continued)

Annual foot check

- There should be an annual screening by a suitably trained health-care professional
- There should be an agreed self-management plan
- The patient should be provided with written and verbal advice
- The patient should also be given appropriate access to a podiatrist when required and emergency contact numbers for use in a crisis.

Managing Stage 2: the high-risk foot

PRESENTATION AND DIAGNOSIS

The diabetic foot enters Stage 2 because it has developed one or more of the risk factors for ulceration: neuropathy, ischaemia, deformity, callus or swelling. These may present clinically or else should be detected at annual review. This is the stage of screening and prevention when patients deemed at risk should be managed by a foot protection team to prevent the onset of active foot disease. Patients with a history of foot ulceration but healed on presentation are deemed as having a high-risk foot for further ulceration. This chapter will describe the principles of a foot protection programme.

The foot should be assessed as described in Chapter 1 and the presence of the above risk factors ascertained. Although patients may have positive symptoms of neuropathy, such as paraesthesiae in both feet and occasionally severe pain (which is addressed at the end of the chapter), neuropathy will usually not result in any symptoms and must be detected by screening. Similarly with ischaemia, pain is often absent in the diabetic patient. In particular, the presentation of ischaemia is different from that in the non-diabetic ischaemic leg. Often the diabetic patient will not have claudication or rest pain. This is because of the distal distribution of the arterial disease, the presence of neuropathy and a poor exercise tolerance.

Thus, screening should be carried out annually so as to detect the onset of risk factors at the earliest opportunity. The foot is then staged, and if either neuropathy or ischaemia is present then the foot is in Stage 2 and classified as either the neuropathic or ischaemic foot. The ischaemic foot may have a varying degree of neuropathy and may then be

Managing the Diabetic Foot, Third Edition. Michael E Edmonds and Alethea VM Foster.
© 2014 John Wiley & Sons, Ltd. Published 2014 by John Wiley & Sons, Ltd.

termed the neuroischaemic foot. Patients with neuropathy or ischaemia are more likely to develop ulceration than patients who have deformity, callus or swelling but have protective pain sensation and an adequate blood supply. Nevertheless, we have regarded the presence of any of the risk factors as indicating a high-risk diabetic foot, which should then enter a foot protection programme.

However, foot protection programmes have determined patients with the loss of one risk factor as at moderate risk compared with patients who have more than one risk factor or a history of previous foot ulceration who are deemed at high risk.

In these programmes, patients at moderate risk should have an agreed and tailored management plan by a podiatrist with review every 3–6 months according to patient needs. Patients at high risk should be reviewed by a specialist diabetic podiatrist who should agree a specific management plan with review every 1–3 months. Both categories of patients should be told of their risk of developing foot problems and provided with written and verbal advice and phone numbers for emergency contacts.

MANAGEMENT

When the foot has been screened and deemed at risk, it is important for the patient to enter a foot protection programme so as to prevent the onset of ulceration. The following components of multidisciplinary management should take place:

- Mechanical control
- Vascular control
- Metabolic control
- Educational control.

As the patient still has intact skin, wound and microbiological control are irrelevant.

Most patients with neuropathy are asymptomatic, but some patients may have an unpleasant painful neuropathy, which is addressed at the end of this chapter. Such patients with painful neuropathy usually do not have ulcers and are still, therefore, Stage 2 patients.

Mechanical control

The main aim of mechanical control is to protect the foot so as to keep the skin intact and protect from ulceration. When the foot is not associated with deformity it may be possible to accommodate it in commercially supplied shoes, stressing the features of good footwear as described in Chapter 2.

It is very important in hospital to protect the heels of those at risk (Fig. 3.1).

In addition to maintaining mechanical control, deformity and callus must be treated as well as dry skin and fissures secondary to neuropathy. Common foot problems, as described in Stage 1, will also need management.

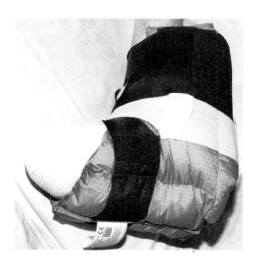

Fig. 3.1 Prevalon pressure-relieving heel protector with pillow style cushioning.

Deformities

Deformities such as hallux valgus, hallux rigidus and hammer toe are associated with an increased risk of elevated foot pressures and subsequent foot ulceration. They should be accommodated in properly fitting footwear and may require special bespoke footwear if the deformity is severe.

Deformities in the neuropathic foot tend to render the sole vulnerable to ulcers, requiring special insoles, whereas in the ischaemic foot the margins of the foot need protection, and appropriately wide shoes should be advised.

Shoes can be divided into four main types:

- Sensible shoes, which are commercially supplied from the 'high-street' shop
- Ready-made, off-the-shelf, orthopaedic stock shoes, which can be extra-depth and/or extra-width (Fig. 3.2). They contain cushioning insoles which are flat non-moulded insoles usually made of microcellular rubber
- Temporary ready-made shoes that can be fitted with prefabricated cushioning insoles (see Chapter 4)
- Customized or bespoke shoes, which accommodate the shape of the foot and can house cradled (moulded) insoles which redistribute weight-bearing from vulnerable pressure areas and at the same time provide a suitable cushion (see Chapter 4).

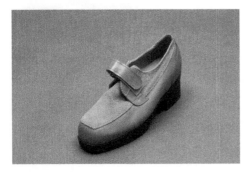

Fig. 3.2 Extra-depth stock shoe.

Table 3.1 **General principles of shoe prescription.**
The patient's choice of colour and style should always be respected as far as possible
For young patients, orthopaedic trainers are often acceptable
Patients need shoes for inside and outside, and may need bespoke shoes or boots for work, if steel toe caps are mandatory
Shoes should be reassessed regularly for excessive wear and the changing needs of patients and problems
Patients should have two pairs so that they are never without a pair

The general principles of shoe prescription are described in Table 3.1. Shoes should be designed with very smooth internal seams or no seams at all and should be fastenable to accommodate for swelling.

Some deformities may be accommodated in 'high-street' footwear with a wide toe box (Fig. 2.2). Trainer styles are useful. Major deformities which result in red pressure marks on the skin or associated callosities will need either ready-made stock shoes (Fig. 3.2) or bespoke shoes. The more abnormal the foot shape, the greater the need for bespoke shoes.

As an alternative to conservative management, prophylactic surgery may sometimes be helpful to correct deformed feet. Operative correction is carried out more freely when the deformity has led to ulceration and not as a purely prophylactic measure. Patients require careful assessment prior to surgery. If there is ischaemia, surgery should not be performed until after the circulation has been restored. Patients should be followed carefully throughout the perioperative and postoperative period. There is danger of precipitating a Charcot foot if the patient is rapidly mobilized too quickly. Careful postoperative care with casts or wound care shoes is necessary to provide protection when Kirschner wires are present. Prophylactic antibiotics may be given. The management of specific deformities will now be discussed.

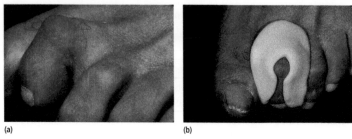

(a) (b)

Fig. 3.3 (a) Clawed second toe. (b) Silicone rubber orthotic to divert pressure from dorsum of claw toe.

Claw toes

Conservative management

Claw toes will be susceptible to ulceration on the dorsal surface (Fig. 3.3a) as well as the apex and will need a shoe with a wide, deep, soft toe box to reduce pressure on the dorsum of the toes. This may be obtainable from the 'high-street' shop, but it may be necessary to supply extra-depth shoes with a cushioning insole, particularly to protect the apices of the toes (see also Chapter 4). A silicone rubber orthotic can be used to divert pressure from the dorsum of the claw toe (Fig. 3.3b).

Surgical management

Arthroplasty of the proximal interphalangeal joint can be performed and the position of the toes maintained by Kirschner wires.

Hammer toes

Conservative management

Hammer toes are susceptible to callus formation and ulceration on the dorsum of the toe. A shoe with a wide, deep toe box will help to reduce pressure. Felt padding is useful in the short term. Silicone devices can be manufactured to off-load sites of high pressure.

Surgical management

If there is a fixed deformity, a proximal interphalangeal joint arthroplasty can be performed. The extensor tendon is exposed and retracted, the medial and lateral ligaments are freed, and the head of the proximal phalanx is transected. The extensor tendon is repaired and can be lengthened. The position of the toe can be maintained with a Kirschner wire.

Mallet toes

Conservative management

These may form callus on the dorsum and the apex of the toe. A silicone toe prop or apical crescent may be useful, together with a shoe that has a wide, deep toe box.

Surgical management

Distal interphalangeal joint arthroplasty corrects mallet toe deformity. The extensor tendon and joint capsule are removed, the collateral ligaments severed and the intermediate phalanx is transected. A Kirschner wire maintains the new position of the joint.

Prominent metatarsal heads

Conservative management

An extra-depth stock shoe with a cushioning insole may suffice. However, in the presence of a very high arch and extremely prominent metatarsal heads, a cradled insole in bespoke shoes will be needed (see Chapter 4).

Surgical management

Surgical management involves resection of one or more metatarsal heads. This is rarely performed except in cases of chronic plantar ulceration or osteomyelitis of the metatarsal head, but may be useful in patients with intermittent plantar ulceration where it is difficult to maintain healing long term. The joint is exposed, collateral ligaments cut through and an oblique cut made in the metatarsal shaft to enable removal of the metatarsal head.

Hallux rigidus

Conservative management

This leads to plantar callus on the first toe. If persistent heavy callus is a problem, then a rocker should be applied to the sole of the shoe to off-load pressure as the foot leaves the ground during the toe-off phase of the gait cycle (Fig. 3.4).

Surgical management

The two possible surgical options are hallux interphalangeal joint arthroplasty or Keller's resectional arthroplasty of the first metatarso-phalangeal

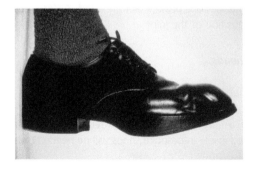

Fig. 3.4 Rocker sole to relieve pressure under the hallux.

joint. In the latter, the collateral ligaments are severed, the base of the proximal phalanx is removed and the joint capsule is closed. Kirschner wires can be used to maintain the new position of the toe.

Hallux valgus

Conservative management
This deformity will need a wide toe box to avoid pressure on the medial convexity. This is a common site of ulceration in the neuroischaemic foot, and extra-width stock shoes will be often required.

Surgical management
Keller's resectional arthroplasty is frequently performed but is unsuitable for young, active patients. An alternative procedure is metatarsal osteotomy.

Fibro-fatty padding depletion

Conservative management
Cushioned insoles, sometimes incorporating silicone or poron inserts, are useful.

Surgical management
Injections of silicone are occasionally used to augment fibro-fatty padding. Percutaneous lengthening of the Achilles tendon may also be performed to reduce pressure over the plantar forefoot, diminishing subsequent callus formation. A triple hemisection technique involves three percutaneous cuts in the tendon through small stab wounds, following which the position of the foot is corrected and maintained in a plaster cast or brace for several weeks.

Callus

Callus, particularly plantar callus, is a characteristic feature of the neuropathic foot (Fig. 3.5). It also occurs in the neuroischaemic foot, but to a much lesser extent. It is the most important pre-ulcerative lesion in Stage 2.

If allowed to become too thick, the callus will press on the soft tissues underneath and cause ulceration. Speckles of blood (Fig. 3.6a) or a deeper layer of whitish, macerated, moist tissue found under the surface of the callus indicate that the foot is close to ulceration and urgent removal of callus is necessary (Fig. 3.6b). Patients should never cut their callus off or use proprietary corn or callus removers. These contain strong acids and allow infection to enter the foot. Instead, the callus should be removed by the podiatrist and regular, sufficiently frequent removal will prevent ulceration.

The easiest way to remove the callus is with a scalpel while ensuring that the fingers of the other hand maintain good skin tension. Sharp debridement should only be performed by experts, as uneven removal can lead to focal points of very high pressure and invasion of the callus by nerve endings and blood vessels which can make future callus removal difficult. If callus reforms repeatedly, this indicates that there

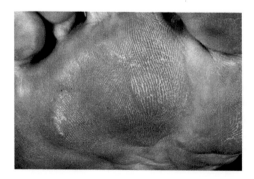

Fig. 3.5 Callus on plantar surface.

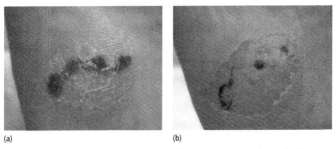

(a)   (b)

Fig. 3.6 (a) Bleeding under neglected callus. (b) The same site after callus has been removed.

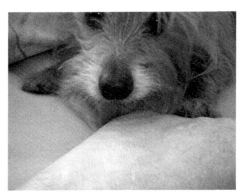

Fig. 3.7 Pet dog chews callus off her owner's feet.

are high pressures acting on the plantar surface of the foot, which need redistribution with footwear before the patient develops ulceration.

An unusual way to remove callus is to have it removed by a pet dog (Fig. 3.7).

Dry skin and fissures

Dry skin should be treated with an emollient such as E45 cream or urea-containing creams such as Calmurid® or Flexitol Heel Balm®. The margins of fissures may be reduced with a scalpel.

Common foot problems

Common foot problems may occur in the Stage 2 foot; treatment is described in Chapter 2. All breaks in the skin that are not healing well in 48 h should be regarded as ulcers and treated as Stage 3. Close observation will be needed, especially if ischaemia is present (see Chapter 4). Healing of such lesions will be slow if the foot is swollen.

Partial nail avulsion (PNA) for onychocryptosis is sometimes needed in patients with a degree of ischaemia. The peripheral circulation should be assessed and revascularization considered to improve the arterial inflow to the foot.

Vascular control

Patients with absent foot pulses should have the ABPI measured to confirm ischaemia. This may be artefactually raised by medial wall calcification, but a low ABPI is low whatever the state of the arterial wall and confirms ischaemia. Podiatrists should always ascertain their patient's vascular status before they cut the toe nails or remove callus, since any injury to the ischaemic foot can result in ulceration.

All diabetic patients with evidence of peripheral vascular disease may benefit from antiplatelet agents: 75 mg aspirin daily; or if this cannot be tolerated, clopidogrel 75 mg daily.

Diabetic patients with peripheral vascular disease should also be given statin therapy. The Heart Protection Study (HPS) has shown that simvastatin reduced the rate of major vascular events in a wide range of high-risk patients, including those with peripheral arterial disease or diabetes. Patients who are above 55 years and have peripheral vascular disease should also benefit from an angiotensin-converting enzyme inhibitor to prevent further vascular episodes (as indicated by the Heart Outcomes Prevention Evaluation (HOPE) study).

Patients with claudication alone should enter an exercise programme. Pharmacological treatment is possible with cilostazol, 100 mg twice daily.

Metabolic control

Even though neuropathy or ischaemia is now present, progression may be checked by treating hyperglycaemia, hypertension, hyperlipidaemia and refraining from smoking as described in Chapter 2. Long-term trials, such as the Diabetes Control and Complications Trial/Epidemiology of Diabetes Interventions and Complications (DCCT/EDIC) Study, the United Kingdom Prospective Diabetes Study (UKPDS), and the Steno-2 Study, have demonstrated microvascular as well as the additional macrovascular benefits of tight glycaemic control. However, the ACCORD trial findings indicated that very tight control should be avoided in middle-aged and elderly patients with long-standing diabetes and cardiovascular disease.

Swelling may complicate both the neuropathic and the neuroischaemic foot. Its main cause will be impaired cardiac and renal function, which should be treated accordingly. Venous insufficiency secondary to local venous disease can cause swelling and should be investigated with Duplex scanning, treated with compression stockings if there is no peripheral arterial disease and referred for a vascular opinion. Patients in end-stage renal failure treated with haemodialysis may have variable degrees of swelling and it is important for their footwear to be adjustable to accommodate fluctuant swelling. Neuropathic oedema may respond to ephedrine starting at a dose of 10 mg t.d.s., but this dose may need to be increased up to 30–60 mg t.d.s.

Educational control

Patients may have lost protective pain sensation and, therefore, they need to protect their feet from mechanical, thermal and chemical trauma. They should compensate for lack of protective pain sensation by establishing a habit of regular inspection of the feet so that problems can be detected quickly and help sought sufficiently early. It is important to educate Stage 2 patients to avoid trauma as far as possible. Patients who go away on holiday are particularly prone to develop foot problems and need special advice.

Patient information

Foot care

Your diabetes has made your feet numb. You may not feel pain if you injure your feet. Please take special precautions to keep your feet safe.

- Do not walk bare footed
- Visit a podiatrist regularly if you have callus. If you miss an appointment, make another quickly
- Never try to remove corns or callus yourself. Corn cures are very dangerous if you have diabetes (Fig. 3.8)
- Be careful not to burn your feet (Fig. 3.9). Always check the temperature of the bath or shower water with your elbow or use a bath thermometer. The water should be below 45°C. Never apply direct heat to your feet. Switch off electric blankets and remove hot water bottles before going to bed
- Position your bed away from wall radiators and hot water pipes
- Never toast your toes in front of the fire
- Prevent dryness in your feet by using a moisture-restoring cream
- If problems develop (splits, blisters, warts, athletes foot or injuries), seek help. Never try to treat the problem yourself, except for simple first aid.

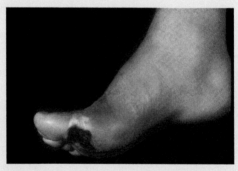

Fig. 3.8 Necrosis of first toe following application of corn cure.

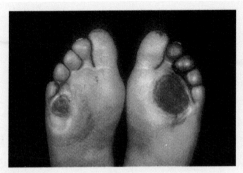

Fig. 3.9 Burns to feet from placing them in very hot water.

Footwear
- Shake out any loose pebbles or grit that may have found its way into the shoes before you put them on
- Run a hand around the insides of the shoes to detect rough, worn places
- When new shoes have been bought, it is best to wear them around the house for 20 min and check for signs of pressure or rubbing, such as redness or blisters. If this does occur, do not wear the shoes again and return them to the shoe shop
- Avoid slippers and slip-on shoes
- Check shoes before wearing to make sure that no sharp objects have gone through the sole (Fig. 3.10a and b)
- If the hospital gives you shoes, please wear them all the time that you are on your feet
- If your shoes are wearing out, get them repaired or replaced in plenty of time
- If shoe problems develop, seek help.

(*Continued*)

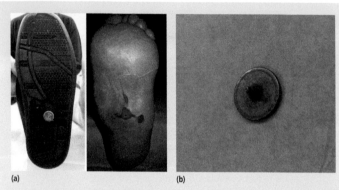

(a) (b)

Fig. 3.10 (a) Ulceration on plantar surface resulting from nail penetrating sole of shoe. (b) Offending nail removed from shoe.

Danger signs

Check your feet every day for:

- Colour change
- Pain or discomfort
- Breaks in the skin or discharge
- Swelling
- Callus.

Holiday foot-care education

The journey

- Wear shoes with adjustable fastening to accommodate swelling
- Arrange a wheelchair if you have foot problems
- Allow plenty of time for your journey
- If in a car or coach, take frequent stops to stretch your legs.

Flying

- Allow plenty of time at the airport
- Do not carry heavy luggage; use a trolley

- Arrange a wheelchair if you have foot problems
- Ask for an aisle seat – walk up and down every half-hour to prevent swelling
- Do not get dehydrated – keep sipping water
- Wear shoes with adjustable fastenings
- Beware of trolleys pushed by other passengers in a hurry.

On arrival
- Hot sand and sharp rocks or broken glass can cause serious injuries. Wear plastic sandals on the beach and in the sea
- Use sun block or very high factor sunscreen or keep in the shade
- Apply cream to dry skin. Products containing urea are very effective for this if normal creams do not help.

First aid
- Take a small first-aid kit on holiday containing plasters, sterile dressings, bandage, tape and antiseptic cream
- Clean and cover all injuries, however slight
- Check them daily. Seek help if they get worse.

Holiday footwear
- Never wear new shoes on holiday. They may cause rubs
- If you have hospital shoes, continue to wear them on holiday
- Wear hose to prevent blisters.

In subtropical or tropical countries
- Backpackers with neuropathy should beware of rats. One of the authors' sons was woken in India by a rat nibbling his toes
- Use insect repellent and mosquito netting to avoid insect bites or stings.

PAINFUL NEUROPATHY

Presentation
The patient develops severe burning pain, worse at night, paraesthesiae and contact discomfort, sometimes rendering it impossible to wear normal clothing. Symptoms may also include interrupted sleep, restless legs, cramps, depression and weight loss. It may be precipitated by optimizing diabetic control or by periods of poor control.

Management

General approach
The patient should be reassured that the intense pain will improve within 2 years. The patient will not become crippled and will not come to an amputation. Sympathetic support is essential, and patients need regular appointments to monitor their pain and try new strategies if previous attempts at relieving pain are ineffective. It is essential to optimize diabetic control. Insulin may be needed. Hyperlipidaemia might be instrumental in the progression of peripheral neuropathy, and thus cardiovascular risk factors should be addressed.

Drugs
In the first instance, simple analgesics such as paracetamol should be tried. For disturbed sleep, hypnotics may be prescribed.

Anticonvulsants
Gabapentin and pregabalin are most frequently used. Gabapentin dosage can be rapidly increased over 7 days to reach 1800 mg as the maximum dose. In some cases, it may be necessary to increase to 3600 mg per day. Occasionally it causes somnolence and dizziness. However, it is generally well tolerated and has no significant interactions

with other drugs. The dosage should be reduced in renal failure. Pregabalin has a similar action to gabapentin with a similar side-effect profile. The dosage can be increased over 2 weeks from 75 mg b.d. to 300 mg b.d. The dosage should be reduced in renal failure. Carbamazepine, valproate and phenytoin may be useful in individual patients. Carbamazepine can be started at 100 mg once or twice daily and increased up to the maximum tolerated dosage (usually 800–1000 mg/day). Sodium valproate (100–500 mg one to three times daily) and phenytoin (100–400 mg one to two times daily) may be helpful.

Tricyclic antidepressants

Imipramine or amitriptyline may relieve burning pain. Therapy should commence with a low dose, gradually increased according to symptomatic response. Imipramine is slightly less effective than amitriptyline but has fewer side-effects. With imipramine, begin at 25–50 mg at night and increase by 25 mg increments on alternate days. The drug should be taken at night both for its relief of pain and for its sedative effect. Tricyclic antidepressants should be used with caution in patients with cardiac disease.

Serotonin and norepinephrine re-uptake inhibitors

Duloxetine hydrochloride at doses of 60–120 mg is effective in the management of neuropathic pain. It has antidepressant effects as well as analgesic effects.

Opioids

Initially, weak opioids, such as dihydrocodeine, may be given. If not helpful, tramadol is an opioid-like, non-narcotic analgesic, which can be prescribed at 50–100 mg at 4–6 h. It is useful either alone or with anticonvulsant therapy when it is used for breakthrough pain. If there is no response to tramadol or it cannot be tolerated, then sustained-release opioids can be used. Controlled-release oxycodone 10–60 mg daily has been effective orally in randomized, double blind, placebo-controlled studies. Alternatively, opioids may be delivered transdermally over 48–72 h through skin patches. These include fentanyl and buprenorphine patches.

Physical methods

Very simple techniques, such as wearing silk pyjamas or nylon tights under clothes, may relieve contact discomfort. A bed cradle holding the bedclothes off the legs may be helpful. Application of cold water may be soothing; some patients even keep a bucket of cold water by the bed in case they wake in pain.

Lidocaine patches have been shown to be as effective as pregabalin in reducing pain. The application of OpSite film to painful areas may reduce pain and contact discomfort. Transcutaneous electrical nerve stimulation machines can be used to block the pain.

Capsaicin is a topical cream which releases substance P, a peptide neurotransmitter involved in pain transmission. Acute release often causes transient burning followed by insensitivity to painful stimuli which lasts several hours. The analgesic effect can take up to 6 weeks to develop.

4

Managing Stage 3:
the ulcerated foot

PRESENTATION AND DIAGNOSIS

Despite screening and prevention, many diabetic patients develop skin breakdown and ulceration and also other active problems in the foot. A foot ulcer is an important sign of systemic disease, which leads to a 50% mortality of diabetic foot patients after 5 years.

In this edition, in addition to ulceration, we have also included in Stage 3 other active diabetic foot problems, such as Charcot osteoarthropathy (which is addressed at the end of this chapter), critical ischaemia, acute ischaemia and the renal ischaemic foot. For Stage 3 is the stage of intervention. It is a pivotal stage when the foot has escaped from preventative treatment and definitive action is required.

The main part of the chapter is devoted to the management of ulceration. A classification of ulcers has not been attempted, as it is necessary to assess each ulcer on its own merits and then plan a specific treatment. Nevertheless, it is essential to differentiate ulceration in the neuropathic foot from that in the ischaemic foot. Furthermore, ulcers commonly develop in the ischaemic foot when there is associated neuropathy, and this type of ischaemic foot is called the neuroischaemic foot and its ulcers called neuroischaemic ulcers.

Neuropathic ulcer

The neuropathic ulcer is usually painless, and the commonest site is the apex of the toe (Fig. 4.1). Ulceration can also occur over the dorsal

Managing the Diabetic Foot, Third Edition. Michael E Edmonds and Alethea VM Foster.
© 2014 John Wiley & Sons, Ltd. Published 2014 by John Wiley & Sons, Ltd.

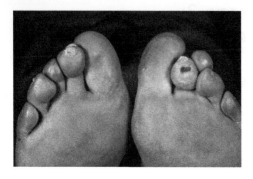

Fig. 4.1 Ulcer at the apex of a clawed second toe. The apex of the second toe on the contralateral foot shows neglected callus.

aspect of the toes due to the pressure of footwear on the flexed interphalangeal joint.

Callus often develops on the plantar aspect of prominent metatarsal heads. It is associated with fibro-fatty padding depletion and failure to remove the callus leads to ulceration (Fig. 4.2a and b). Removal of callus may often reveal ulcers (Fig. 4.3a and b). Ulcers on the plantar aspect of the heel are usually caused by acute trauma, in particular treading on foreign bodies.

On initial observation, a neuropathic ulcer may seem shallow. It is always important to probe an ulcer as this may reveal hidden depths (Fig. 4.4a and b), and also reveal a sinus down to bone suggesting osteomyelitis.

Neuroischaemic ulcer

Ulceration in the neuroischaemic foot usually occurs on the margins of the foot over a bony prominence. The first sign of ischaemic ulceration may be a red mark, which is difficult to see in dark skin. This then leads to formation of a bulla (Fig. 4.5). The bulla can develop into a shallow ulcer with a base of sparse pale granulations or yellowish closely adherent slough (Fig. 4.6). In ischaemia there is often a halo of erythema

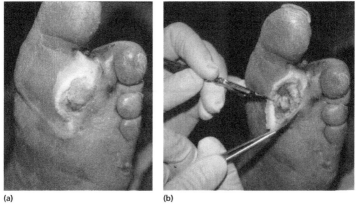

Fig. 4.2 (a) Callus over the forefoot has been left too long as it was not painful. (b) Debridement by the podiatrist reveals tissue breakdown – the birth of a neuropathic ulcer.

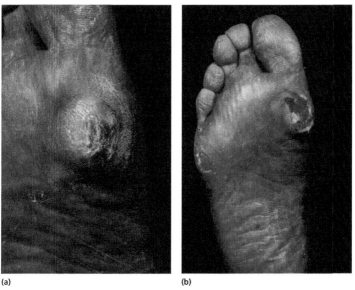

(a)   (b)

Fig. 4.3 (a) Heavy callus overlying neuropathic ulcer. (b) Callus has been removed to reveal neuropathic ulcer.

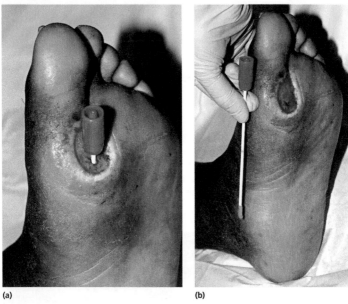

(a)   (b)

Fig. 4.4 (a) An apparently shallow ulcer but with deep track as shown by inserted wound swab. (b) The extent of the tracking is demonstrated by the length of wound swab that could be probed along the track.

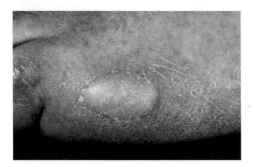

Fig. 4.5 Bulla on lateral margin of neuroischaemic foot.

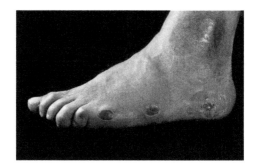

Fig. 4.6 New ischaemic ulcers resulting from bullae on lateral margin of foot.

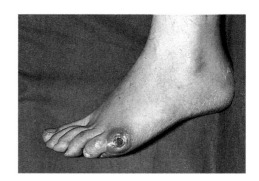

Fig. 4.7 An ischaemic ulcer on the margin of the foot with a halo of erythema.

around the ulcer (Fig. 4.7). Initially, pressure over bony prominences leads to partial thickness ulceration and eventually full-thickness ulceration with exposed tendon and bone.

Ulcers occur on the medial surface of the first metatarso-phalangeal joint (Fig. 4.8), over the lateral aspect of the fifth metatarso-phalangeal joint, but the commonest sites are the apices of the toes (Fig. 4.9) and also beneath toe nails if allowed to become overly thick (Fig. 4.10).

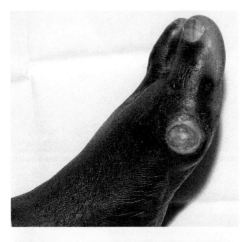

Fig. 4.8 Ischaemic ulceration over the first metatarso-phalangeal joint.

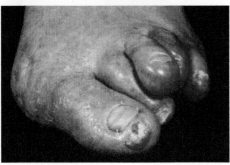

Fig. 4.9 Ischaemic ulceration on apex of first toe.

MANAGEMENT

All of the components of multidisciplinary management are important in Stage 3:

- Mechanical control
- Wound control
- Microbiological control

- Vascular control
- Metabolic control
- Educational control.

The aim is to heal ulcers within the first 6 weeks of their development. This is the time for aggressive management and is a window of opportunity that should be taken seriously.

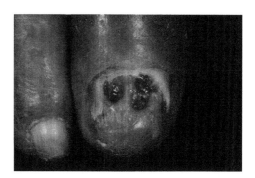

Fig. 4.10 Subungual ulcer. The nail had grown too thick. It is cut back to reveal the ulcer.

Mechanical control

Ideally, ulcers should be managed with rest and avoidance of pressure. However, total non-weight-bearing is rarely practical, and ambulatory methods have been developed.

In the neuropathic foot the overall aim is to redistribute plantar pressures, whereas in the neuroischaemic foot it is to protect the vulnerable margins of the foot. Thus, mechanical control will be considered separately in the neuropathic and neuroischaemic foot.

Neuropathic foot

The most efficient way to redistribute plantar pressure is by the application of some form of cast. If casting techniques are not available, temporary ready-made shoes with a cushioning insole can be supplied. These can take the form of dressing shoes or weight-relief shoes, and felt pads may also be used. General measures such as the use of crutches, wheelchairs and Zimmer frames may be necessary.

Heel ulcers will need specific off-loading techniques such as a pressure-relieving heel protector in bed or a pressure relief ankle foot orthosis (PRAFO).

When the neuropathic ulcer has healed, the patient should be fitted with a cradled insole and bespoke shoes to prevent recurrence. Occasionally, extra-depth, ready-made orthopaedic shoes with flat cushioning insoles may suffice in the absence of very high pressure areas.

Casts

Various casts are available, and their use is governed by local experience and expertise. Techniques include the removable cast walker such as Aircast, the total contact cast and the Scotchcast boot.

Removable cast walker

Prefabricated walking casts have become popular because of the potential problems with total contact casts. The Aircast (Fig. 4.11) is a bivalved cast and the halves are joined together with Velcro strapping. The Aircast is lined with four air cells which can be inflated with a hand pump through four valves to ensure a close fit. Care must be taken that the brace does not impinge on the borders of the foot. The removable cast can be simply adapted with a heat gun applied to the outer shell, which is then softened and bent out to accommodate deformity. Felt padding may be stuck on to the lining of a removable cast to off-load discrete areas.

Removable casts are supplied with flat-bed insoles which can be replaced by cradled insoles. As the name suggests the removable cast is removable, so patients can check their ulcers and remove the cast in bed. However, this very fact that makes the cast seem potentially safe also renders it unsuitable for those patients who may find it difficult to wear the cast continuously. The removable cast can be rendered irremovable (the 'instant total contact cast') by wrapping fibreglass tape around it, and this technique can be applied to other removable walking braces.

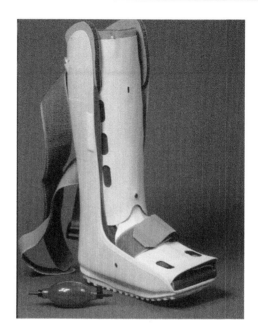

Fig. 4.11 Aircast.

Total contact cast

The total contact cast is an efficient method of redistributing plantar pressure. However, it is not without its complications and should be reserved for indolent plantar ulcers that have not responded to other treatments. Previously, plaster of Paris bandage was used, but now fibreglass casting tape is applied over minimal padding (Fig. 4.12).

The procedure is as follows:

• A layer of stockinette should be applied to the patient's lower leg. The length of the stockinette should be twice the distance from knee to toes and the excess should be gathered up over the knee and later folded down over the cast to cover any roughness. Cast padding is

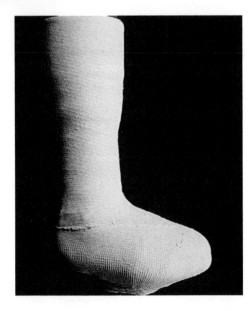

Fig. 4.12 Total contact cast.

placed between the toes to prevent rubs. The distal end of the stockinette is closed with tape, and any creases in the stockinette are cut out and taped flat

- Pieces of adhesive felt, 7 mm thick, are applied over bony prominences, including medial and lateral malleoli, and tibial crest (and a prominent tuberosity of the navicular or styloid process)

- A thin layer of cast padding is applied to the entire area below the knee, with thicker layers at the proximal end of the cast and the area over the toes as these are the areas where rubs most frequently occur

- Fibreglass casting tape is wrapped around the foot and leg starting 3 cm below the cast padding and rubbed gently on to the contours and then reinforced with several layers of fibreglass tape

- The excess stockinette which was gathered up over the knee at the beginning of the procedure is rolled down to cover the outer fibreglass layer. Rubbing the stockinette provides a smooth finish
- If the cast is applied to the neuropathic foot with a postoperative wound, it may be necessary to cut a window in the cast at the site of the wound in order to observe it closely.

Common mistakes are to make the cast too lightweight, to handle the fibreglass tape with the finger tips instead of the flats of the hands, or to apply the cast to a plantar-flexed foot. It is dangerous to enclose an insensitive foot in a closed cast without careful education of the patient. Patients should monitor their body temperature and blood glucose daily.

The instructions given to our patients are shown in Table 4.1.

Often there is rapid resolution of swelling once the leg is in the cast, which then may become loose on the patient's leg. Casts should be initially removed after 1 week for wound inspection. They should be then renewed and removed at regular intervals. Once the ulcer is healed,

Table 4.1 Instructions for patients fitted with a total contact cast.
Ring immediately:
If your temperature rises above 37.5°C
If your blood glucose rises above 15 mmol/L
If you feel unwell, tired, hot, shivery, with flu-like symptoms
If you feel pain or discomfort in your foot or leg
If your cast becomes loose, tight, stained, wet, soft, cracked or smelling badly
Never poke or pour anything down your cast
Never try to remove your cast yourself
Walk as little as possible

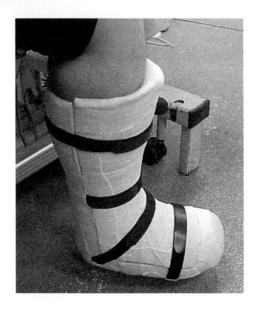

Fig. 4.13 Bivalved cast with Velcro strapping.

the patient should be assessed for cradled insoles and bespoke shoes but should remain in the total contact cast until the new shoes are ready. The patient will then be ready for rehabilitation as follows:

- A removable, bivalved cast should be made by cutting out the front of the total contact cast and then holding the two halves in place with a bandage or Velcro strapping (Fig. 4.13). However, the removable bivalved cast is less efficient than the total contact cast, and putting the patient into a removable cast may be an alternative to bivalving
- The patient may walk for a few steps each day in their new shoes and insoles around the house, but the rest of the time they should wear the removable cast
- Very gradually, the patient can build up the amount of time they spend in the shoes and decrease the time spent in the cast

- If blistering or ulceration occurs, the patient should return to the clinic at once
- The patient should ideally receive rehabilitation from the physiotherapist to build up wasted muscles.

Patients should not fly in total contact casts because of the danger of developing deep vein thrombosis. If the patient needs to travel by plane, then the total contact cast should be removed and the patient fitted with a removable cast for the journey.

Problems associated with total contact casting are showed in Table 4.2.

Scotchcast boot

This is a simple removable boot made of stockinette, felt and fibreglass tape which is effective in redistributing plantar pressure (Fig. 4.14). A large sock worn over the cast offers some protection to the toes. It is useful for patients with neuroischaemic feet or cast phobia.

Table 4.2 **Problems with casts.**
Risk of iatrogenic lesions (rubs, pressure sores, infections) which may be undetected
Cast often heavy and uncomfortable and reduces patient's mobility
Problems with knee, hip and spine due to leg length disparity. This can be prevented with a shoe raise on the contralateral side
Patient may not drive a car in a cast
The leg may develop immobilization osteoporosis
Danger of fracture and the development of a Charcot foot when coming out of a cast if patient walks too far too soon
A few patients develop a cast phobia and will not wear them. One of our patients borrowed the neighbour's electric saw and removed her cast (but fortunately not her leg)!

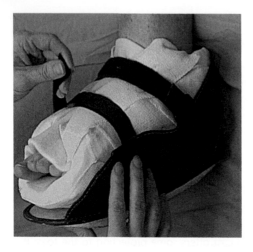

Fig. 4.14 Scotchcast boot.

The procedure is as follows:

- A layer of stockinette is applied to the lower limb from mid-calf to 10 cm distal to the toes
- Felt, 7 mm thick, is applied to the sole of the foot extending to the tips of the toes, up the back of the heel and up each side of the foot
- Cast padding is wrapped around the foot over the felt
- Overlapping strips of fibreglass tape cover the sole of the foot, and more fibreglass tape is wrapped around the foot
- Fibreglass is trimmed away below the malleoli, round the back of the heel and along the sides of the foot. The fibreglass covering the dorsum of the foot is lifted away
- The stockinette is folded back over the foot from both ends and the entire foot is wrapped in Elastoplast tape
- If a removable boot is required, the dorsal area is cut open, the raw edges are sealed with Elastoplast, a strip of felt is used as a protective tongue and the boot is held on with ready-made straps or Velcro fastening.

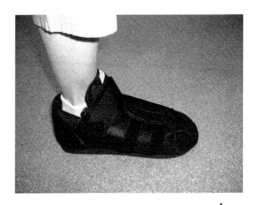

Fig. 4.15 Wound care shoe.

Temporary shoes

When it is not possible to provide a cast, ready-made temporary shoes with cushioning insoles that can accommodate dressings or weight-relief shoes may be helpful.

Dressing or wound care shoes

The Darco boot provides closed toe protection and room for bulky dressings. It can also be fitted with a cushioning insole (Fig. 4.15).

Weight-relief shoes

These take various forms according to the area of the foot which is off-loaded.

- The OrthoWedge shoe off-loads pressure from the metatarsal heads and toes using a rocker bottom wedge (Fig. 4.16)
- The Forefoot relief shoe transfers weight from forefoot to hindfoot with 10 degrees of dorsiflexion built into the shoe. A semi-rigid heel counter provides stability
- The HeelWedge shoe eliminates weight-bearing on the posterior end of the foot, which is put into a plantar-flex mode to facilitate

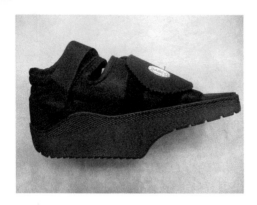

Fig. 4.16 OrthoWedge forefoot off-loading shoe.

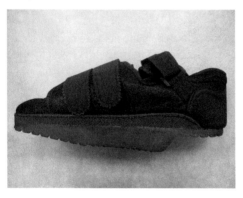

Fig. 4.17 HeelWedge off-loading shoe.

off-loading of the heel area. Weight is transferred from heel to mid-foot and forefoot (Fig. 4.17).

Felt padding
Semi-compressed adhesive felt padding is often used to divert pressures from ulcers but can prevent complications from being detected unless lifted regularly.

Crutches

Young patients with neuropathic ulcers may do well with crutches. However, patients with postural hypotension may be unsteady. Patients with neuropathy of the hands or Dupuytren's contracture may find hand-held crutches difficult to manage. Untrained patients can risk falls, especially on stairs, so crutches should always be fitted by a physiotherapist.

Knee scooters

This is an alternative to crutches, placing the weight of the body on the scooter's knee pad (Fig. 4.18).

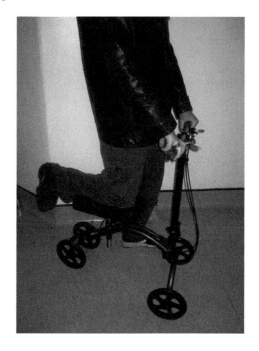

Fig. 4.18 Knee scooter.

Wheelchairs
A lightweight folding wheelchair can be of great help in achieving maximal off-loading.

Zimmer frames
Many patients who cannot cope with crutches find that a Zimmer frame is more helpful, being lightweight and providing more stability.

Electric carts and buggies
Small electrically powered carts and buggies with rechargeable batteries are used by diabetic foot patients with great success.

Cradled (or moulded) insoles
These are designed to be total contact insoles to redistribute weight-bearing away from the vulnerable pressure areas and at the same time provide a suitable cushioning. To make a cradled insole, a plaster cast is taken of the foot to represent its overall contours including the sole. The cast is filled with a foam to make a last, over which the insoles are moulded.

Fitting
An extra-depth orthopaedic stock shoe can sometimes accommodate a bespoke insole if the foot itself has a reasonably normal shape. Otherwise customized or bespoke shoes will be needed to accommodate the shape of the foot and to house cradled (moulded) insoles. A variety of polyethylene foams, microcellular rubbers and ethylene-vinyl acetates are used to construct cradled or moulded insoles, which are usually made of two or three layers of differing densities, with the most compressible layer at the foot–insole interface.

Materials
Closed-cell polyethylene foam (e.g. Plastazote):
- Easily mouldable
- Cushions
- Bottoms out.

Open-cell polyurethane rubber (e.g. Poron) or closed-cell synthetic rubber (e.g. Neoprene):
- Not mouldable
- Excellent shock absorption
- Good long-term resilience, will not bottom out
- Firm density.

Ethylene-vinyl acetate (EVA; e.g. Nora or Evalon range of different densities of EVAs):
- Mouldable
- Resilient
- Elastic.

Design

Various designs of cradled or moulded insoles are in use.

EVA insoles have a top layer of low-density EVA for cushioning, followed by two to four layers of medium-density EVA and a base layer of high-density EVA, the most dense and rigid layer acting as a cradle. Under particularly high pressure regions, areas of the insole can be excavated to form a 'sink' which is filled in with pressure-relieving material (Fig. 4.19).

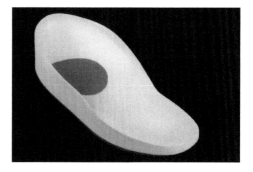

Fig. 4.19 Cradled insole with excavated sink filled with Neoprene to accommodate plantar deformity.

The Tovey insole uses a high-density Plastazote material for the cradle. Pressure areas are marked on this and these areas are cut away to be filled in with Neoprene cushioning. The insole is covered with an upper layer of Neoprene cushioning.

Alternatively, composite insoles can be made with an upper layer of low-density Plastazote and a lower layer of polyurethane rubber. Discrete areas of very high pressure can be compensated by insertion of 'sinks' of Poron into the Plastazote.

Neuroischaemic foot

Ulcers in the neuroischaemic foot usually develop around the margins of the foot. Many of these lesions are caused by a tight shoe or a slip-on style shoe which leads to frictional forces on the vulnerable margins of the foot. A 'high-street' shoe that is sufficiently long, broad and deep and fastens with a lace or strap high on the foot may be all that is needed to manage neuroischaemic ulceration (Fig. 4.20).

Alternatively, a ready-made stock shoe which is wide-fitting may be suitable. In the first instance, a temporary shoe such as a Darco boot may be used if dressings are bulky. Following healing, an extra-width orthopaedic stock shoe may be worn.

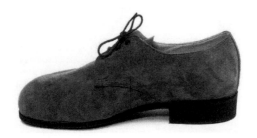

Fig. 4.20 A 'high-street' shoe suitable for an undeformed neuroischaemic foot.

Surgery as part of mechanical control

Diabetic neuropathic patients who present with ulceration often have deformity of the foot which has precipitated the initial ulceration. Such patients often need surgical debridement, decompression or excision of ulcers and in addition can benefit at the same time from surgical correction of the deformity. Previously, the standard approach was to accommodate such deformity in appropriate footwear, but it is now possible to correct the deformity surgically as well as heal the ulcers. The potential dangers of surgery on the ischaemic foot and possibility of triggering Charcot osteoarthropathy in the neuropathic foot were discussed in Chapter 3 and also apply to the Stage 3 foot. In the case of the ischaemic foot, revascularization should be considered before undertaking reconstructive surgery. The following techniques are available:

- Ulcer excision is a possible alternative to conservative pressure-relieving therapy. When indolent neuropathic ulceration develops over an underlying bony prominence, removal of bone and excision of the ulcer may enable the edges of the fresh surgical wound to be approximated. When this is not possible, local flaps may be used or the wound left to heal by secondary intention
- Procedures already discussed for correction of hammer toe, claw toe, mallet toe, metatarsal head resection and Achilles tendon lengthening can also be used to heal existing ulcers or prevent recurrence of ulcers. Fig. 4.21a and b shows, on X-ray, surgical correction of a prominent first metatarso-phalangeal joint due to plantar-flexed first ray deformity associated with osteomyelitis and ulceration under the first metatarsal head in a neuropathic foot
- Achilles tendon lengthening may relieve pressure over the forefoot
- Partial calcanectomy is useful when calcaneal bone can be probed in a heel ulcer.

Further details of these operations are described in the companion volume to this book: *A Practical Manual of Diabetic Foot Care*, second edition (Blackwell Publishing, 2008).

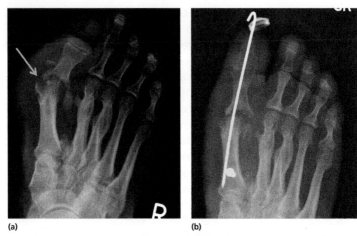

Fig. 4.21 (a) Destruction of first metatarsal head (arrow) associated clinically with ulceration under prominent first metatarso-phalangeal joint due to plantar-flexed first ray deformity. (b) Excision arthroplasty, dorsiflexion osteotomy of first metatarso-phalangeal joint and Kirschner wire.

Wound control

Wound control of the neuropathic and neuroischaemic ulcer is centred upon sharp debridement. This is probably the most efficient way to remove associated biofilm, which contains multiple bacterial species and forms polymicrobial communities.

Debridement

Neuropathic ulcer

Debridement is the most important part of wound control. It removes the cellular burden of dead and senescent cells. Ulcers also need maintenance debridement at repeated visits to the clinic to accelerate wound

Table 4.3 Rationale for the debridement of neuropathic ulcers.

Debridement removes callus, thus lowering plantar pressures. It enables the true dimensions of the ulcer to be perceived

Drainage of exudate and removal of dead tissue renders infection less likely

Debridement enables a deep swab to be taken for culture

Debridement encourages healing, restoring a chronic wound to an acute wound

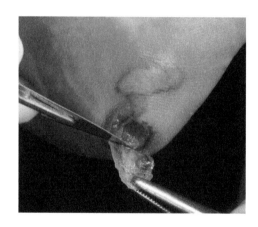

Fig. 4.22 'Scalpel and forceps' debridement technique.

healing. The rationale is described in Table 4.3, and the procedure is as follows:

• Remove all callus surrounding ulcer with a sterile scalpel
• Cut away all slough and non-viable tissue. It is helpful to grip the material to be cut with a pair of forceps and to apply gentle traction so that the material is under tension (Fig. 4.22) while it is being cut. It is almost impossible to remove moist slough with a scalpel blade unless this manoeuvre is performed. Dry gauze may be directly applied

to moist slough to remove moisture and thus render it easier to grip. The forceps are also useful for probing an ulcer to ensure its true dimensions

- Probe ulcer (if probe reaches bone, this is indicative of osteomyelitis – regard as Stage 4 foot)
- Take deep swab and tissue samples (not surface callus) and send for culture without delay
- Clean ulcer with sterile normal saline or with antiseptic such as Prontosan
- Apply sterile dressing held in place with light bandage – not too tight. Tubular bandage is useful
- Review at weekly intervals and repeat the procedure as maintenance debridement (but ensure the patient knows that if problems develop they should return to clinic immediately).

Outpatient debridement should be regarded as a minor surgical procedure. Control of cross-infection is important.

- Pre-prepared sterile packs contain a disposable instrument tray, sterile field, scalpel handle, blunt forceps and scissors. The contents of the packs are laid out on the top shelf of a two-storey trolley and sterile scalpel blades, dressings, saline and any other necessary materials are added as needed
- The bottom shelf of the trolley has dressings, conforming bandages, saline ampoules, tubular bandage and hypoallergenic tape. When the patient has left the clinical area, the patient's chair and trolley are cleaned with an antiseptic solution containing 2.1% sodium chlorite.

When a neuropathic ulcer has been present for more than 3 months without healing, despite regular debridement and good management, and where bone is exposed in the base of the ulcer, then surgical resection of underlying bone is probably the best way to achieve rapid healing.

Table 4.4 **Rationale for debridement of neuroischaemic ulcers.**
It enables the true dimensions of the ulcer to be perceived
Drainage of exudate and removal of dead tissue renders infection less likely
Debridement enables a deep swab to be taken for culture

Neuroischaemic ulcer

The rationale for debridement is described in Table 4.4, and the procedure is as follows:

- Vascular status should be quantified by measuring the ABPI before debridement. Only very cautious debridement should be performed if the foot is very ischaemic (ABPI <0.5)
- Some ischaemic ulcers develop a halo of thin glassy callus that dries out, becomes hard and curls up (Fig. 4.23a and b). It is necessary to smooth off these areas as they can catch on dressings and cause trauma to underlying tissue
- If the foot is very sensitive, it may be necessary to anchor the area being debrided with forceps while cutting takes place so as not to cause painful dragging of the scalpel blade through the slack tissues
- If a subungual ulcer beneath a thickened toe nail is suspected, the nail should be very gently cut back or layers of nail can be pared away with a scalpel to expose and drain the ulcer.

Supplementary techniques of wound control
Maggots (larvatherapy)

The larvae of the green bottle fly (*Lucilia sericata*) are sometimes used to debride ulcers, especially in the neuroischaemic foot. Sterile maggots should be obtained from a medical maggot farm (Fig. 4.24). Larvae can achieve atraumatic physical removal of necrotic material. Larvae produce secretions that have antimicrobial activity against Gram-positive cocci, including methicillin-resistant *Staphylococcus aureus* (MRSA).

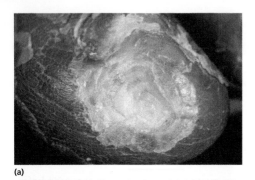

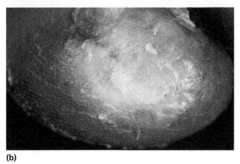

Fig. 4.23 (a) An ischaemic ulcer with halo of thin glassy callus. (b) The halo has been cut away without causing trauma.

Negative pressure wound therapy

Negative pressure wound therapy (NPWT) is commonly used to achieve closure of postoperative diabetic foot wounds (Fig. 4.25a–d). Debrided heel ulcers also often respond to NPWT. It is important to apply NPWT on wounds that have been thoroughly debrided and do not contain slough or necrotic tissue. The pump applies continuous negative pressure of 125 mmHg through a tube and foam sponge which are applied to the wound and sealed in place with a plastic film to create a vacuum. The sponge is replaced every 2 or 3 days. Exudate from the wound is sucked along the tube to a disposable collecting chamber. The NPWT stimulates

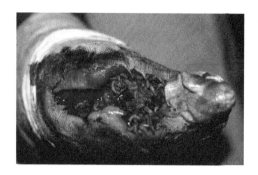

Fig. 4.24 Maggots in a wound.

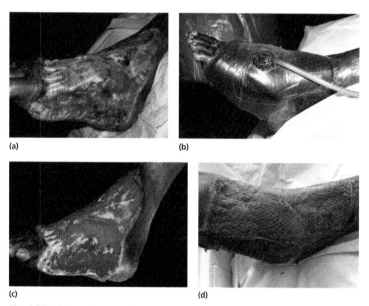

(a)

(b)

(c)

(d)

Fig. 4.25 (a) Extensive wound on dorsal and lateral aspect of left foot. (b) Negative pressure sponge shown before suction applied. (c) Wound granulating after negative pressure wound therapy. (d) Skin graft successfully applied.

granulation, which can form even over bone and tendon. Recently, installation tubes have been added to facilitate irrigation with wound chemotherapeutic agents. NPWT is increasingly used to treat postoperative wounds in the diabetic neuropathic foot and also in the ischaemic foot when it is especially useful if revascularization is not possible.

Skin graft

To speed the healing of ulcers which have a clean granulating wound bed, a split skin graft may be harvested and applied to the ulcer. The donor site is usually the thigh, and this is infiltrated with local anaesthetic. The graft is taken with a special knife, meshed and applied to the wound with sutures or clips. It is treated with NPWT for 5 days to prevent an accumulation of fluid beneath the graft site and then sprayed with iodine for a further 5 days (Fig. 4.26a). Careful follow-up of skin grafts will be needed (Fig. 4.26b) as plantar grafts often develop callus.

Hydrosurgery

It is possible to debride wounds using a high velocity stream of sterile saline. The Venturi effect creates a localized vacuum across the operating window, which simultaneously holds, cuts and removes tissue, while aspirating debris from the operating site (Fig. 4.27a and b).

Hyperbaric oxygen

Studies involving relatively small groups of patients have shown that hyperbaric oxygen accelerates the healing of ischaemic diabetic foot ulcers. Adjunctive systemic hyperbaric oxygen therapy has been shown to reduce the number of major amputations in ischaemic diabetic feet. In a recently performed double-blinded trial the healing of ischaemic diabetic foot ulcers was accelerated.

Dressings

Sterile, non-adherent dressings should cover all open diabetic foot lesions to protect them from trauma, absorb exudate, reduce infection

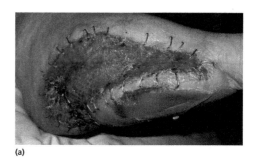

(a)

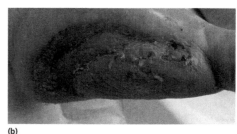

(b)

Fig. 4.26 (a) Partial-thickness skin graft sprayed with iodine and clips in situ. (b) Skin graft has contracted and wound has healed.

and promote healing. There is no hard evidence from large studies that any dressing is better or worse than any other. Also, we are not convinced that moist wound healing is particularly applicable to the diabetic foot. However, the following dressing properties are essential: ease and speed of lifting, ability to be walked on without disintegrating, good exudate control and prevention of drying out of the ulcer.

Dressings should be lifted every day to ensure that problems or complications are detected quickly, especially in patients who lack protective pain sensation. Dressings should be chosen according to the state of the wound. The types of dressings used in diabetic foot patients and their relevant features are described below.

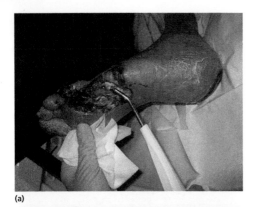

(a)

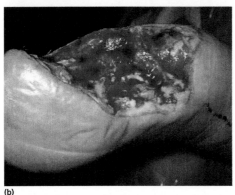

(b)

Fig. 4.27 (a) Versajet™ hydrosurgery used to debride sloughy wound. (b) Wound has progressed and is granulating well.

Wound contact dressings

- Simple non-adherent dressings consisting of polyester or viscose materials are useful. More recently available products include soft polymer dressings composed of a soft silicone polymer held in a non-adherent layer

- Low-adherence dressings are used as a primary dressing on lightly exuding or granulating wounds.

Absorbent dressings
- These are helpful for exudate control. They can be used as primary dressings and applied directly to the wound but also may be used as secondary absorbent layers in the management of heavily exuding wounds.

Hydrogels
- Consist of a starch polymer with 96% water
- Promote autolysis and debridement by rehydrating the wound
- Can absorb wound exudate
- May cause maceration
- Risk of changing dry necrosis into wet necrosis
- We do not favour moist wound healing in the diabetic foot and see no strong indication for hydrogel therapy.

Foams
- Hydrophilic polyurethane gel or silicone-film-coated foam
- Can absorb wound exudate
- Non-occlusive
- Non-adherent
- Bulky – may need specially roomy shoe to accommodate
- Conforms to contours
- Cushioning effect
- May be preformed for application to particularly difficult areas, such as the heel cup.

Alginates
- Non-woven composites of fibres from calcium alginate and a cellulose-like polysaccharide
- Highly absorbent

- The alginates form a gel when in contact with the wound surface which can be lifted off with dressing removal or rinsed away with sterile saline
- Drying out of dressing may prevent wound drainage and dessicate the wound bed
- Calcium alginate is a good haemostatic agent
- Daily removal is time consuming
- Not to be used on infected or necrotic wounds.

Hydrocolloids
- Composed of an absorbent hydrocolloid matrix on a vapour-permeable film or foam backing
- Designed to be left on for several days
- Daily changing prevents dressing from acting optimally
- Can be used only in patients with protective pain sensation
- Not for heavily exuding wounds.

Films
- Permeable to water vapour and oxygen but not to water or microorganisms
- Transparent, so wound inspection can be achieved without disturbing the wound
- Cannot absorb exudate, which will collect under the film and may irritate underlying tissue
- Should not be used on exuding, infected or necrotic wounds
- Rarely appropriate for diabetic feet.

Hydrophilic fibre dressings
- Non-woven pad or ribbon made of hydrocolloid (carboxymethylcellulose) fibres
- Absorb wound fluid and form a gel
- Non-adherent
- Conform to the wound

- Used on light–moderately exuding wounds
- Contra-indicated for dry eschar wounds.

Kerraboot

A transparent boot which allows easy inspection of the lower limb and free drainage of exudate from a wound.

- Enables easy inspection of the ulcer and lower limb
- Easy removal
- Rapid re-dressing.

Fastening dressings

- Hypoallergenic tape and tubular bandages are useful. Only small amounts of tape should be applied to the skin. Encircling the entire toe with tape should be avoided in case it swells
- Conventional bandaging may cause excessive tightness.

Topical therapy

Topical antimicrobial agents may benefit poorly healing wounds which have signs suggesting infection, such as friability of granulation tissue (see Chapter 5). These can be divided into antiseptics, antimicrobials, cleansing agents and oxidizers. They are available in several formulations, including dressings, ointments and sprays.

Antiseptics

Honey

Honey can be incorporated into sheet dressings or topical applications. Medical-grade Manuka honey has antibacterial properties. Honey facilitates autolytic and mechanical debridement.

Iodine

Iodine is effective against a wide spectrum of organisms in a variety of formulations, including solutions, alcoholic tinctures, powder sprays and impregnated dressings. At high concentrations, it can be toxic to human cells, but bacteria are more sensitive to these effects than human cells such as fibroblasts. Thus, iodine may be useful for antisepsis without impairing wound healing.

Two types of iodine are available – Povidone-iodine and Cadexomer iodine as a paste:

- Povidone-iodine is effective in antibacterial prophylaxis, particularly in burn patients
- Cadexomer iodine consists of microspheres formed from a three-dimensional lattice of cross-linked starch chains (cadexomers). It decreases bacterial load and has been used with success in the diabetic foot ulcer. Secondary dressing is required.

Silver

Silver versions of most dressing types are available that release silver ions which have antimicrobial properties against Gram-negative and Gram-positive organisms. *In vitro*, they are effective in killing *Staphylococcus aureus*, including MRSA, and *Pseudomonas* species. Silver sulphadiazine has been used in antibacterial prophylaxis in wounds and in skin graft donor sites.

Antimicrobial

Gentamicin

Gentamicin-impregnated collagen sponges have been recently used in the treatment of diabetic foot ulcers.

Mupirocin

Mupirocin is active against Gram-positive bacteria, including MRSA. To avoid the development of resistance, mupirocin should not be used for longer than 10 days.

Metronidazole

Topical preparations can be used to treat anaerobes and reduce odour from the wound.

Cleansing agents

Saline
Saline can be used as a wound cleansing agent. It does not interfere with microbiological samples and is not damaging to granulating tissue.

Prontosan
This is a useful cleansing agent. It contains betaine, an effective surfactant to penetrate, clean and remove wound debris and biofilm, and also poly-hexanide, a powerful antimicrobial agent that can reduce bioburden.

Oxidizers

Potassium permanganate
This is an oxidizing agent and liberates nascent oxygen. It thereby acts as a potent antiseptic agent against bacteria and fungi. The feet are soaked in potassium permanganate baths.

Hydrogen peroxide
Hydrogen peroxide can be useful in very necrotic and sloughy wounds.

Advanced wound-healing products
When ulcers do not respond to basic treatment, advanced products to facilitate wound healing may have to be put into practice. These are expensive treatments and should only be used when basic treatments have failed.

Advanced wound-healing products include:
- Growth factors
- Skin substitutes
- Extracellular matrix proteins
- Protease inhibitors
- Vaso-active compounds
- Platelet therapies and stem cells.

Growth factors

Various growth factors have been applied to diabetic foot ulcers, including platelet-derived growth factor (PDGF) and human epidermal growth factor.

PDGF is used in the form of a gel, and trials have shown significantly improved healing rates compared with controls. Increased rate of mortality secondary to malignancy has been observed in patients treated with 3 or more tubes of PDGF. Recombinant human epidermal growth factor has shown enhanced healing of chronic diabetic foot ulcers.

Skin substitutes

Dermagraft is a bioengineered living human dermis. It contains human fibroblast cells which are obtained from neonatal foreskin and cultivated on a three-dimensional polyglactin scaffold. Controlled trials have shown significant healing in neuropathic ulcers treated with Dermagraft.

Apligraf is a bioengineered, bilayered, skin substitute consisting of human fibroblasts embedded in bovine collagen and covered by human keratinocytes. Controlled studies have shown significantly increased healing rates in neuropathic ulcers.

Bilayered cellular matrix (BCM) is a porous collagen sponge containing co-cultured allogeneic keratinocytes and fibroblasts derived from human neonatal foreskin. In a multicentre, controlled, parallel-group pilot study, patients with chronic, diabetic, neuropathic foot ulcers were randomized to receive either standard care (moist saline gauze cover for up to 12 weeks ($n = 20$)) or active treatment ($n = 20$). By 12 weeks, 7 of 20 wounds (35%) treated with BCM showed complete healing compared with 4 of 20 wounds (20%) treated with standard care. Mean rates of wound closure were greater for BCM-treated wounds compared with standard care (1.8% per day versus 1.1% per day, $p = 0.0087$).

Extracellular matrix proteins

The extracellular matrix (ECM) plays an important role in tissue regeneration and is the major component of the dermal skin layer. Recognition of the importance of the ECM in wound healing has led to the development of wound products that aim to stimulate or replace the ECM. These tissue-engineered products consist of a reconstituted or natural collagen matrix that mimics the structural and functional characteristics of native ECM. A variety of animal- and human-derived products are available. A number of studies have been performed in patients with diabetes and lower extremity ulcers (foot, ankle or leg) using animal- and human-derived products which promote wound healing of diabetic foot ulcers compared with conventional treatments.

Products derived from animal sources

These products may consist of the tissue scaffold only such as Unite® BioMatrix Collagen Wound Dressing or may be combined with synthetic materials to create a composite product such as Integra® Bilayer Matrix Wound Dressing. This is a non-living, 2 mm thick matrix composed of chondroitin-6-sulfate and bovine type 1 collagen together with a semipermeable polysiloxane (silicone layer). It acts as a scaffold to facilitate the migration of macrophages, fibroblasts and lymphocytes to initiate angiogenesis from the dermal wound bed and to create granulation tissue for support of local tissue or a split skin graft.

OASIS® Wound Matrix is derived from the pig small intestine submucosa. This consists of a natural collagenous, three-dimensional ECM that acts as a framework for cytokines and cell adhesion molecules for tissue growth.

Products derived from human sources

Donated human cadaver skin (allografts) undergoes various processes to remove the cells and deactivate or destroy pathogens; examples include AlloDerm® Regenerative Tissue Matrix and Graftjacket® Regenerative Tissue Matrix. These provide a thin, fenestrated acellular matrix that supports regeneration of host tissue with a single application in most cases.

Hyaff is an ester of hyaluronic acid, which is a major component of the ECM. Hyaff-based autologous dermal and epidermal grafts derived from skin biopsy have shown increased healing in dorsal foot ulcers.

Protease inhibitors

Promogran is a protease inhibitor that consists of oxidized regenerated cellulose and collagen. It inhibits proteases in the wound and protects endogenous growth factor. In a 12-week study of 184 patients, 37% of Promogran-treated patients healed compared with 28% of saline-gauze-treated patients, a non-significant difference.

Vaso-active compounds

In a study of diabetic patients with peripheral arterial disease, there was a better ulcer outcome and a greater number of patients healed with intact skin or decreased ulcer area of 50% in the patients who were randomized to dalteparin, a low molecular weight heparin, compared with the placebo group ($p = 0.042$).

Platelet therapies and bone marrow cultured cells

Some preliminary work suggests that autologous platelet-rich plasma (a limited volume of plasma enriched in platelets that is derived from the patient's whole blood) and topically applied autologous bone-marrow cultured cells can heal human chronic wounds that are recalcitrant to other treatments.

Special wounds

In addition to the neuropathic and neuroischaemic ulcer, there are special wounds which need particular approaches to treatment:

- Decubitus ulcer
- Puncture wound
- Chemical and thermal traumatic wound
- Animal bites
- Iatrogenic ulcer
- Artifactual ulcer
- Malignant ulcer
- Ulcer overlying the Achilles tendon
- Bullae.

Decubitus ulcer

All patients with neuropathic or neuroischaemic feet are at risk of decubitus ulcers. These may develop after a period of illness or immobilization, after a severe hypoglycaemic episode, whilst resting on a trolley, or even on the operating table. The heels are particularly vulnerable sites.

The first sign of a heel sore is localized erythema. If pressure is not relieved, a blister develops which fills with serosanguinous fluid. The base of the blister becomes blue and then black. If pressure remains unrelieved, necrosis may develop (Fig. 4.28).

Heel ulcers can be off-loaded by a foam wedge, a PRAFO or heel protector. The latter has a built-in pillow-style cushioning which provides a soft support surface. It is easy to apply and stays on the patient's foot. It reduces foot rotation inside the boot (Fig. 3.1).

The PRAFO (Fig. 4.29) is a ready-made orthotic device that has a washable fleece liner with an aluminium and polypropylene adjustable frame and a non-slip walking neoprene base. It is used to relieve pressure over the posterior aspect of the heel and maintain the ankle joint in a suitable position. It is important to make sure that it does not rub and ulcerate very fragile skin, which is seen in some diabetic patients with ischaemia.

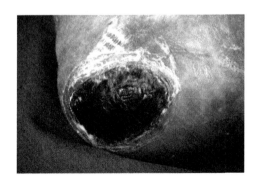

Fig. 4.28 Decubitus heel ulcer with necrosis.

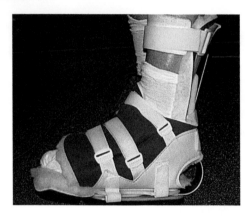

Fig. 4.29 The pressure relief ankle foot orthosis (PRAFO) relieves pressure on the back of the heel.

Regular turning and repositioning of immobile patients to relieve continuous local ischaemia over pressure points is crucial in the prevention and management of diabetic heel ulcers. Special pressure-relieving mattresses are also useful.

Puncture wound

These may appear as pinpoint injuries usually caused by a foreign body that may inoculate bacteria at the base of the injury (Fig. 4.30a and b). Puncture wounds can be very deceptive. Initial assessment reveals a very small break in the skin and often no signs of infection. However, there may be a nidus of infection at the base of the wound, which eventually reveals itself, as infection extends to the surface several days later. The foot should be X-rayed, but some objects, such as splinters of wood, are not radio-opaque. Ultrasound examination may then be useful. Any foreign body should be removed. Close follow-up is required and prophylactic antibiotics are advised.

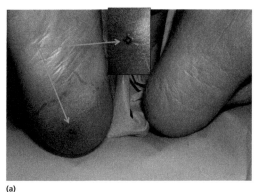
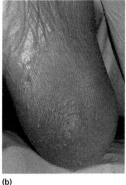

(a) **(b)**

Fig. 4.30 (a) Puncture wound (arrows) on plantar surface of heel with surrounding erythema. Green pen line shows initial extent of erythema which has progressed. Inset shows close up of puncture wound. (b) Healing wound with resolution of oedema.

Chemical and thermal traumatic wound

Chemical trauma may originate from proprietary remedies such as corn cure and callus removers, which contain strong acids, and from undiluted antiseptics applied directly to wounds.

Thermal traumas include burns from hot baths or showers, hot water bottles and electric blankets, hot sand on beaches, poultices, fires and radiators. Patients are also susceptible to cold trauma. Frostbite in diabetic patients who stay outside in wintry conditions (one patient worked in a meat market and stayed in a walk-in deep freezer for too long) can cause severe tissue damage.

Partial-thickness burns are allowed to heal by secondary intention. Extensive wounds need skin grafting. Full-thickness burns should be referred to specialist burn centres. These are very susceptible to infection and antibiotics are prescribed as for ulcers.

Animal bites

Dog, cat and rat bites and scratches, bee and wasp stings and insect bites may cause marked swelling and lead to ulceration. This may become secondarily infected.

Iatrogenic ulcer

Iatrogenic ulcers are caused by tape applied to atrophic skin and ripped off, by overtight bandages and by bulky dressings which are not accommodated properly in footwear. Ulcers can be caused by capillary blood samples taken from the toe instead of the finger, and severe and indolent ulceration can follow cortisone injections into the heel.

Artifactual ulcer

A very small minority of patients deliberately cause ulcers and prevent them from healing (Fig. 4.31). Most patients are young and female and may have a history of 'brittle diabetes' or eating disorders.

This is a difficult condition to treat, and involvement of a psychiatrist with a special interest in artifactual disorders may be useful. Patients are aware of what they are doing but have little insight into their motives. They injure themselves with impunity because of neuropathy. Tamper-free dressings or casts which cannot be removed by the patient may

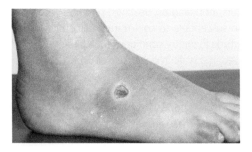

Fig. 4.31 Artifactual ulcer caused by application of lavatory cleaner.

provide the best opportunity for short-term healing, but the long-term outlook is bleak. Confrontation and admonishment are unhelpful as patients will just go elsewhere for their care.

Malignant ulcer

Melanoma
Any pigmented lesion which enlarges, develops satellite lesions or an irregular edge, erosions or ulceration may be a malignant melanoma. Some melanomas are not associated with pigment (Fig. 4.32).

Subungual melanoma
There is a brown to black band at a breadth of 3 mm or more with vari-egated borders. The hallux is most commonly involved, and there can be extension of pigment into the proximal or lateral nail fold.

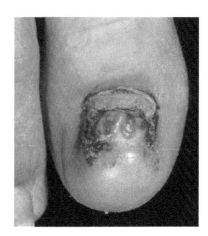

Fig. 4.32 Amelanotic malignant melanoma which is not pigmented.

113

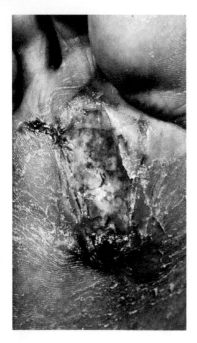

Fig. 4.33 Ulcer following application of a proprietary wart remedy which proved to be a squamous cell carcinoma.

Non-melanoma skin cancer

Squamous cell carcinoma may occasionally masquerade as an indolent diabetic foot ulcer (Fig. 4.33). Rarely, a basal cell carcinoma may develop in an indolent diabetic foot ulcer or scar from previous ulcer or surgery. All lesions suspected to be melanomas or skin cancer should be referred urgently to a dermatologist.

Ulcer overlying the Achilles tendon

This is a notoriously difficult site to heal. Ulceration is usually triggered by unsuitable footwear or from pressure in an immobile patient. When tendon is exposed in the base of the ulcer this may need to be surgically removed. NPWT can achieve granulation over the tendon.

Bullae

Bullae are superficial fluid-filled sacs that develop when the skin is traumatized. There is controversy over the procedure of de-roofing bullae. Our practice is to drain tense bullae and all bullae more than 1 cm in diameter.

Microbiological control

The Stage 3 patient is at great risk of infection as there is a clear portal of entry for invading bacteria. In the presence of neuropathy and ischaemia, the inflammatory response is impaired. The patient lacks protective pain sensation that would otherwise automatically force them to rest. This state of affairs is a recipe for disaster unless effective microbiological surveillance is carried out.

We use the following plan for neuropathic and neuroischaemic ulcers based on many years of clinical experience and significant amputation reduction.

- As clinical signs of infection can be greatly diminished in the diabetic foot, close attention is paid to the results of microbiological investigations which are undertaken after debridement, at the first visit and at each subsequent visit. All ulcers undergo sharp debridement to remove callus and slough. Ideally, a tissue specimen is collected for microbiology. It is sometimes difficult and painful to take a tissue specimen in the ischaemic foot, and a deep ulcer swab taken from the base of the wound is a suitable alternative. The cultures give an indication of the bacteria that are present. These bacteria may progress from colonization to active infection. Antibiotics are prescribed more readily for the neuroischaemic foot as untreated infection can lead rapidly to necrosis and major amputation

- Neuropathic ulcer: at the first visit, if the base of the ulcer is clean and a healthy pink colour, and there is no cellulitis, discharge or sinus present, then debridement, cleaning with Prontosan, application of dressing, off-loading and daily inspections will suffice
- Neuroischaemic ulcer: at the first visit, if the ulcer is superficial, oral amoxicillin 500 mg t.d.s. and flucloxacillin 500 mg q.d.s. to cover Gram-positive organisms are prescribed. (If the patient is penicillin allergic, clarithromycin 500 mg b.d. is prescribed. If the patient is taking a statin, then temporarily stop it and restart the day after clarithromycin treatment has finished.) If the ulcer extends to the subcutaneous tissue, then ciprofloxacin 500 mg b.d. or trimethoprim 200 mg b.d. to cover Gram negatives and metronidazole 400 mg t.d.s. to cover anaerobes are added to the above therapy
- The patient is reviewed within 1 week, together with the result of the ulcer swab
- If the neuropathic ulcer is healing well, treatment is continued without antibiotics
- If the ulcer has not improved and the swab is positive, the patient is treated with the appropriate antibiotic according to culture antibiotic sensitivities. In some cases of severe ischaemia, antibiotics are continued until the ulcer is healed.

At every patient visit, it is important to take an ulcer swab and examine for local signs of infection, cellulitis or osteomyelitis. If these are found, the patient has entered Stage 4 and action taken as in Chapter 5.

Vascular control

When a patient presents with an ulcer, it is important to establish whether the foot is ischaemic or not. This is decided by the presence or absence of palpable pulses. The diabetic ischaemic lower limb presents differently from a non-diabetic ischaemic limb. Often the patient has no history of claudication, and rest pain may be absent because of a coexisting neuropathy.

The modern approach to the ischaemic foot is to encourage early referral and prompt assessment with modern non-invasive investigations. This is best carried out in a diabetic foot clinic which can see the ischaemic patient without delay and investigate and treat in a joint diabetic foot/vascular surgical clinic which has rapid access to angiography and then angioplasty if indicated. If angioplasty is not possible, arterial bypass to the distal arteries, previously thought to be unduly risky with poor patency rate, has been shown to be an important part of diabetic limb salvage.

Scenarios of the diabetic ischaemic foot

The ischaemic foot includes the neuroischaemic foot, the critically ischaemic foot, acutely ischaemic foot and renal ischaemic foot. Infection often complicates the neuroischaemic foot and the combination of ischaemia and infection leads to necrosis in a 'diabetic foot attack'. In the critically ischaemic, acutely ischaemic and renal ischaemic foot, it is ischaemia itself that leads to necrosis and a 'diabetic foot attack'.

Neuroischaemic foot

This foot is characterized both by ischaemia from narrowing of leg and foot arteries and by neuropathy that predisposes to ulceration. The perfusion pressure may be adequate enough to preserve the tissues intact in the absence of trauma and ulceration but cannot be increased sufficiently to heal an ulcer if it develops.

Critically ischaemic foot

Ischaemia is so severe that the integrity of the tissues of the foot is compromised by a global reduction in limb perfusion. Pain may be present in the foot, although this depends on the degree of ischaemia and neuropathy. This pain is relieved by hanging the foot over the side

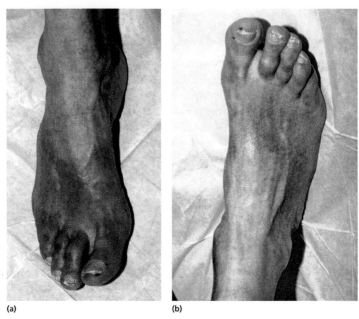

(a)   (b)

Fig. 4.34 (a) Critical ischaemia with rubor of foot on dependency. (b) Foot becomes pale on elevation.

of he bed. The skin is shiny and taut. The foot is red on dependency and becomes pale on elevation (Fig. 4.34a and b). The critically ischaemic foot will progress eventually to localized areas of ulceration and necrosis and become directly a Stage 5 foot.

Acutely ischaemic foot

There is sudden onset of pallor, paraesthesiae, numbness and eventually paralysis and the foot becomes extremely cold. The severity of pain will depend on the degree of neuropathy.

Renal ischaemic foot

This foot is characterized initially by digital tissue loss that seems to develop spontaneously and then proceeds to necrosis in a patient with renal impairment.

Assessment of ischaemia

Initially the ABPI should be measured, supplemented by assessment of the Doppler waveform. Further tests, such as measurement of transcutaneous oxygen tension and toe pressure, may be helpful to decide when to perform invasive investigations with a view to revascularization.

Ankle Brachial Pressure Index

If arteries are calcified, ABPI may be artifactually raised but the test is still important as long as one understands its interpretation.

Thus, if the ABPI is 0.5, then it is low and indicates severe ischaemia, whether the foot arteries are calcified or not. Indeed, if it is calcified, the true ABPI may be lower. In critical ischaemia, the ankle pressure is usually less than 70 mmHg.

However, one should always pay attention to the Doppler waveform, either in audible or visible form. The normal waveform is pulsatile (Fig. 4.35a) with a positive forward flow in systole followed by a short reverse flow and a further forward flow in diastole, but in the presence of arterial narrowing the waveform shows a reduced forward flow and is described as damped (Fig. 4.35b).

Transcutaneous oxygen tension

This measurement is a non-invasive method for monitoring arterial oxygen tension and reflects local arterial perfusion pressure. It is measured on the dorsum of the foot. A reading below 30 mmHg indicates critical ischaemia, but levels can be falsely lowered by swelling and cellulitis. Levels between 30 and 50 mmHg indicate moderate ischaemia. A level above 50 mmHg is associated with healing.

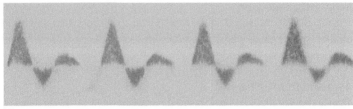

(a)

(b)

Fig. 4.35 (a) Doppler waveform from normal foot showing normal triphasic pattern. (b) Doppler waveform from neuroischaemic foot showing damped pattern.

Toe pressure

A toe pressure below 30 mmHg is consistent with critical ischaemia. Values between 30 and 50 mmHg indicate moderate ischaemia.

Vascular intervention

The degree of ischaemia is thus assessed both clinically and with non-invasive haemodynamic investigations. However, there is no complete consensus on the haemodynamic criteria to differentiate the neuroischaemic, the critically ischaemic and acutely ischaemic foot, and these are essentially diagnoses made from clinical examination and the Doppler waveforms.

Imaging the arteries of the lower limb

Visualization of the lower limb arteries is a crucial first step. Duplex ultrasound, computed tomography angiography (CTA) and magnetic resonance angiography (MRA) are used to image the lower limb arterial vessels of diabetic patients. The acutely ischaemic foot needs immediate imaging, and the critically ischaemic foot requires urgent imaging within 24–48 h. The neuroischaemic foot should be imaged as soon as possible, but usually within 1 week.

Duplex angiography
Duplex angiography combines the features of Doppler waveform analysis with ultrasound imaging to produce a picture of arterial flow dynamics and morphology (Fig. 4.36). The Duplex angiogram will show sites of arterial disease from the iliac arteries downwards.

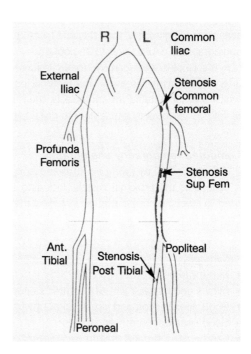

Fig. 4.36 Print-out of Duplex examination showing stenoses in the left common femoral artery, superficial femoral (Sup Fem) artery and posterior tibial (Post Tibial) artery.

Advantages:
- No radiation used
- Avoidance of contrast
- Portability
- Well tolerated
- High spatial resolution
- Demonstrates vessel wall as well as lumen.

Disadvantages:
- User dependent with inter-observer variability
- Vessels obscured by calcified plaque
- Difficult to appreciate overall anatomy.

If the Duplex indicates stenoses or occlusions which are considered suitable for angioplasty, then the next investigation is digital subtraction angiography (DSA) leading to angioplasty.

If the Duplex angiography reveals lesions at the common femoral artery or extensive disease in the femoral, popliteal and tibial regions, which are not suitable for angioplasty, then further imaging with CTA or MRA is performed with a view to distal bypass surgery.

Computed tomography angiography

CTA is performed by giving an intravenous injection of contrast agent; it delineates the proximal vessels, including the aorta. It can also be used to assess the distal arteries, including the patency of arterial grafts (Fig. 4.37).

Advantages:
- Non-invasive
- Allows good assessment of eccentric stenoses
- Good opacification and visualization of vessels distal to occlusion
- Good visualization of iliac arteries
- Can be used in patients with pacemakers.

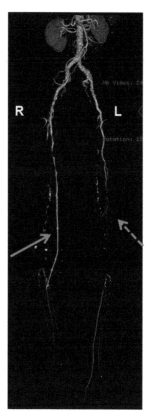

Fig. 4.37 CT angiography. On the right there is a superficial femoral artery to posterior tibial artery bypass graft (arrow), which is stenosed proximally but graft remains patent. There are stenoses of the origins of the peroneal and tibial vessels. On the left there is occlusion of the distal superficial femoral artery as it exits Hunter's canal (broken arrow) with several small collaterals present at this level. Flow reconstitutes distally at the level of the tibial and peroneal arteries, immediately distal to the trifurcation.

Disadvantages:

- Requires use of radiation and iodinated contrast
- Calcification, often seen in diabetic patients, can cause overestimation of stenosis.

Magnetic resonance angiography

There are two techniques of MRA:

- Time-of-flight MRA is dependent on a non-contrast enhanced flow-sensitive magnetic resonance sequence. It is slow, lasting up to 2 h, to cover the area from the bifurcation of the aorta to the distal lower extremity.
- Gadolinium-enhanced MRA involves an intravenous injection of gadolinium contrast and a fast imaging that follows the passage of the contrast bolus through the arteries. It is much less nephrotoxic than conventional contrast (Fig. 4.38a and b).

Advantages:

- No need for an intra-arterial catheter
- Nephrotoxic contrast can be avoided
- Non-invasive
- No radiation involved.

Disadvantages:

- Metallic implants and pacemakers are contraindications
- Claustrophobia
- Risk of contrast-related nephrogenic systemic fibrosis in patients with low glomerular filtration rate (GFR) of less than 30 mL/min
- Longer image acquisition time than CTA.

Angiography and angioplasty

If Duplex ultrasound reveals lesions that are deemed suitable for angioplasty then patients proceed to DSA, which permits clear visualization of vascular structures by subtracting superimposed bone and soft-tissue densities and angioplasty. In the rare cases of iliac disease, further imaging may be necessary either by retrograde femoral angiography or by MRA.

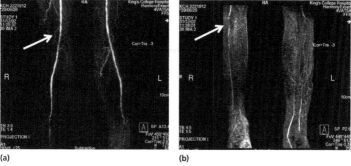

Fig. 4.38 (a) Magnetic resonance angiography. There is diffuse atheromatous disease of both superficial femoral arteries with an area of focal narrowing at the mid-level on the right (arrow). Both popliteal arteries are severely diseased. (b) On the right there is a single vessel, the anterior tibial artery, extending to the level of the plantar arch and it is severely diseased in the proximal aspect (arrow). There is reconstitution of the posterior tibial artery at ankle level. On the left there is an occlusion of the tibio-peroneal trunk with collaterals filling the more distal anterior and posterior tibial arteries.

Transfemoral angiography

Angiography is a safe procedure with few complications. Pre-procedure investigations should include:

- Full blood count, including a platelet count
- Blood coagulation indices
- Serum electrolytes, creatinine and estimated GFR (eGFR)
- Blood grouping.

Metformin may aggravate renal failure induced by contrast media. Patients taking metformin should stop this 2 days before the procedure and restart 2 days after, or when renal function returns to normal.

All patients should have their renal function assessed prior to angioplasty. Patients with chronic renal insufficiency have been shown to be protected against contrast-media-induced renal nephropathy by administering acetylcysteine. Although not strictly evidence based, acetylcysteine can be used in patients with significant baseline renal dysfunction, namely GFR less than 45 mL/min. Acetylcysteine should be prescribed at 600 mg orally b.d. for 1 day pre-procedure and 1 day post-procedure. It is important to keep the patient well hydrated. Renal function should be rechecked 24 h post-procedure.

Blood coagulation indices should also be measured. If the patient is on warfarin then it must be stopped at least 3 days prior to the procedure and the patient changed to fractionated subcutaneous heparin, or if the GFR is less than 20 mL/min then unfractionated heparin should be given intravenously. The unfractionated heparin infusion is stopped 2 h before the procedure and the fractionated heparin the night before.

Insulin-dependent patients are placed first on the list in outpatient angiography and have their insulin after the procedure is finished. Blood glucose in patients admitted to hospital can be controlled with sliding-scale intravenous insulin pump and intravenous 10% glucose.

Post-angiography, patients should be monitored closely, recording blood pressure and pulse. With the modern use of narrow-gauge catheters, bleeding from the femoral artery injection site is now extremely uncommon.

In the unlikely event of bleeding, the pulse rate may not respond in the usual way to loss of intravascular volume because of autonomic neuropathy; therefore, tachycardia may not be present. However, blood pressure will drop and an urgent blood count together with cross-matching for at least six pints of blood should be performed. Full resuscitation should immediately be carried out with haemodynamic monitoring. Most cases of bleeding resolve with blood replacement and tamponade themselves off spontaneously. A mass may become palpable in the lower abdomen, but this may not appear until 5–6 hours after the procedure. Continued hypotension despite adequate blood replacement is an indication for surgical exploration.

Angioplasty

Considerable advances have been made to establish angioplasty as the initial approach to revascularization. Two techniques are described: percutaneous transluminal angioplasty (PTA) and subintimal angioplasty, when a wire is put in a false lumen and then re-enters the true lumen. Angioplasty is tolerated well and can be carried out in very elderly patients. Advances have included novel dedicated steerable guide wires and long, small-diameter, balloon-tipped catheters such that stenoses and occlusions in tibial and plantar arteries can be treated (Fig. 4.39a–e).

One problem associated with angioplasty is restenosis. In this event, angioplasty is easily repeatable to achieve straight-line flow to the foot. However, recently, drug-eluting balloons that deliver antiproliferative agents such as Paclitaxel have been used to dilate stenoses and reduce the rate of restenosis. Also, as well as balloons, stents have been used to treat stenoses and occlusions. Both self-expanding and balloon-expandable stents are available in bare metal or fabric-covered types, the latter acting as a barrier to prevent the ingrowth of intimal hyperplasia. Also, drug-eluting stents have led to improved patency in stenosed infra-popliteal arteries and arterial graft stenoses (Fig. 4.40a and b).

In suitable patients it is now possible to carry out transfemoral angiography and angioplasty as an outpatient procedure. A small-bore needle is used, and after the procedure the puncture site is closed by a special 'Perclose' technique, which is a suture-mediated closure of the arterial access site. This allows the patient to sit up after 2 h and to walk in 4 h.

Contraindications to day-case angiography include:
- Myocardial infarction/cerebrovascular event within last 6 months
- Severe cardiac/respiratory disease
- Major surgery within the last month
- Warfarin therapy
- Renal failure.

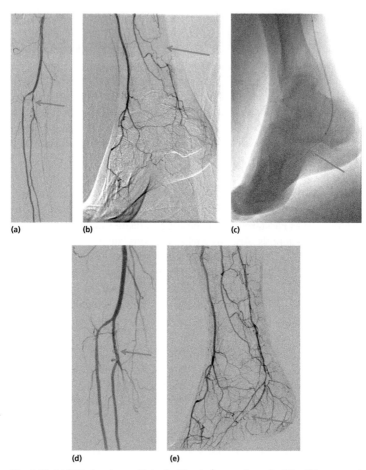

(a)   (b)   (c)

(d)   (e)

Fig. 4.39 (a) DSA showing multiple significant stenoses (arrow) of the tibio-peroneal trunk. (b) The posterior tibial artery (arrow) is heavily diseased with multiple critical stenoses and occlusions. (c) Guide wire (arrow) inserted to posterior tibial artery. (d) Tibio-peroneal trunk (arrow) has been angioplastied. (e) Posterior tibial artery recanalized by angioplasty to the medial plantar arch (arrow).

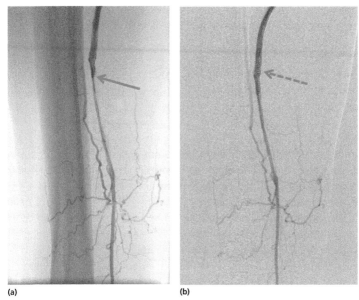

(a)   (b)

Fig. 4.40 (a) Femoral angiography showing severe stenosis of calcified posterior tibial artery (arrow) distal to a graft anastomosis. (b) The tight stenosis was crossed with a guide wire and a drug-eluting stent was placed across the distal anastomosis and posterior tibial artery distal to the anastomosis (broken arrow). This resulted in significant improvement in flow through the graft and posterior tibial artery distal to graft.

Arterial bypass

If lesions are too widespread for angioplasty then arterial bypass may be necessary. However, this is a major, sometimes lengthy, operation and is not without risk. It is more often reserved to treat extensive tissue destruction that cannot be managed without the restoration of pulsatile blood flow to the foot (see Chapter 6). However, in some patients, angioplasty may not be technically feasible. Arterial surgery will be needed for disease of the common femoral artery and long occlusions of the superficial femoral artery, popliteal and tibial arteries.

Distal bypasses are more successful if they are relatively short and are carried out from the popliteal region to the ankle or foot. Thus, in cases of femoral and tibial disease, hybrid procedures involving initially angioplasty above the knee and a distal bypass below the knee are performed.

Pain relief

In general, the neuroischaemic foot is not painful; however, in a few cases when neuropathy is mild the patient suffers pain from the ulcer as well as rest pain, particularly at night.

- An opioid such as dihydrocodeine, alone (30 mg every 4–6 h) or in combination with a non-opioid analgesic – paracetamol, to constitute co-dydramol (dihydrocodeine 10 mg, paracetamol 500 mg, two tablets every 4–6 h) – may be useful in moderate pain
- Tramadol (50–100 mg every 4–6 h) is an opioid derivative, which is often less sedating and less constipating than codeine
- Tricyclic antidepressants, for example dothiepin 50–100 mg at night, are useful at relieving rest pain in bed.

When pain is severe, it is important to give regular morphine therapy. The initial dose of modified-release preparations, devised for twice-daily administration, is 10–20 mg every 12 h if no other analgesic or paracetamol has been previously prescribed. However, if it is replacing a weaker opioid analgesic, for example co-dydramol, the initial dose should be 20–30 mg every 12 h. The doses should be gradually increased but the frequency kept at every 12 h. If breakthrough pain occurs between the 12-hourly doses, then morphine, as oral solution (Oramorph 5–20 mg every 4 h) or standard formulation tablets such as Sevredol 10–50 mg every 4 h, can be given. An opioid derivative, oxycodone, is useful in relieving moderate to severe pain. A further approach is to use skin patches containing opioids which are delivered transdermally and can last from 48–72 h. These include fentanyl and buprenorphine patches.

- When using any opioid-like drugs, beware of respiratory depression, to which diabetic patients with autonomic neuropathy can be susceptible
- Also, opiates will be retained by patients in renal failure, often leading to drowsiness
- It is preferable to avoid non-steroid anti-inflammatory drugs and cyclo-oxygenase-2 inhibitors as they may cause renal impairment and worsen cardiac function, leading to congestive heart failure
- If patients do come to major amputation, then a lumbar epidural block with bupivacaine should be started 48 h beforehand to relieve perioperative pain.

Metabolic control

It is important to make sure that there is no systemic, metabolic or nutritional disturbance to retard healing of the ulcer.

The patient needs the following assessments and treatment:

- Full blood count to exclude anaemia
- Serum electrolytes, serum creatinine and eGFR to assess renal function
- Liver function tests to obtain baseline of liver enzymes before starting possible antibiotic therapy and to measure serum albumin as an indicator of nutrition (<3.5 g/L indicates malnutrition and dietary advice should be obtained)
- Wound healing and neutrophil function are impaired by hyperglycaemia, which should be controlled as tightly as possible. Type 2 patients on oral hypoglycaemic therapy with suboptimal control that cannot be corrected should be started on insulin
- Hyperlipidaemia, hypertension and smoking should be actively treated. Patients with neuroischaemic ulcers should be on statin therapy as well as antiplatelet therapy. Patients who are older than 55 years and

have peripheral vascular disease should also benefit from an angiotensin-converting enzyme inhibitor to prevent further vascular episodes (as indicated by the Heart Outcomes Prevention Evaluation (HOPE) study)

- When managing hypertension in the presence of leg ischaemia, it is important to achieve a fine balance between maintaining a pressure that improves perfusion of the ischaemic limb while reducing the blood pressure enough to limit the risk of cardiovascular complications. However, beta-blockers, such as bisoprolol, have been shown to increase survival in cardiac failure and are not contraindicated in patients with neuroischaemic feet

- Many patients with diabetic foot problems will have evidence of cardiac failure. Aggressive treatment with angiotensin-converting enzyme inhibitors, diuretics, beta-blockers and aldosterone antagonists will improve tissue perfusion and also reduce swelling of the feet

- Renal impairment may also be present, and it is important to control fluid balance. These patients are very susceptible to dehydration. A short period of nausea and vomiting may lead to significant renal impairment and patients will need urgent replacement with intravenous fluids. These patients have very little renal reserve, and infection also leads to deterioration of renal function. Just as these patients are susceptible to dehydration and pre-renal failure, they are also liable to go rapidly into fluid overload by the administration of excess intravenous fluids. This will lead to peripheral oedema, which impairs healing.

Educational control

Patients who lack protective pain sensation need to know that foot ulcers are an important problem but that they will heal with optimal care. The following educational material – aimed directly at patients – seeks to clarify common misconceptions about ulcers and their management. It is important to judge how much information the patient can take on board to allow maximum cooperation between patient and the diabetic foot team. This is difficult in patients with psychiatric disease and cognitive disabilities, when the approach must be specifically tailored to the patient.

Patient information

Foot ulcers
- Foot ulcers can be a very serious problem. It is essential to heal them quickly
- Nerve damage from diabetes can reduce pain; therefore, a foot ulcer may not be painful, so it is easy to ignore. Most serious health problems are painful or make patients feel ill. By the time a foot ulcer hurts or gives symptoms of illness it has seriously damaged your foot
- To give your ulcer the best chance of healing quickly, please follow this advice.

Rest
- When you walk, every step is like hitting your ulcer with a hammer. It helps to use crutches, a Zimmer or a wheelchair to take the weight right off your ulcer
- Special shoes and insoles, plaster casts or removable braces can take the load off your foot if it is essential for you to walk a little.

Treating your ulcer
- Ulcers gather debris and dead tissue around them, and some develop hard skin
- Unless ulcers are cleaned by cutting away all the debris and hard skin, they can become choked and they will not heal quickly
- It can be helpful to clean up the edges until they bleed a little. This gives the ulcer a fresh start. You should never try to do this for yourself; it is the job of the doctor or podiatrist.

(*Continued*)

Dressings
- Keep your ulcer covered by a dressing to keep it clean and warm
- It will need a quick check every day to be sure it is healing well and not infected.

Danger signs
These are the danger signs and the questions you must always ask yourself when checking your foot:

1 Swelling – has your shoe become tight?
2 Colour change – is there redness of the skin around the ulcer? Are there bluish marks like bruises or is the skin going black?
3 Has the ulcer itself changed colour?
4 Discharge – has your ulcer become wet where it was dry before? Is there blood or pus discharging from it?
5 Have you developed any new ulcers or blistering?
6 Has your ulcer become painful or uncomfortable or is your foot throbbing?
7 Do you feel unwell with fever, flu-like symptoms or poorly controlled diabetes?
- If the answer to any question is yes, then the foot should be checked the same day either by your doctor or the diabetic foot clinic
- If you cannot reach your feet or see them clearly, ask your family or a friend to help you with checking and dressing your foot ulcer, or your doctor can ask a nurse to help you.

CHARCOT OSTEOARTHROPATHY

This is an acute osteoarthropathy, with bone and joint destruction that occurs in the neuropathic foot. It commonly presents in the midfoot but also occurs in the forefoot and hindfoot. The prognosis for the hindfoot is much more serious, with a high risk of instability of the ankle. However, with a modern approach, embracing rapid diagnosis and early intervention, many Charcot feet can be healed and deformity prevented.

It is extremely important to have a high index of suspicion when a patient presents with a hot, swollen foot. There may be a history of minor trauma such as tripping, twisting the ankle or walking over rough surfaces such as cobbles. About 30% of patients complain of pain or discomfort. Rarely, pain may be very severe. Charcot osteoarthropathy may follow injudicious mobilization after surgery, a period of bed rest or casting.

Patients who develop Charcot osteoarthropathy usually have evidence of a peripheral neuropathy, autonomic neuropathy and a good blood supply to the lower limb. Diabetic patients with renal transplants have an increased risk of Charcot osteoarthropathy. Rarely, in diabetes, the knee and wrist can also be affected by Charcot osteoarthropathy.

Charcot osteoarthropathy can be divided into two phases:
- Active phase
- Non-active phase.

Early presentation of active Charcot osteoarthropathy

This is characterized by unilateral erythema and swelling (Fig. 4.41). The foot is at least 2°C hotter than the contralateral foot as measured with a skin thermometer. When patients present early in the acute active phase, the X-ray may be normal. Further investigations are then necessary. Initially, a technetium methylene diphosphonate bone scan can detect early evidence of bone damage by demonstrating focal areas of increased uptake of radionuclide. Recently, single-photon emission computed tomography (SPECT) together with conventional computed

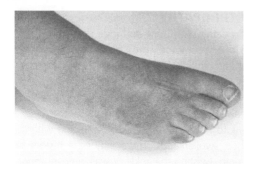

Fig. 4.41 Swelling and erythema in acute onset Charcot osteoarthropathy.

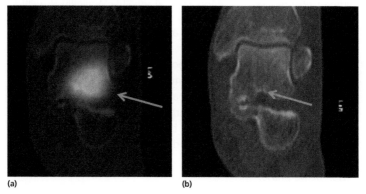

(a)   (b)

Fig. 4.42 (a) SPECT/CT showing fusion of SPECT and CT images revealing increased radionuclide uptake in the talus (arrow). (b) CT shows fracture (arrow) of talus as cause of increased radionuclide uptake.

tomography (CT) known as SPECT/CT, can be carried out in addition to the conventional bone scan (Fig. 4.42a and b). If positive, then a magnetic resonance imaging (MRI) examination will portray in more detail the nature of the bony damage, including bone oedema (Fig. 4.43a and b). Patients awaiting these investigations should be treated as if the diagnosis has been confirmed.

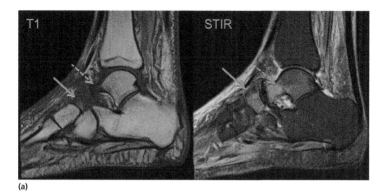

(a)

(b)

Fig. 4.43 (a) MRI: T1 sequence shows reduced signal in the talus (broken arrow) and navicular (arrow) bones. STIR sequence shows increased signal in the talus (broken arrow) and navicular (arrow) indicating bone marrow oedema. (b) MRI: T1 sequence shows improved signal in the talus (broken arrow) and navicular (arrow) bones. STIR sequence shows minimal signal in the navicular (arrow) and reduced signal in the talus (broken arrow), demonstrating partial resolution of previous bone oedema.

Differential diagnosis of active Charcot osteoarthropathy

It is important to differentiate between the red, hot, swollen appearance of Charcot osteoarthropathy and the red, hot, swollen cellulitic foot. Cellulitis is more likely in the presence of an ulcer, which may show typical signs of infection. Infection severe enough to cause generalized redness, warmth and swelling will usually cause local signs such as discolouration of the wound bed and discharge from the ulcer.

The swelling of Charcot osteoarthropathy responds more rapidly to elevation than does that of the infected foot. In a recent series of 25 Charcot feet with acute presentation, CRP was normal in 47% of the cases and only moderately elevated in the remainder. However, infection and Charcot osteoarthropathy can sometimes be present concurrently in the same foot. If in doubt, treat for both. Gout and deep vein thrombosis may also masquerade as Charcot osteoarthropathy but can be excluded by measurement of serum uric acid (which is usually raised in gout) and Duplex vein scan.

Late presentation of active Charcot osteoarthropathy

In the late presentation, deformity can present in the forefoot, midfoot, hindfoot and ankle. This is accompanied by swelling, warmth, and a temperature 2°C greater than the contralateral foot. Advanced radiological changes show fragmentation, fracture, new bone formation, subluxation and dislocation. These often develop very rapidly, within a few weeks of the onset, and sometimes within a few days.

A specific forerunner to the development of joint disruption in the Charcot foot is fracture. This can occur painlessly in the neuropathic foot. However, neuropathic fractures may precipitate Charcot osteoarthropathy, and it is impossible at the outset to predict those fractures which will or will not develop this complication. There has often been a delay in diagnosis of the fractures that lead to Charcot osteoarthropathy.

The midfoot is the commonest site of presentation of Charcot osteoarthropathy and is recognized clinically by the medial convexity and

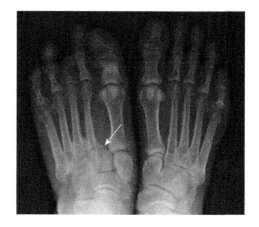

Fig. 4.44 Lisfranc's tarso-metatarsal joint dislocation (arrow) in left foot which also shows amputation of third toe and old fracture of proximal phalanx of first toe. Also note arterial calcification.

rocker bottom deformities. The medial convexity is associated with the classical Lisfranc's tarso-metatarsal fracture–dislocation (Fig. 4.44). The rocker bottom deformity develops when there is disintegration and displacement of the cuneiforms or the proximal tarsal bones, resulting in collapse of the midfoot. Rocker bottom deformity is frequently associated with plantar ulceration. Fractures of the base of the first metatarsal may precipitate Charcot osteoarthropathy in the midfoot.

When the hindfoot is involved, the early presentation is of a swollen ankle. Later, there is severe structural deformity and instability of the ankle joint (Fig. 4.45). This can lead to a flail ankle on which it is impossible to walk. Ulceration can often develop over the malleoli.

Treatment of active Charcot osteoarthropathy

Whether an early or late presentation, the foot is initially immobilized in a non-weight-bearing plaster cast. The cast is checked after 1 week and replaced if it has become loose due to reduction of swelling. It is regularly checked and replaced as necessary. The patient should use crutches and be encouraged to avoid weight-bearing on the affected

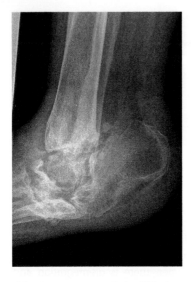

Fig. 4.45 Severe disorganization and disruption of the hindfoot and ankle joint.

side. In many cases it is difficult to be completely non-weight-bearing because the patient has multiple co-morbidities, including loss of proprioception, postural hypotension, high body mass index and, in some cases, neuropathy of the upper limbs, all of which can make it difficult to use crutches.

Furthermore, a wheelchair existence is often impractical in many home environments. Also, total immobility has disadvantages in itself, with loss of muscle tone, reduction in bone density and loss of body fitness. An alternative treatment is a prefabricated walking cast, such as the Aircast, described earlier in this chapter. A moulded insole should replace the standard insole provided with the cast by the manufacturer. However, the hindfoot Charcot is probably best treated in a total contact cast.

Patients may also receive treatment with bisphosphonates or calcitonin. However, these agents have not been shown to alter significantly the natural history of the condition.

When patients present early, and the X-ray is normal, prompt immobilization should keep the X-ray normal and prevent deformity. Casting is continued until the swelling has resolved and the temperature of the affected foot is within 2 °C of the contralateral foot. When patients present with established X-ray changes, including fracture, immobilization in a plaster cast is continued until there is no longer evidence on X-ray of continuing bone destruction, and the foot temperature is within 2°C of the contralateral foot.

Deformity in Charcot osteoarthropathy can predispose to ulceration, particularly on the plantar surface of the rocker bottom deformity. It may also occur on the medial convexity. These ulcers may become infected and lead to osteomyelitis. This may be difficult to distinguish from neuropathic bone and joint changes, as on X-ray, bone scan or MRI the appearances are similar.

Surgical reconstruction of the unstable hindfoot

If conservative care is unsuccessful, and the patient has a 'flail ankle', which is often associated with intractable ulceration over the malleoli, then operative stabilization, either external or internal, may be necessary.

External stabilization

A Taylor spatial frame is applied at operation and secured by pins through the bones of the foot. The wires within the frame are adjusted daily to gradually change the shape of the foot, particularly the soft tissues (Fig. 4.46). When this has been achieved the patient may then undergo internal stabilization. Infection around the pin site may be a complication in diabetes.

Internal stabilization

This can be carried out with intramedullary rods and special screws (Fig. 4.47). Following reconstructive ankle surgery, the lower limb is usually

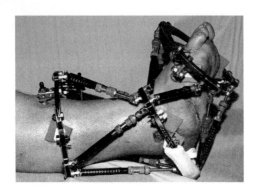

Fig. 4.46 Taylor spatial frame providing external stabilization of Charcot ankle.

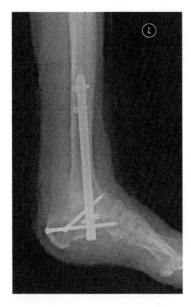

Fig. 4.47 Internal stabilization of the hindfoot with intramedullary rod and screws.

managed in a cast and is non-weight-bearing for 3 months. A removable cast is then supplied as the patient gradually becomes ambulant. When skin temperatures have remained normal and the patient is fully ambulant, a bespoke boot provides long-term stability.

Treatment of non-active Charcot osteoarthropathy

The foot is no longer warm and red. There may still be swelling but the difference in skin temperature between the feet is usually less than 2°C. The X-ray shows fracture healing, sclerosis and bone remodelling. The patient must now be rehabilitated and gradually progressed from cast treatment to suitable footwear. When the patient comes out of the cast there will be wasting of the calf muscles and joint stiffness and they will need physiotherapy. The patient needs close observation to detect any relapse, which will be evident from further swelling and heat in the foot. It is important not to reactivate bony destruction by excessively rapid mobilization or protracted weight-bearing in the early stages of rehabilitation.

Extremely careful rehabilitation should be the rule, beginning with just a few short steps in the new footwear. The patient rests for the remainder of the day and monitors the foot. If there is no increase in warmth, swelling and redness then they can walk a few more steps the next day, and very carefully build up to a reasonable amount of walking.

Finally, the patient may progress to bespoke footwear with moulded insoles. The rocker bottom foot with plantar bony prominence is a site of very high pressure. If ulceration does occur, an exostectomy may be needed.

When rehabilitating patients with hindfoot Charcot osteoarthropathy, a Charcot restraint orthotic walker (CROW) may be used, followed by an ankle–foot orthosis (AFO) with bespoke footwear.

The CROW is a bespoke bivalved total contact device which externally fixates the ankle (Fig. 4.48a and b). The yellow corrugations contain EVA to strengthen the device without increasing the bulk. The rigid,

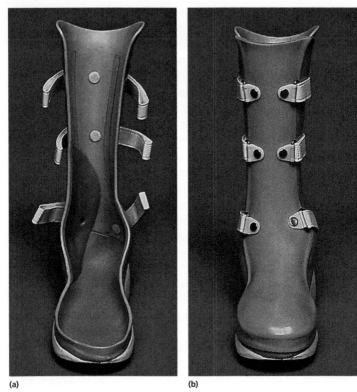

(a)   (b)

Fig. 4.48 (a) Anterior view of the CROW with removal of the front piece to show interior. (b) CROW with front piece attached.

durable outer shell is constructed out of polypropylene and is lined with EVA. There is a bespoke moulded insole to accommodate any existing deformity and to redistribute plantar pressures. A rocker bottom, crepe sole is attached to facilitate roll-off during walking. It is used after swelling is controlled and progressive destruction halted by total contact casting.

The AFO is a device used to stabilize the foot and ankle. There are two main forms of AFO: the traditional conventional metal and leather calliper and the newer thermoplastic types, which are more cosmetic.

Follow-up of patients with Charcot foot

Patients need follow-up in a multidisciplinary diabetic foot service. Occasionally there may be a relapse in an already stabilized foot. This will present with erythema, swelling and warmth. The patient should be treated as if they were again in the acute phase.

Many patients will eventually develop Charcot osteoarthropathy in both feet. All patients with unilateral Charcot osteoarthropathy should, therefore, be taught to check their feet and ankles regularly for hot spots and danger signs.

Managing Stage 4: the infected foot

PRESENTATION AND DIAGNOSIS

The diabetic patient enters Stage 4 because the foot is now infected and microbiological control has been lost. Diabetic foot ulcers are very susceptible to infection, which is the main pathology that destroys most diabetic feet. Infection in the diabetic foot is thus a medical emergency. In the presence of neuropathy and ischaemia, signs and symptoms of infection may be minimal, but nevertheless the pathology proceeds rapidly. The end stage of tissue death is quickly reached and there is a limited window of opportunity for intervention. It is one of the greatest challenges for the health-care professional to diagnose infection early and to prescribe the most efficacious antibiotics with the help of frequent microbiological specimens.

At no other stage in the natural history of the diabetic foot is early diagnosis and intervention so important. Twenty-four hours of undiagnosed and untreated infection can destroy the diabetic foot. Diabetic foot patients who experience repeated crises from the rapid onset of infection need a special form of easily accessible care provided by a multidisciplinary diabetic foot clinic.

There is a reduced host response to infection, particularly in diabetic patients with impaired renal and liver function. White blood count and body temperature may be normal even in severe infections. Only 50% of episodes of severe infections will provoke a fever or leucocytosis. However, serum CRP is a good indicator of the extent of infection and tissue destruction, and a subsequent fall in its level during treatment is a useful monitor of resolution of infection. Levels of CRP above 200 mmol/L indicate severe infection either from a bacteraemia or extensive tissue destruction needing surgical debridement.

Managing the Diabetic Foot, Third Edition. Michael E Edmonds and Alethea VM Foster.
© 2014 John Wiley & Sons, Ltd. Published 2014 by John Wiley & Sons, Ltd.

Infection can be an important complication of the neuropathic foot and also the ischaemic foot. Although all four categories of the ischaemic foot can become infected, it is the neuroischaemic foot that carries the main burden of infection.

Presentation of infection

Every diabetic patient with a foot ulcer should be assessed for the presence of infection. The most common manifestation is cellulitis, defined as an infection of skin and subcutaneous tissue and presenting as redness or erythema. However, Stage 4 covers a spectrum of presentations under the general heading of infection. Clinically, three distinct stages of diabetic foot infection may be recognized:

- Infection of the ulcer itself, namely local infection with cellulitis less than 2 cm from ulcer
- Infection spreading more than 2 cm from the ulcer, referred to as spreading infection
- Infection into the deep tissues, called severe deep infection.

Each of these presentations may be complicated by osteomyelitis. The severity of infection should be properly assessed after debridement of callus and necrotic tissue, based on its extent and depth and the presence of any systemic findings.

All patients presenting with clinical signs of infection should have an X-ray of the foot to detect possible

- Osteomyelitis
- Gas in the deep tissues
- Foreign body.

It is usually possible to make an accurate diagnosis after clinical assessment and X-rays. Further investigations may be necessary. Grey-scale ultrasound is useful to image soft tissue infections and collections of fluids (Fig. 5.1) and MRI helpful to detect anatomical location and extent of infection.

Local infection

This refers to infection in the ulcer bed and cellulitis within 2 cm of the ulcer. This may present with purulent discharge, but often the classical signs of infection redness, heat, pain and loss of function are diminished. Thus, the signs of infection may be very subtle and early warning signs of infection and signs of deterioration should be sought in all diabetic patients, especially those with breaks in the skin.

Local signs that an ulcer has become infected include:

- The base of the ulcer changes from healthy pink granulation to yellowish or grey tissue and becomes moist (Fig. 5.2)

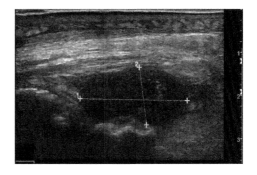

Fig. 5.1 Grey-scale ultrasound. There is a 2.6 cm × 1.4 cm echogenic collection at the plantar aspect of the foot.

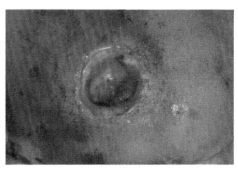

Fig. 5.2 Local infection. The base of the ulcer has changed from pink to grey.

- Ulcer stops healing
- Develops unpleasant smell
- Ulcer becomes painful
- Sinuses develop in an ulcer
- Edges may become undermined
- Bone or tendon becomes exposed.

Spreading infection

Infection has progressed to spreading erythema, at least 2 cm from the ulcer. There is usually swelling and lymphangitis in addition to local signs of infection (Fig. 5.3). The portal of entry of infection may be a corn, callus, blister, fissure or any other skin break. Puncture wounds may be complicated by cellulitis. Bacteria are inoculated at the base of the puncture wound and then track back towards the surface of the skin, with infection eventually manifesting itself as a cellulitis. Systemic symptoms and signs may be present when the foot has extensive diffuse cellulitis but not necessarily so, because of a reduced inflammatory response.

It is important to note that cellulitis in the pigmented (e.g. Afro-Caribbean) foot can be difficult to detect, but careful comparison with the other foot may reveal a tawny hue (Fig. 5.4). In the neuroischaemic foot, it may be difficult to differentiate between the erythema of cellulitis and the redness of ischaemia. However, the redness of ischaemia is usually in a cool skin, although not always so and is most marked on dependency, while the erythema of inflammation is associated with a warm foot. Erythematous inflammation of the feet also occurs in eczema, which is characterized by crusting and scaling. This is not seen in cellulitis. Erythema also occurs in response to traumas, including insect stings.

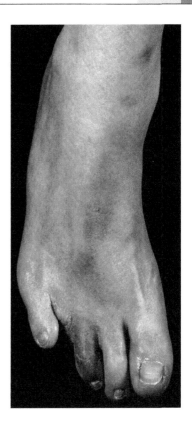

Fig. 5.3 Cellulitic third toe with lymphangitis indicating spreading infection. The fourth toe has been amputated.

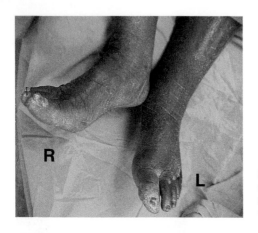

Fig. 5.4 Cellulitis in dark skin showing tawny appearance in the left foot.

Severe deep infection

This refers to extensive deep soft tissue infection complicating an ulcer (Fig. 5.5). In the presence of neuropathy, pain and throbbing may be absent, but if present this is a danger sign, usually indicating deep infection within the tissues. Palpation may reveal fluctuance, suggesting abscess formation, but this is rare in the diabetic foot because poor white cell function cannot localize the infection to create an abscess. Many inexperienced surgeons are unaware of this and feel that the only indication for operation is fluctuance with abscess formation. However, there is often widespread subcutaneous, fascial and tendinous sloughing, which is not obvious on clinical examination of the foot. Such sloughing eventually liquefies and disintegrates and needs surgical debridement.

Severe infection can also present as a bluish–purple discolouration when there is inadequate supply of oxygen to the soft tissues. This is caused by increased metabolic demands of infection and a reduction of blood flow to the skin, secondary to a septic vasculitis of the cutaneous circulation. Blue discolouration can occur in either the neuropathic or the neuroischaemic foot, particularly in the toes, and in the neuroischaemic foot must not be automatically attributed to worsening ischaemia (Fig. 5.6a and b). In very severe cases of infection, bluish–purplish

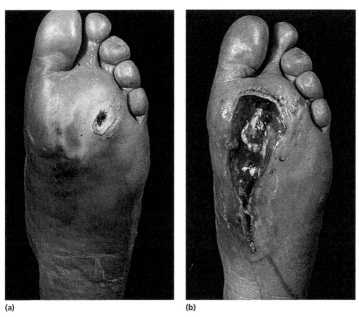

(a) (b)

Fig. 5.5 (a) Deep ulcer with subcutaneous sloughing visible. (b) Extent of debridement necessary to remove all necrotic tissue down to healthy bleeding tissue. (c) The wound is healed at 10 weeks.

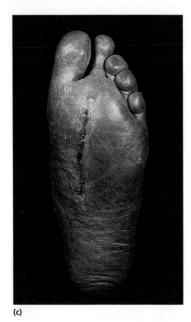

(c)   **Fig. 5.5** (*Continued*)

discolouration of the skin often appears as purple blebs indicating subcutaneous necrosis (Fig. 5.7). Severe subcutaneous infection by Gramnegative and anaerobic bacteria produces gas, which can be detected by palpating crepitus and can be seen on X-ray (Fig. 5.8). In extreme cases there is widespread destruction of tissues with bullae formation indicative of a classical necrotizing fasciitis.

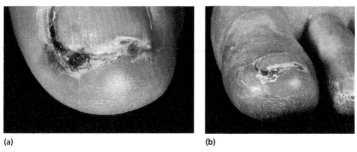

(a)   (b)

Fig. 5.6 (a) Blue discolouration in the first toe of neuroischaemic foot secondary to infection. (b) Blue toe has become pink after treatment of infection with antibiotics.

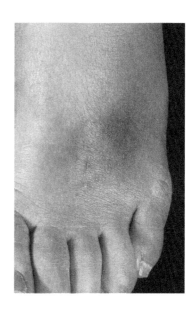

Fig. 5.7 Purplish discolouration indicating subcutaneous necrosis.

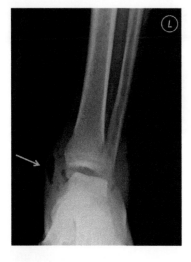

Fig. 5.8 Gas (arrow) in the tissues in severe soft tissue infection.

Systemic infection

All stages of infection, local, spreading and severe, may also be associated with a bacteraemia, leading to systemic signs of infection. Signs of systemic infection include drowsiness, shivering, tachycardia, reduced body temperature (<35 °C) or raised body temperature (>37 °C) and hypotension. Any body temperature that is raised above 37 °C is significant in a diabetic patient. However, systemic signs and symptoms are notoriously absent in many severe infections of the diabetic foot. When a fever is present it usually indicates a severe infection that has tracked into the deep spaces of the foot. Among patients hospitalized for late infections, only 12–35% have significant fever and only 50% of episodes of severe cellulitis will provoke a fever or leucocytosis. However, serum CRP is a more reliable indicator of systemic infection, although it reflects inflammatory systemic activity over the previous 24 h and thus may not mirror the true extent of inflammation at the time the blood is taken.

Osteomyelitis

Osteomyelitis can complicate any of the above infective presentations. It is caused by contiguous spread of infection from ulcer to bone. Clinically, osteomyelitis may be suspected when a sterile probe inserted into the base of the ulcer penetrates to bone. This may happen in an apparently clean, uninfected ulcer, but osteomyelitis must still be suspected. It may also present as obvious fragmentation of the bone within the ulcer bed that is easily visible. A sign that an underlying joint is infected is the drainage of viscous, bubbly synovial fluid that is clear and sometimes has a yellowish tinge. Chronic osteomyelitis of a toe has a swollen, red, sausage-like appearance.

Osteomyelitis is most commonly diagnosed on X-ray. Although in the initial stages, plain X-ray may be normal, loss of cortex, lucency of bone fragmentation and bony destruction on X-ray indicate the development of osteomyelitis (Fig. 5.9). However, these changes may take 10–14 days to develop. MRI scanning may detect early changes. It is the best

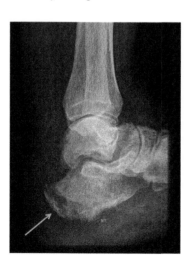

Fig. 5.9 Osteomyelitis with loss of bone density and cortical outline of the displaced calcaneum (arrow).

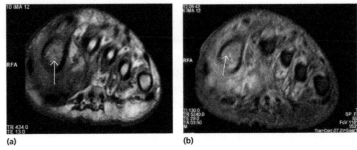

Fig. 5.10 (a) Osteomyelitis in the first metatarsal head. T1 sequence shows reduced signal in the fatty marrow of the first metatarsal head (arrow) compared with other metatarsal heads. (b) Increased uptake on STIR sequence indicating oedema in first metatarsal head (arrow) compared with other metatarsal heads. This is more pronounced than in other metatarsal heads.

imaging technique to diagnose osteomyelitis and can demonstrate oedema and abscesses in bone (Fig. 5.10a and b).

Osteomyelitis may be confirmed by a positive bone culture or bone biopsy from an aseptically obtained bone sample showing bacteria, bone death, inflammation and repair. Bone biopsy may also be valuable for defining the pathogenic organisms, and for determining the antibiotic susceptibilities of such organisms. Bone biopsy is often not very practical, and then the diagnosis is made on clinical and radiological grounds.

MANAGEMENT

There are three crucial decisions when managing infected diabetic feet: first, to confirm the presence of infection so as to start rapidly antibiotic therapy; second, to select appropriate initial antibiotic therapy; and third, to determine whether the patient needs surgical debridement to remove infected tissue. Often, the latter is a very difficult decision. Diabetic feet can be severely infected and need operative removal of infected sloughing tissue and drainage of abscess yet may not on the surface exhibit the signs of such pathologies.

It is vital to achieve:
- Microbiological control
- Wound control
- Vascular control
- Mechanical control
- Metabolic control
- Educational control.

If infection is not controlled, it can spread with alarming rapidity, and can cause extensive tissue necrosis, taking the foot into Stage 5 or Stage 6.

Microbiological control

General principles
The development of infection constitutes a foot care emergency, which requires referral to specialized foot care team within 24 h. The underlying principles are to diagnose infection, culture the bacteria responsible, treat aggressively with antibiotic therapy and consider the need for debridement and surgery. When managing these very difficult and unstable feet, decision making should be guided by symptoms and signs of infection, results of properly taken ulcer swabs and tissue cultures, and past and present knowledge of individual patients.

The microbiology of the diabetic foot is unique. Infection can be caused by Gram-positive, Gram-negative and anaerobic bacteria, singly or in combination (Table 5.1). As there is a poor immune response of the diabetic patient to sepsis, even bacteria regarded as skin commensals may cause severe tissue damage.

Group A streptococcus is a rare isolate from ulcers, but when present it can cause severe systemic upset and Group B streptococcus is an important pathogen in the diabetic foot. MRSA is associated with the whole spectrum of clinical presentations of diabetic foot infections and

Table 5.1 Bacteria isolated from the diabetic foot.

Gram-positive

Staphylococcus aureus

Streptococcus (often Group B)

Enterococcus

Anaerobes

Bacteroides

Clostridium

Peptostreptococcus

Peptococcus

Gram-negative

Proteus

Klebsiella

Enterobacter

Escherichia coli

Pseudomonas aeruginosa

Citrobacter

Morganella morganii

Serratia

Acinetobacter

commonly occurs in patients who have been in hospital. There is a strain of MRSA that is found in the community, so-called community-acquired MRSA. This has been associated with outbreaks in groups of individuals with close contact in institutions such as prisons but can then be transferred to hospitals. These MRSA do not have the multi-resistance of the hospital-acquired MRSA but nevertheless can rapidly progress to severe infections. Approximately two-thirds possess the Panton–Valentine leukocidin toxin, which acts to form pores in the cell membrane of mononuclear cells and polymorphonuclear cells and can lead to severe tissue necrosis.

When Gram-negative bacteria such as *Citrobacter*, *Serratia* and *Pseudomonas* are isolated from an ulcer swab, they should not be regarded automatically as insignificant. Recently, Gram-negative bacteria have acquired various resistance patterns through the development of certain enzymes, and this is relevant to the choice of antibiotic therapy.

These include extended spectrum beta lactamases known as ESBLs (extended-spectrum beta lactamases). By this means, they have developed resistance to extended-spectrum (third-generation) cephalosporins (e.g. ceftazidime, cefotaxime and ceftriaxone) but not to carbapenems (e.g. meropenem or imipenem). ESBL enzymes are most commonly produced by two bacteria: *Escherichia coli* and *Klebsiella pneumoniae*. Another group of lactamases are AmpC β-lactamases, which are typically encoded on the chromosomes of many Gram-negative bacteria, notably *Citrobacter*, *Serratia* and *Enterobacter* species, where expression is usually inducible. Carbapenems are the only reliable beta-lactam drugs for the treatment of severe *Enterobacter* infections.

Anaerobes are commonly found in deep infections and can act synergistically with Gram-positive and Gram-negative aerobes to cause severe tissue destruction.

When a positive culture is found, it is necessary to focus antibiotic therapy according to sensitivities. Good communication with the microbiologist is advised. Useful antibiotics are shown in Table 5.2.

Table 5.2 Antibiotics for treating the infected foot (doses for normal renal function).

Microorganism	Antibiotic treatment	
	Oral	**Intravenous**
Streptococcus (incl. Groups A, B, C and G)	Amoxicillin 500 mg–1 g t.d.s. Clindamycin 150–450 mg q.d.s. Clarithromycin 500 mg b.d. Co-amoxiclav 625 mg t.d.s.	Amoxicillin 500 mg–1 g t.d.s. Clindamycin 150–600 mg q.d.s. Clarithromycin 500 mg b.d. Co-amoxiclav 1.2 g t.d.s.
Staphylococcus aureus	Flucloxacillin 250–500 mg q.d.s. Clarithromycin 500 mg b.d. Clindamycin 150–450 mg q.d.s. Rifampicin 600–1200 mg daily in 2–4 divided doses Sodium fusidate 500 mg t.d.s.	Flucloxacillin 250 mg–2 g q.d.s. Clarithromycin 500 mg b.d. Clindamycin 150–600 mg q.d.s.
Anaerobes	Metronidazole 400 mg t.d.s. Clindamycin 150–450 mg q.d.s. Co-amoxiclav 625 mg t.d.s.	Metronidazole 500 mg t.d.s. Clindamycin 150–600 mg q.d.s. Co-amoxiclav 1.2 g t.d.s.

Table 5.2 (Continued)		
Microorganism	**Antibiotic treatment**	
	Oral	**Intravenous**

Gram negatives	Ciprofloxacin 250–750 mg b.d.
	Cefadroxil 500 mg–1 g b.d.
	Trimethoprim 200 mg b.d.
		Ciprofloxacin 100–400 mg b.d.
		Ceftriaxone 1–4 g daily (not active against *Pseudomonas*)
		Ceftazidime 1–2 g t.d.s.
		Ertapenem 1 g daily (not active against *Pseudomonas*)
		Gentamicin 5 mg/kg/day) (according to levels)
		Piperacillin–tazobactam (Tazocin) 2.25–4.5 g t.d.s.
		Meropenem 500 mg–1 g t.d.s.
		Ticarcillin/clavulanate 3.2 g t.d.s.
		Tigecycline 100 mg loading dose then 50 mg b.d.
		Colistin:
		  <60 kg,
		  50 000–75 000 units/kg in 3 divided doses
		  >60 kg, 1–2 million units every 8 h

(Continued)

Table 5.2 (Continued)

Microorganism	Antibiotic treatment	
	Oral	Intravenous
MRSA	Sodium fusidate 500 mg t.d.s. Trimethoprim 200 mg b.d. Rifampicin 600–1200 mg daily in 2–4 divided doses Doxycycline 200 mg first day then 100 mg daily Linezolid 600 mg b.d.	Vancomycin 1 g b.d. (according to levels) Teicoplanin loading dose: <70 kg, 400 mg every 12 h for 3 doses, then 400 mg daily >70 kg, 6 mg/kg every 12 h for 3 doses then 6 mg/kg daily Daptomycin 4–6 mg/kg daily Linezolid 600 mg b.d. Synercid (quinupristin 150 mg/ dalfopristin 350 mg) 7.5 mg/ kg t.d.s. (through central line)

Recently, daptomycin has been used for the treatment of Gram-positive infections, including MRSA. Tigecycline is active against Gram-positive and Gram-negative organisms, including some anaerobes, although it has not been recommended for the treatment of foot infections in patients with diabetes. *Pseudomonas* infections have become increasingly difficult to treat, and it is sometimes necessary to resort to antibiotics such as timentin (ticarcillin/clavulanic acid), colistin or fosfomycin. If *Stenotrophomonas maltophilia* is regarded as a significant organism in a diabetic foot infection, then co-trimoxazole is the optimum therapy, although it is associated with rare but serious side-effects, particularly in the elderly.

Antibiotics alone do not always treat foot infections successfully. Severe infection in the diabetic foot may be accompanied by deep soft tissue sloughing which spreads along the fascial planes and needs early extensive surgical debridement as well as concomitant antibiotic therapy. At initial presentation, it is important to prescribe a wide spectrum of antibiotics because it is impossible to predict the organisms from the clinical appearance. It is therefore vital to send swabs or tissue for culture from the ulcer after initial debridement without delay in all Stage 4 patients. If the patient undergoes operative debridement, then deep tissue from the operating theatre should also be sent straight away to the laboratory. Ulcer swabs or tissue should be taken at every follow-up visit for close microbiological surveillance. Blood cultures should be sent if there is any fever or systemic toxicity.

Antibiotic treatment

General principles
Usually, therapy is commenced with wide spectrum therapy which is then focused according to the culture results. We believe it is advisable to cover both Gram-positive and Gram-negative organisms with initial empirical therapy. Infection in the neuroischaemic foot is often more serious than in the neuropathic foot; therefore we regard a positive ulcer swab or tissue in a neuroischaemic foot as having serious implications, and this influences antibiotic policy. Antibiotic treatment is discussed both as initial and follow-up treatment and covers treatment of the locally infected ulcer, spreading infection from the ulcer and the foot with severe deep infection. Treatment of osteomyelitis is also discussed. Diabetic patients with renal impairment are particularly susceptible to infection and their antibiotic dosages will need to be reduced in renal failure (Table 5.3). However, dosages for vancomycin and the aminogly-cosides gentamicin, amikacin and tobramycin should be obtained from local antibiotic protocols.

Table 5.3 Antibiotic dosage in renal failure and renal replacement therapies.

Antibiotic	Dose for normal renal function	Impairment		
		Mild eGFR 20–50 mL/min	**Moderate eGFR 10–20 mL/min**	**Severe eGFR <10 mL/min**
Amoxicillin	IV/po 500 mg–1 g t.d.s.	IV/po No adjustment	IV/po No adjustment	IV/po 250 mg–1 g t.d.s.
Benzylpenicillin	IV 2.4–14.4 g daily in 4–6 divided doses	IV No adjustment	IV 600 mg–2.4 g q.d.s.	IV 600 mg–1.2 g q.d.s.
Cefadroxil	po 500 mg–1 g b.d.	po No adjustment	po No adjustment	po 500 mg–1 g daily
Ceftazidime	IV 1–2 g t.d.s.	IV 1 g b.d.	IV 500 mg–1 g daily	IV 500 mg–1 g 48 hrly
Ceftriaxone	IV 1–4 g daily	IV No adjustment	IV No adjustment	IV No adjustment maximum 2 g daily
Cefuroxime	IV 750 mg–1.5 g t.d.s. po 125–500 mg b.d.	IV 750 mg–1.5 g t.d.s. po No adjustment	IV 750 mg–1.5 g b.d. or t.d.s. po No adjustment	IV 750 mg–1.5 g b.d. or daily po No adjustment
Ciprofloxacin	IV 100–400 mg b.d. po 250–750 mg b.d.	IV/po No adjustment	IV/po 50–100% of normal dose	IV/po 50% of normal dose

Antibiotic	HD	CAPD	HDF/high flux	CAV/VVHD
Amoxicillin	IV/po 250 mg–1 g t.d.s.	IV/po 250 mg–1 g t.d.s.	IV/po 250 mg–1 g t.d.s.	IV/po Dose as in normal renal function
Benzylpenicillin	IV 600 mg–1.2 g q.d.s.	IV 600 mg–1.2 g q.d.s.	IV 600 mg–1.2 g q.d.s.	IV 600 mg–2.4 g q.d.s.
Cefadroxil	po 500 mg–1 g daily	po 500 mg–1 g daily	po 500 mg–1 g daily	po Dose as in normal renal function
Ceftazidime	IV 500 mg–1 g every 24–48 h	IV 500 mg–1 g daily	IV 500 mg–1 g every 24–48 h	IV 2 g t.d.s.
Ceftriaxone	IV Dose as in normal renal function: maximum 2 g daily	IV Dose as in normal renal function: maximum 2 g daily	IV Dose as in normal renal function: maximum 2 g daily	IV 2 g b.d. or daily
Cefuroxime	IV 750 mg–1.5 g b.d. or daily po Dose as in normal renal function	IV 750 mg–1.5 g b.d. or daily po Dose as in normal renal function	IV 750 mg–1.5 g b.d. or daily po Dose as in normal renal function	IV 750 mg–1.5 g t.d.s. or bd po Dose as in normal renal function
Ciprofloxacin	IV 200 mg b.d. po 250–500 mg b.d.	IV 200 mg b.d. po 250 mg b.d. or t.d.s.	IV 200 mg b.d. po 250–500 mg b.d.	IV 200–400 mg b.d. po 500–750 mg b.d.

(Continued)

Table 5.3 (Continued)

Antibiotic	Dose for normal renal function	Impairment		
		Mild eGFR 20–50 mL/min	**Moderate eGFR 10–20 mL/min**	**Severe eGFR <10 mL/min**
Clarithromycin		**eGFR 30–50 mL/ min**	**eGFR 10–30 mL/ min**	
	IV 500 mg b.d.	IV No adjustment	IV 250–500 mg b.d	IV 250–500 mg b.d.
	po 500 mg b.d.	po No adjustment	po 250–500 mg b.d.	po 250–500 mg b.d.
Clindamycin	IV 150–600 mg q.d.s. po 150–450 mg q.d.s.	IV No adjustment po No adjustment	IV No adjustment po No adjustment	IV No adjustment po No adjustment
Co-amoxiclav		**eGFR 30–50 mL/ min**	**eGFR 10–30 mL/ min**	
	IV 1.2 g t.d.s.	IV No adjustment	IV 1.2 g b.d.	IV 1.2 g stat followed by 600 mg t.d.s. or 1.2 g b.d.
	po 625 mg t.d.s.	po No adjustment	po No adjustment	po No adjustment
Colistin	IV <60 kg: 50 000–75 000 units/kg t.d.s. >60 kg: 1–2 million units t.d.s.	IV 1–2 million units t.d.s.	IV 1 million units every 12–18 h or 50% of normal dose	IV 1 million units every 18–24 h or 30% of normal dose

Antibiotic	HD	CAPD	HDF/high flux	CAV/VVHD
Clarithromycin	IV 250–500 mg b.d. po 250–500 mg b.d.	IV 250–500 mg b.d. po 250–500 mg b.d.	IV 250–500 mg b.d. po 250–500 mg b.d.	IV 250–500 mg b.d. po 250–500 mg b.d.
Clindamycin	IV/po Dose as in normal renal function	IV/po Dose as in normal renal function	IV/po Dose as in normal renal function	IV/po Dose as in normal renal function
Co-amoxiclav	IV 1.2 g stat followed by 600 mg t.d.s. or 1.2 g b.d. po Dose as in normal renal function	IV 1.2 g stat followed by 600 mg t.d.s. or 1.2 g b.d. po Dose as in normal renal function	IV 1.2 g stat followed by 600 mg t.d.s. or 1.2 g b.d. po Dose as in normal renal function	IV 1.2 g b.d. po Dose as in normal renal function
Colistin	IV 1 million units every 18–24 h or 30% of normal dose	IV 1 million units every 18–24 h or 30% of normal dose	IV 1 million units every 18–24 h or 30% of normal dose	IV 2 million units every 48 h

(*Continued*)

Table 5.3 (Continued)

Antibiotic	Dose for normal renal function	Impairment		
		Mild eGFR 20–50 mL/min	**Moderate eGFR 10–20 mL/min**	**Severe eGFR <10 mL/min**
Daptomycin	IV 4–6 mg/kg daily	**eGFR 30–50 mL/ min** IV No adjustment **eGFR 20–30 mL/ min** IV 4 mg/kg/ 48 h	IV 4 mg/kg/ 48 h	IV 4 mg/ kg/48 h
Doxycycline	po 200 mg First day then 100 mg daily	po No adjustment	po No adjustment	po No adjustment
Ertapenem	IV 1 g daily	**eGFR 30–50 mL/ min** IV No adjustment	**eGFR 10–30 mL/ min** IV 50–100% of normal dose	IV 50% of normal dose
Flucloxacillin	IV 250 mg–2 g q.d.s.	IV No adjustment	IV No adjustment	IV No adjustment up to a total dose of 4 g daily
	po 250–500 mg q.d.s.	po No adjustment	po No adjustment	po No adjustment

Antibiotic	HD	CAPD	HDF/high flux	CAV/VVHD
Daptomycin	IV 4 mg/kg every 48 h	IV 4 mg/kg every 48 h	IV 4 mg/kg every 48 h	IV 4–6 mg/kg every 48 h
Doxycycline	po Dose as in normal renal function	po Dose as in normal renal function	po Dose as in normal renal function	po Dose as in normal renal function
Ertapenem	IV 50% of the dose used in normal renal function	IV 50% of the dose used in normal renal function	IV 50% of the dose used in normal renal function	IV 50% of the dose used in normal renal function
Flucloxacillin	IV/po Dose as in normal renal function (up to a total dose of 4 g IV daily)	IV/po Dose as in normal renal function (up to a total dose of 4 g IV daily)	IV/po Dose as in normal renal function (up to a total dose of 4 g IV daily)	IV/po Dose as in normal renal function

(*Continued*)

Table 5.3 (Continued)

Antibiotic	Dose for normal renal function	Impairment		
		Mild eGFR 20–50 mL/min	Moderate eGFR 10–20 mL/min	Severe eGFR <10 mL/min
Meropenem	IV 500 mg–1 g t.d.s.	IV 500 mg–2 g b.d.	IV 500 mg–1 g b.d. or 500 mg t.d.s.	IV 500 mg–1 g daily
Metronidazole	IV 500 mg t.d.s. po 400 mg t.d.s.	IV No adjustment po No adjustment	IV No adjustment po No adjustment	IV No adjustment po No adjustment
Rifampicin	po 600–1200 mg daily in 2–4 divided doses	po No adjustment	po No adjustment	po 50–100% of normal dose
Sodium fusidate	IV 500 mg t.d.s. po 500 mg t.d.s.	IV No adjustment po No adjustment	IV No adjustment po No adjustment	IV No adjustment po No adjustment
Synercid (quinupristin 150 mg/ dalfopristin 350 mg)	IV 7.5 mg/kg t.d.s.	IV 5–7.5 mg/ kg b.d. or t.d.s.	IV 5–7.5 mg/ kg b.d. or t.d.s.	IV 5 mg/kg b.d. or t.d.s.
Tazocin (piperacillin/ tazobactam)	IV 2.25–4.5 g t.d.s.	IV No adjustment	IV 4.5 g b.d. or t.d.s. or 2.25 g q.d.s.	IV 4.5 g b.d. or 2.25 g t.d.s.

Antibiotic	HD	CAPD	HDF/high flux	CAV/VVHD
Meropenem	IV 500 mg–1 g daily	IV 500 mg–1 g daily	IV 500 mg–1 g daily	IV 1 g b.d. or 0.5–1 g t.d.s.
Metronidazole	IV/po Dose as in normal renal function	IV/po Dose as in normal renal function	IV/po Dose as in normal renal function	IV/po Dose as in normal renal function
Rifampicin	po 50–100% of the dose used in normal renal function	po 50–100% of the dose used in normal renal function	po 50–100% of the dose used in normal renal function	po Dose as in normal renal function
Sodium fusidate	IV/po Dose as in normal renal function	IV/po Dose as in normal renal function	IV/po Dose as in normal renal function	IV/po Dose as in normal renal function
Synercid (quinupristin 150 mg/ dalfopristin 350 mg)	IV 5 mg/kg b.d. or t.d.s.	IV 10–20 mg/ kg/day in 2 divided doses	IV 5 mg/kg b.d. or t.d.s.	IV 5–7.5 mg/ kg b.d. or t.d.s.
Tazocin (piperacillin/ tazobactam)	IV 4.5 g b.d. or 2.25 g t.d.s.	IV 4.5 g b.d. or 2.25 g t.d.s.	IV 4.5 g b.d. or 2.25 g t.d.s.	IV 4.5 g b.d. or t.d.s or 2.25 g q.d.s.

(Continued)

Table 5.3 (Continued)

Antibiotic	Dose for normal renal function	Impairment		
		Mild eGFR 20–50 mL/min	Moderate eGFR 10–20 mL/min	Severe eGFR <10 mL/min
Teicoplanin	IV loading dose according to weight then 400–600 mg daily	IV No adjustment	IV Give normal loading dose, then 200–400 mg every 24–48 h	IV Give normal loading dose, then 200–400 mg every 48–72 h
Tigecycline	IV Loading dose of 100 mg then 50 mg b.d.	IV No adjustment	IV No adjustment	IV No adjustment
Trimethoprim		**eGFR 30–50 mL/ min**	**eGFR 15–30 mL/ min**	**eGFR <15 mL/min**
	po 200 mg b.d.	po No adjustment	po Normal dose for 3 days then half normal dose	po Half normal dose. Monitor levels if eGFR <10 mL/min

With reference to Ashley C., Currie A. (eds) (2009) *The Renal Drug Handbook*, 3rd edition, Radcliffe Publishing, Oxford.
British National Formulary March 2013.
b.d.: twice daily; CAPD: continuous ambulatory peritoneal dialysis; CAV/VVHD: continuous arteriovenous/venovenous haemodialysis; eGFR estimated glomerular filtration rate; HD: intermittent haemodialysis; HDF: haemodiafiltration; IV: intravenous; po: by mouth; q.d.s.: four times daily; stat: immediately; t.d.s.: three times daily.

Antibiotic	HD	CAPD	HDF/high flux	CAV/VVHD
Teicoplanin	IV Give normal loading dose, then 200–400 mg every 48–72 h	IV Give normal loading dose, then 200–400 mg every 48–72 h	IV Give normal loading dose, then 200–400 mg every 48–72 h	IV Give normal loading dose, then 200–400 mg every 24–48 h
Tigecycline	IV Dose as in normal renal function	IV Dose as in normal renal function	IV Dose as in normal renal function	IV Dose as in normal renal function
Trimethoprim	po 50% of the dose used in normal renal function	po 50% of the dose used in normal renal function	po 50% of the dose used in normal renal function	po 50% of the dose used in normal renal function

Clostridium difficile

We recommend the aggressive use of antibiotics in Stage 4, but keep a very close surveillance for side-effects, particularly vomiting and diarrhoea. If this does occur, it is advisable to stop the antibiotics, at least for a short period, to prevent the development of *Clostridium difficile* colitis. Faeces should be sent for culture, but therapy should be started immediately with either vancomycin 125 mg q.d.s. orally (intravenous vancomycin does not treat *Clostridium difficile*) or metronidazole 400 mg t.d.s. orally. We advise our patients to eat live yoghurt when taking antibiotics. In severe cases of *Clostridium difficile* infection there is abdominal pain associated with diarrhoea and often a raised white blood cell count and fever. Patients may need hospitalization and intravenous fluids. A useful diagnostic investigation is an abdominal CT scan which will reveal loops of oedematous large bowel.

When patients with foot infections develop diarrhoea with a high white blood cell count and fever, it is difficult to know whether the fever and raised white cell count are due to either worsening of the foot infection or the onset of diarrhoea secondary to *Clostridium difficile*. Close examination of the foot will determine whether infection here has worsened. If this is not the case, then the high white cell count and fever are likely to be due to colitis and the antibiotics should be stopped immediately.

Fungal bacteraemia

Another cause of a high white cell count and fever in a diabetic patient taking antibiotics is fungal bacteraemia, especially in patients with an indwelling intravenous line. Blood cultures should be taken from vein and from the line. Positive blood cultures from the line indicate that the line is the source of infection. It should be removed and the tip sent for culture. Most systemic fungal infections are due to Candida albicans, which is the most common pathogen, followed by *Torulopsis glabrata* and *Aspergillus*. Patients with fungaemia may develop endophthalmitis and patients should undergo ophthalmological examination to detect this complication. Treatment failure occurs in about 20–30% of patients with candidaemia, and the death rate in patients can be high. It is important to diagnose early and intervene promptly with correct dosing of antifungal agents. These comprise the following groups:

- Echinocandins
- Azoles
- Amphotericin.

Echinocandins
Echinocandins include anidulafungin, micafungin and caspofungin. The initial dose of caspofungin is 70 mg on day 1; subsequent dosing is 50 mg/day. It may increase up to 70 mg/day if tolerated and if initial clinical response is inadequate.

Azoles
Fluconazole, often in high doses, can be given for candida infection. Treatment of systemic infections should consist of 800 mg followed by 400 mg/day. During severe illness, continuing the 800 mg/day dosing should be considered. *Candida krusei* and *Candida glabrata* are often resistant to fluconazole, and with the advent of repeated or long-term fluconazole therapy/prophylaxis even *Candida albicans* may be resistant.

Amphotericin
Amphotericin is a very effective agent but has significant toxicities. Infusion-related reactions include hypotension, fever and tachycardia, and dosing should be preceded by a 1 mg test dose followed by infusion over 4 h. Nephrotoxicity can develop in up to 30% of patients. Liposomal amphotericin (Ambisome) is less potent, but there is a marked reduction in nephrotoxicity that allows much higher dosing.

Route of administration of antibiotics

In diabetic foot patients, tunnelled lines may be associated with metastatic infections, including discitis and also systemic fungal infections. For this reason, we try to avoid them in our patients. Recently, we have used peripherally inserted central catheter (PICC) lines as the main route of intravenous access, both in the home and in hospital. The site of insertion of PICC lines in the antecubital fossa needs special hypoallergenic dressings. Many dressings cause an allergic reaction and it is important to protect the skin with a barrier cream. Migration of the line out of the antecubital fossa is a frequent problem (Fig. 5.11) but can be reduced by stabilization devices. It is important to flush the line with normal saline after injecting the antibiotic, otherwise the PICC line may block, but it can usually be unblocked by installation of urokinase. PICC lines are increasingly used to facilitate the administration of intravenous antibiotics at home.

In patients with very poor venous access and who are having haemodialysis three times weekly, vancomycin and the aminoglycosides can be given intravenously at the time of dialysis. Also, meropenem at a dosage of 2 g at each dialysis can be given intravenously, three times weekly.

Historically, we have used intramuscular injections of antibiotics for patients in the community and still do so for short courses.

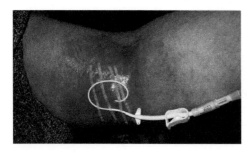

Fig. 5.11 PICC line showing allergic reaction to film dressing previously applied. Line has migrated from its insertion and is being held temporarily by steri-strips pending new line insertion in opposite arm.

Antibiotic therapy of local infection, spreading infection, severe deep infection

Local infection in the neuropathic foot and ischaemic foot

Initial treatment
Local infections with limited cellulitis (less than 2 cm from ulcer) can generally be treated with oral antibiotics on an outpatient basis:
- Give amoxicillin 500 mg t.d.s., flucloxacillin 500 mg q.d.s. or alternatively co-amoxiclav 625 mg t.d.s. In the ischaemic foot, metronidazole 400 mg t.d.s. and ciprofloxacin 500 mg b.d. may be added if the ulcer is sloughy, to cover anaerobes and Gram-negative bacteria.
- If the patient is allergic to penicillin, substitute clarithromycin 500 mg b.d. for amoxicillin and flucloxacillin. If the patient is taking a statin, then temporarily stop it and restart the day after antibiotic treatment has finished.
- The patient should be reviewed within 1 week.

Follow-up plan
- If no signs of infection and no organisms isolated, stop antibiotics. However, if severely ischaemic and ABPI <0.5 and there is no possibility of revascularization, consider continuing antibiotics until healing.
- If no signs of infection but organisms are isolated, focus antibiotics according to sensitivities. If MRSA is cultured, consider oral therapy with two of the following: sodium fusidate 500 mg t.d.s., rifampicin 600 mg b.d., trimethoprim 200 mg b.d. and doxycycline 100 mg daily, according to sensitivities. Linezolid is a possible alternative and has good activity against Gram-positive organisms, including MRSA.
- If signs of infection but no organisms are isolated, re-culture and continue the same antibiotics.

- If signs of infection are still present and organisms are isolated, focus antibiotics according to sensitivities.
- The patient should be reviewed at least weekly.

Spreading infection in the neuropathic foot and ischaemic foot

Initial treatment
- The patient should be treated with systemic antibiotics, usually in the hospital, but occasionally at home, via PICC line according to the general condition of the patient.
- Infection can be treated with ceftriaxone 1 g daily intravenously and oral metronidazole 400 mg t.d.s. or piperacillin–tazobactam 4.5 g t.d.s. intravenously as initial empirical treatment. If the intravenous route is not possible then give ceftriaxone 1 g daily intramuscularly in 3.5 mL of 1% lidocaine.
- The intramuscular route should not be used in those patients taking anticoagulants.
- If the patient is allergic to penicillin, give vancomycin 1 g b.d. intravenously or teicoplanin intravenously or intramuscularly. If the patient is less than 70 kg, give 400 mg teicoplanin intravenously 12 hourly for three doses and then intravenously or intramuscularly daily according to renal function. If the patient is heavier than 70 kg, then give 6 mg/kg intravenously 12 hourly for three doses and then continue intravenously or intramuscularly daily according to renal function. Oral ciprofloxacin and metronidazole should be given with vancomycin or teicoplanin.
- On admission, the foot should be urgently assessed as to the need for surgical debridement.

Follow-up plan
- The infected foot should be inspected daily to gauge the initial response to antibiotic therapy and to assess whether surgical debridement is necessary.

- The culture results from specimens taken from the foot at presentation should be examined. Appropriate antibiotics should be selected when sensitivities are available. See Table 5.2.
- If no organisms are isolated, and yet the foot remains severely cellulitic, then a repeat deep swab or tissue should be taken, but antibiotic therapy, as above, should be continued.
- Intravenous antibiotic therapy can be changed to the appropriate oral therapy when the signs of cellulitis have resolved.
- Regular deep swabs or tissue should be taken so as to keep close microbiological surveillance and antibiotics adjusted according to culture sensitivities.

Severe deep infection in the neuropathic and ischaemic foot

Initial treatment
- Admission for intravenous antibiotics is the treatment of choice for this serious condition.
- It is important to give wide-spectrum antibiotic therapy. Previously we used quadruple antibiotic therapy: amoxicillin 500 mg t.d.s. intravenously, flucloxacillin 500 mg q.d.s. intravenously, metronidazole 500 mg t.d.s. intravenously and ceftazidime 1 g t.d.s intravenously. We still believe that this is the most effective treatment, but in respect to antibiotic stewardship we now use piperacillin–tazobactam 4.5 g t.d.s. intravenously as initial empirical treatment. Flucloxacillin 500 mg q.d.s. intravenously may be added to this regime. If MRSA is strongly suspected, then substitute vancomycin for flucloxacillin. With either empirical treatment, if the patient shows systemic signs of infection then one intravenous dose of gentamicin should be considered at 5 mg/kg, although this dose should be reduced appropriately in renal failure.
- If the patient is allergic to penicillin, then vancomycin 1 g b.d. intravenously plus ciprofloxacin 400 mg b.d. intravenously and metronidazole 500 mg t.d.s. intravenously should be given.

- On admission, the foot should be urgently assessed as to the need for surgical debridement by a team experienced in assessing infected diabetic feet and proficient in diabetic foot surgery (see 'Wound control' section).

Follow-up plan This is the same as for spreading infection.

Osteomyelitis

Initial treatment
- Osteomyelitis is usually associated with soft tissue infection. At first, antibiotics will be given for the infected foot as above.
- After diagnosing osteomyelitis, antibiotic selection may be guided by the results of deep swabs or tissue, but it is useful to choose oral antibiotics with good bone penetration, such as sodium fusidate 500 mg t.d.s., rifampicin 600 mg b.d., clindamycin 300 mg q.d.s. and ciprofloxacin 500 mg b.d.

Follow-up plan
- Antibiotics should be given for at least 12 weeks. During this time, the ulcer should have regular debridement, and bone fragments at the base of ulcer can be easily removed.
- Such conservative therapy is often successful and is associated with resolution of cellulitis and healing of the ulcer.
- However, if after 3 months' treatment the ulcer persists, with continued probing to bone which is fragmented on X-ray, we favour resection of the infected bone, conserving as much of the foot anatomy as possible.

Wound control

The neuropathic foot

Diabetic foot infections are almost always more extensive than would appear from initial examination and surface appearance. It is wise to perform an initial debridement in the diabetic foot clinic so that the true dimensions of the lesion can be revealed and tissue samples obtained for culture. Often, callus may be overlying the ulcer and this must be removed to reveal the extent of the underlying ulcer and allow drainage of pus and removal of infected sloughy tissue (Fig. 5.12a–d). Infection should respond to intravenous antibiotics, but the patient needs daily

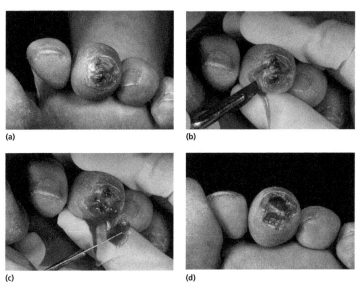

(a) (b)

(c) (d)

Fig. 5.12 (a) Debridement in the foot clinic. Cellulitic toe with apical callus. (b) Sharp debridement to remove callus. (c) Pus is drained. (d) The true dimensions of the lesion when probed to bone, are exposed.

review to detect evidence of spread. An outline of any area of cellulitis may be drawn on the foot so that extension of the cellulitic area can be detected quickly.

In severe episodes of infection, the ulcer may be complicated by extensive infected sloughing subcutaneous tissue, including tendon and fascia. At this point, the tissue is not frankly necrotic but has started to break down and liquefy. It is best for this tissue to be removed operatively. The definite indications for urgent surgical intervention are:

- Large area of infected sloughy tissue (Fig. 5.13a and b).
- Localized fluctuance and expression of pus (Fig. 5.14a and b).

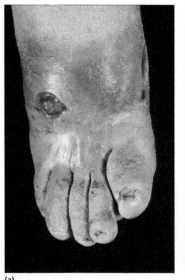
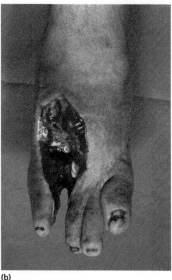

(a)   (b)

Fig. 5.13 (a) Severe cellulitis associated with deep infection. (b) Same foot after surgery to remove infected tissue.

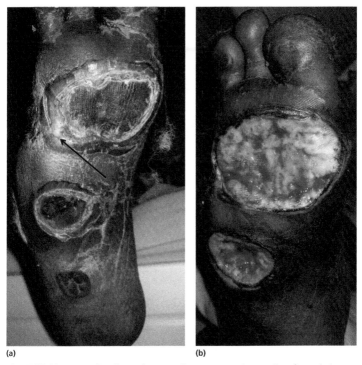

(a)   **(b)**

Fig. 5.14 (a) Pus exuding from plantar surface; arrow points to site of pus drainage. (b) Postoperative appearance following debridement of infected tissue.

- Crepitus with gas in the soft tissues on X-ray. However, air immediately adjacent to an ulcer may have entered the foot through the ulcer and is of less importance than gas in the deep tissues of the foot or leg.
- Purplish discolouration of the skin, indicating subcutaneous necrosis (Fig. 5.15a and b).

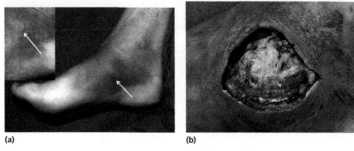

(a)   (b)

Fig. 5.15 (a) Cellulitic foot with patch of purple discolouration (arrows) also shown in inset. (b) Same foot after debridement showing extent of subcutaneous necrosis.

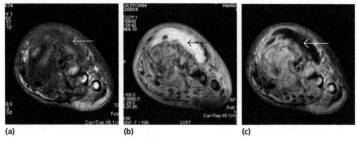

(a)   (b)   (c)

Fig. 5.16 (a) T1 sequence shows inflammatory mass (arrow) but normal uptake in dorsum of foot. (b) STIR sequence shows high signal due to inflammatory mass on dorsum (arrow). (c) Collection of fluid (arrow) on the dorsum (post gadolinium).

There are two other indications for surgery in the management of the neuropathic foot, namely osteomyelitis that has not responded to conservative measures and the development of collections of fluid or pus that are difficult to detect clinically. MRI may be useful to look for the presence of osteomyelitis and also to detect collections of fluid (Fig. 5.16a–c). Intravenous injection of gadolinium-containing contrast agent heightens the sensitivity of the diagnosis of these clinical features as gadolinium concentrates in areas of inflammation. However, MRI has limitations and can show a number of false-positive diagnoses.

The ischaemic foot
In severe infections, surgical debridement may also be necessary, and similar criteria as for the neuropathic foot are used in the decision to operate. Any surgical debridement needs to be accompanied by an assessment of the arterial perfusion to the foot to evaluate the healing potential of surgical wounds. All of these patients will need urgent vascular investigation.

Perioperative care of neuropathic and ischaemic patients
On admission, these patients should be regarded as medical and surgical emergencies. The infected diabetic foot may require immediate surgical intervention.

Preparation for surgery
The following investigations should be carried out:
- Full blood count and cross-matching
- Serum electrolytes, creatinine and eGFR
- Blood glucose
- Liver function tests
- Electrocardiogram
- Chest X-ray.

Often, it is difficult to assess how much debridement will be necessary, and in some cases it may need to be accompanied by toe or ray amputation. Therefore, consent for these procedures should be obtained prior to operation.

An intravenous insulin sliding scale (Table 5.4) should be started. It is important to avoid veins in the lower limb as insertion of an intravenous cannula into the veins of the foot can lead to ulceration, especially if the tip of the cannula goes into the subcutaneous tissues (Fig. 5.17).

Table 5.4 Insulin sliding scale. Adjust volume of fluids according to clinical state of patient. 50 units soluble human insulin in 50 mL 0.9% sodium chloride.

Blood glucose (mmol/L)	Infusion rate (units/h)
<4	0.5
4.1–9	1
9.1–15	2
15.1–19.9	4
>20	review and call doctor
Fluids	
If blood glucose >11 mmol/L give sodium chloride 0.9%	
If blood glucose ≤11 mmol/L give glucose 5%	

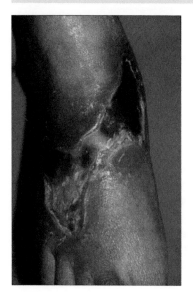

Fig. 5.17 Cellulitis and necrosis on dorsum of foot at infected intravenous cannula site.

The anaesthetist must be aware that virtually all of these patients will have autonomic as well as peripheral somatic neuropathy, and respiratory reflexes may be diminished. Postoperative respiratory arrests have been reported. Careful anaesthetic attention, particularly in the recovery room, is necessary.

Debridement of the foot is not a rapid procedure, such as incision and drainage for abscess; therefore, the anaesthetist should anticipate at least 40–50 min operating time.

During surgery

- It is important that a meticulous wound exploration is carried out, with removal of infected sloughy tissue, including tendons and fascia and laying open of all sinuses. It is rare to find a well-defined abscess
- The usual presentation is of heavily infected sloughy, grey tissue that needs to be removed down to healthy, bleeding tissue
- Wide excision is necessary; small incisions with drains should be avoided
- Fragmented infected and non-bleeding bone should be removed
- Deep infected tissue should be sent urgently to the microbiology laboratory
- The wound should not be sutured but left to heal by secondary intention. A proflavine pack may be inserted into the wound.

In addition to debridement, it may be necessary to perform a formal digital or ray amputation to establish drainage. The following techniques are used:

- Partial digital amputation may be performed for apical infection/osteomyelitis. Plantar and dorsal skin flaps are fashioned and the toe is disarticulated at the interphalangeal joint. If the toe is infected the wound may be left open for delayed wound closure
- Hallux amputation may include removing the metatarsal head and a portion of the shaft in addition to the hallux (Faraboeuf procedure) to assist closure and render future ulceration less likely

- Amputation of the lesser toes should be performed through the metatarso-phalangeal joint
- Ray amputation is performed for infection of a toe with limited spread to the forefoot and involves removal of toe and part or all of its corresponding metatarsal
- Open transmetatarsal, Lisfranc and Chopart's partial foot amputations are performed for extensive forefoot infections.

Further details of these operations are described in the companion volume to this book: *A Practical Manual of Diabetic Foot Care,* second edition (Blackwell Publishing 2008).

After surgery

- Continue the intravenous insulin pump postoperatively until infection is resolving. Then transfer to short-acting subcutaneous insulin three times daily with long-acting subcutaneous insulin at night
- Most surgical wounds, especially cavity wounds, are now treated with NPWT. This is usually continued until the cavity wound has filled in and is granulating, when either split skin grafts can be applied or otherwise the wound be left to heal by secondary intention. Recently, it has been possible to combine NPWT with instillation of chemotherapeutic agents
- Previously, wound irrigation with a sodium hypochlorite solution (Milton) was useful for the sloughy postoperative neuropathic foot. We no longer routinely use this. However, it may be useful in situations where availability of other antiseptics and antibiotics is limited. At present our cleansing fluid is Prontosan, which contains betaine surfactant and polyhexanide
- When there is an initial fever preoperatively, the patient's temperature is a useful indication of progress. A steady fall in temperature is expected over the subsequent 3–4 days. If this does not occur, then uncontrolled infection should be suspected. Postoperatively, regular estimations of serum CRP are made. Initially, this level may rise in

response to surgery but should then fall if the infection has been controlled and the foot wound is beginning to heal

- At operation, it is sometimes difficult to remove all infected tissue. It is important to inspect the wound every day after the operation and if signs of infection recur then the patient may need further surgical intervention. Signs that the foot is settling include a decrease in erythema, less swelling and a pink wound
- Patients will need bed rest, and it is wise to give prophylactic anticoagulation. Antithrombotic stockings should not be used on ischaemic feet. If used on a neuropathic foot, they should be folded back from the toe nails.

Vascular control

It is important to explore the possibility of revascularization in the infected ischaemic foot. Improvement of perfusion will not only help to control infection but will also promote healing of wounds if operative debridement is necessary.

Duplex angiography is usually carried out first. If this reveals lesions suitable for angioplasty or stenting then the patient goes forward to DSA as described for the foot in Stage 3. If the DSA needs to be performed urgently and the patient has previously been on warfarin then it may be necessary to reverse its activity by administering vitamin K parenterally. Angioplasty is indicated in the treatment of single or multiple stenoses or short segment occlusions. If Duplex angiography does not show lesions suitable for angioplasty then either CTA or MRA may be carried out before arterial bypass.

If the infection is responding to conservative treatment, with resolution of cellulitis on intravenous antibiotics, then arterial bypass, with its inherent risks, is probably not indicated. However, if operative debridement is necessary with amputation of a toe or ray, then arterial bypass may be necessary to achieve full wound healing.

Mechanical control

Patients with infected feet should not walk; they should be on bed rest and use crutches or a wheelchair for trips to the bathroom. Heels should be protected with special heel protectors and regular frequent turning in bed. After operative debridement in the neuropathic foot, off-loading of the postoperative wound may be achieved by casting techniques, including Scotchcast boots and total contact casts. It may be necessary to cut a window in the cast (a 'windowed total contact cast') at the site of the wound in order to observe it closely. In the neuroischaemic foot, non-weight-bearing is advised until the wound is healed.

Metabolic control

It is important to make sure that there is no systemic, metabolic or nutritional disturbance to impair the response to infection and retard healing of wounds. Full blood count, serum electrolytes and serum creatinine and liver function tests should be checked. If serum albumin is <3.5 g/L, supplementary feeding with high-energy drinks should be instituted under the supervision of a dietician.

In severe infections, considerable metabolic decompensation may occur. Full resuscitation is urgently required with intravenous fluids and intravenous insulin sliding scale, which is often necessary to achieve good blood glucose control whilst the patient is infected. This is followed by a basal-bolus regimen of three times a day short-acting subcutaneous insulin before meals and long-acting subcutaneous insulin at night.

These are complex patients, and cardiac and renal function should be assessed. Echocardiography will identify patients with left ventricular dysfunction. This is expressed as the ejection fraction, and a value less than 35% increases the risk of surgery. Close observation and monitoring of cardiovascular and renal function are essential to maintain correct electrolyte and fluid balance. Ischaemic patients should be regularly taking statins, angiotensin-converting enzyme inhibitors and antiplatelet agents, and these should be continued if the patient is admitted to hospital. Aspirin should not be stopped before angiography or angioplasty, although if the patient is taking aspirin and clopidogrel then the latter may be stopped.

High blood glucose is associated with reduced white blood cell function, which improves when the blood glucose is lowered.

Controlling the great quartet of risk factors – hyperglycaemia, hypertension, hyperlipidaemia and smoking – is still important for Stage 4 patients.

Educational control

It is important for patients to know the warning signs of infection and to understand what to do once they have developed an infection.

Patient information

Warning signs of infection

If a wound becomes

- Wetter than usual with increased amounts of discharge on the dressing
- Discoloured with redness, blueness or darker colour, or red streaks on the leg

you should be worried about infection.

Other signs of infection include

- Swelling around the ulcer
- If your foot becomes warmer than the other foot.

If you cannot see your foot clearly then someone will need to help you to check your foot for danger signs of infection.

The earlier an infection is treated the easier it is to control it. Always seek help the same day, as early as possible.

(*Continued*)

What to do when you have an infection

Your foot has developed an infection. This is a very serious problem which can destroy your foot.

- You should take your antibiotics regularly
- Please stay in bed or on a sofa with your feet up
- If in bed, your heels need to be protected. Also, make sure your feet are not pressing against the end of the bed
- If you are allowed to sit out of bed on a chair, put your feet up on a stool covered by a pillow
- Contact the doctor or nurse at once if your leg becomes more painful or if you feel hot, shivery or unwell
- Some people with diabetes are particularly prone to develop infection. When you have recovered from this infection it will be necessary for you to keep a close eye on your feet in future, to prevent further episodes.

6

Managing Stage 5: the necrotic foot

PRESENTATION AND DIAGNOSIS

This is the end stage of the natural history of the diabetic foot. It is characterized by the presence of necrosis (gangrene), threatening the loss of the limb. Early diagnosis and intervention, even at this late stage, can save limbs. Necrosis can involve skin, subcutaneous and fascial layers. In the skin it is easily evident, but in the subcutaneous and fascial layers it is not so apparent. Often, the bluish–black discolouration of skin is the 'tip of an iceberg' of massive necrosis which occurs in subcutaneous and fascial planes, so-called necrotizing fasciitis (Fig. 6.1a and b).

The two great drivers to necrosis are infection leading to wet necrosis (Fig. 6.2) and ischaemia leading to dry necrosis (Fig. 6.3). Progress towards necrosis can be rapid and devastating, and this potentially catastrophic situation has been termed a 'diabetic foot attack'. Purplish–black discolouration of the skin also occurs after bruising and is sometimes difficult to differentiate from early necrosis in the very ischaemic foot, although extensive bruising is usually associated with a history of trauma. Blood within a blister on a toe gives the toe a black appearance. Blue–black cyanosed toes and feet are seen in severe cardiac and respiratory failure. Shoe dye and the application of henna will result in black discolouration of the skin.

Wet necrosis

In wet necrosis, the tissues are grey, black, brown, white or greenish, moist and often malodorous (Fig. 6.2). Adjoining tissues are infected and pus may discharge from the ulcerated demarcation line between necrosis and viable tissue.

Managing the Diabetic Foot, Third Edition. Michael E Edmonds and Alethea VM Foster.
© 2014 John Wiley & Sons, Ltd. Published 2014 by John Wiley & Sons, Ltd.

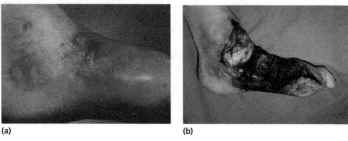

(a) (b)

Fig. 6.1 (a) Cutaneous necrosis on medial surface of foot indicating severe underlying tissue destruction. (b) After debridement with extensive removal of necrotic tissue.

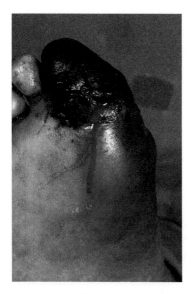

Fig. 6.2 Wet necrosis resulting from infection in a neuropathic foot.

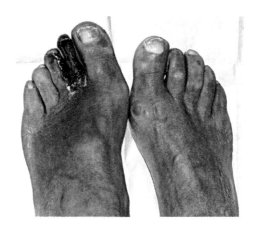

Fig. 6.3 Dry necrosis in a critically ischaemic foot.

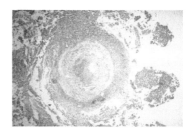

Fig. 6.4 Septic vasculitis. Cross-section of digital artery showing lumen almost totally occluded by septic thrombus.

Wet necrosis is secondary to a septic vasculitis (Fig. 6.4), associated with severe soft tissue infection and ulceration, and is the commonest cause of necrosis in the diabetic foot.

In the neuropathic foot, necrosis is almost invariably wet, and is caused by infection complicating a digital, metatarsal or heel ulcer, and leading to a septic vasculitis of the digital and small arteries of the foot. The walls of these arteries are infiltrated by polymorphs, leading to occlusion of the lumen by septic thrombus (Fig. 6.4). Wet necrosis is also prominent in the infected neuroischaemic foot and has a similar pathology to septic vasculitis. However, in the neuroischaemic foot, reduced arterial perfusion to the foot resulting from atherosclerotic occlusive disease of the leg arteries is also an important predisposing factor.

Dry necrosis

Dry necrosis is hard, blackened, mummified tissue and there is usually a clean demarcation line between necrosis and viable tissue. It may be difficult to diagnose in the Afro-Caribbean patient.

Dry necrosis can be seen usually in three situations in the ischaemic foot, namely critical ischaemia, acute ischaemia and the renal ischaemic foot. It can also result from emboli to the toes.

Critical ischaemia

Peripheral arterial disease usually progresses steadily in the diabetic patient, but eventually a severe reduction in arterial perfusion results in vascular compromise of the tissues of the foot, leading to a state of critical ischaemia. The final reduction in blood supply is caused by a thrombotic event or more rarely an embolic event on top of the existing atherosclerotic disease. Toes may become cyanosed and may progress to necrosis unless the foot is revascularized (Fig. 6.3).

Acute ischaemia

Blue discolouration leading to necrosis of the toes is also seen in acute ischaemia, which is usually caused either by thrombosis complicating an atherosclerotic stenosis in the superficial femoral or popliteal artery, or by emboli from proximal atherosclerotic plaques in the aorta, iliac, femoral or popliteal arteries. Emboli may also come from the heart in atrial fibrillation or after myocardial infarction.

It presents as a sudden onset of pain in the leg associated with pallor of the foot, quickly followed by mottling and slatey grey discolouration (see Fig. 1.20). The diabetic patient may not get paraesthesiae because

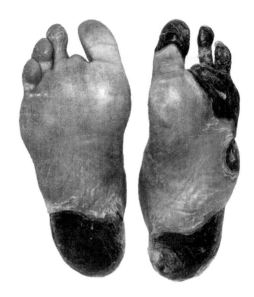

Fig. 6.5 Necrosis in the renal foot.

of sensory neuropathy, which reduces the severity of ischaemic pain and may delay presentation.

Renal ischaemic foot

Digital necrosis is a problem in patients with advanced diabetic nephropathy and can occur in the absence of severe peripheral arterial disease and infection. It may be precipitated by trauma and can spread to involve the midfoot and hindfoot (Fig. 6.5).

Emboli to the toes

Another cause of necrosis, particularly to the toes, are emboli (Fig. 6.6) to the digital circulation often originating from atherosclerotic plaques in the aorta and leg arteries. Occasionally, emboli are dislodged from arterial plaques during angioplasty. The initial sign may be bluish or

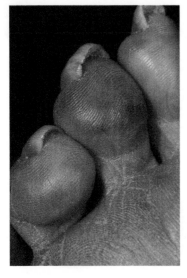

Fig. 6.6 Purple discolouration of fourth toe secondary to embolus.

purple discolouration that is quite well demarcated but which quickly proceeds to necrosis. If it escapes infection, it will dry out and mummify. Microemboli present with painful petechial lesions in the foot that do not blanch on pressure. Rarely, emboli which are dislodged at angioplasty may cause acute ischaemia.

MANAGEMENT
Patients should be admitted immediately for urgent investigations and multidisciplinary management. It is important to achieve:
- Wound control
- Microbiological control
- Vascular control
- Mechanical control
- Metabolic control
- Educational control.

Wound control

Neuropathic foot

In the neuropathic foot, operative debridement is almost always indicated for wet necrosis. Although necrosis may not be associated with a definite collection of pus, there is usually sloughing of subcutaneous and fascial tissue that needs to be removed with the necrotic tissue.

In addition, a formal amputation may be necessary, and this includes:

- Partial or total amputation of necrotic toes
- Ray amputation
- Transmetatarsal amputation
- Chopart or Lisfranc partial foot amputations
- Symes amputation.

Further details of these operations are described in the companion volume to this book: *A Practical Manual of Diabetic Foot Care*, second edition (Blackwell Publishing 2008). Postoperatively, wounds are treated with NPWT. In the neuropathic foot, there is a good arterial circulation and the wound should heal as long as infection is controlled.

Very occasionally patients may not be suitable for operation or refuse it and the aim would then be to convert wet necrosis into dry by conservative treatment and intravenous antibiotics.

Ischaemic foot

The neuroischaemic foot is often complicated by wet necrosis, and this should be removed urgently when it is associated with severe spreading sepsis. This should be done whether pus is present or not (Fig. 6.7a–c).

In cases when the limb is not immediately threatened, and the necrosis is limited to one or two toes, it may be possible to control infection with intravenous antibiotics and proceed to urgent revascularization and then digital or ray amputation.

The critically ischaemic foot is characterized by dry necrosis. The ideal treatment is removal of the necrotic digit after revascularization.

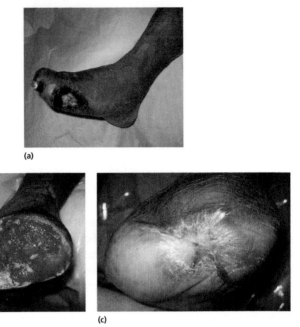

Fig. 6.7 (a) Wet necrosis of forefoot secondary to infection and ischaemia.
(b) Granulating wound after NPWT of metatarsal amputation site. (c) Healed wound.

Similarly, dry necrosis is also a feature of the renal ischaemic foot and can be removed surgically after revascularization. If angioplasty or bypass is not possible, then a decision must be made either to amputate the toes in the presence of ischaemia or to allow the toes to shrivel up and autoamputate. Surgical amputation should be undertaken if the circulation is not severely impaired, as indicated by an ABPI >0.5 or a transcutaneous oxygen tension >30 mmHg. The recent use of the NPWT promptly applied to such amputation wounds has encouraged healing in ischaemic limbs even though they could not be revascularized.

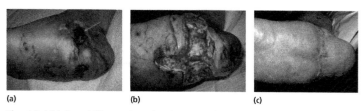

(a)   (b)   (c)

Fig. 6.8 (a) Infected Charcot foot showing area of wet necrosis (arrow). (b) Foot has been debrided to remove necrotic and sloughy tissue. (c) Healed foot after NPWT and intravenous antibiotics.

Operative debridement

The preparation and principles of operative debridement are similar to that described in Stage 4. Patients will need a full blood count, serum electrolytes and creatinine, blood grouping, chest X-ray and an electrocardiogram (ECG). Consent should be obtained for the most extensive debridement anticipated, including digital or ray amputation.

It is important to remove all necrotic and sloughy tissue, down to bleeding tissue, as well as opening up all sinuses (Fig. 6.8a–c). Deep necrotic tissue should be sent for culture immediately. Wounds should not be sutured. Postoperatively, wounds are treated with NPWT to encourage granulation, after which skin grafting may be the best way to achieve healing of large tissue deficits. Ischaemic wounds are extremely slow to heal even after revascularization, and wound care needs to continue on an outpatient basis in the diabetic foot clinic; but with patience, outcomes may be surprisingly good.

Free tissue transfer

Debridement of necrotic lesions of the foot often leads to severe tissue deficits. Management of these soft tissue deficits is complex, and skin grafts, local flaps and free tissue transfer have been used. Free flaps can comprise skin, fascial or muscle flaps. A flap commonly used for lower limb defects is the anterolateral thigh perforator free flap, which is a septocutaneous flap based on perforators that originate from the descending branch of the lateral circumflex femoral system. The arteriovenous pedicle accompanies the transferred tissue and is anastomosed usually to a pedal or tibial vessel. These serve as the inflow tract for the free flap, and anastomosis is achieved using microsurgical techniques.

Autoamputation

Careful sharp debridement is performed along the demarcation line between necrosis and viable tissue to debulk dead tissue, drain pockets of pus and prevent accumulation of debris. Dry sterile dressings are used to separate necrotic toes from their fellows. This provides an ideal culture medium for bacteria, and infection and necrosis can spread. Patients should not bathe to ensure that necrotic tissues are kept dry, since moistening necrosis may encourage infection.

Such ischaemic feet with dry necrosis may remain at Stage 5 for many months and are followed up until the necrotic toe drops off to reveal a healed stump. With recent improved techniques of revascularization and wound care, most necrotic toes are successfully amputated and autoamputation is now rare.

Microbiological control

Wet necrosis

The microbiological principles of managing wet necrosis are similar to those of the management of infection in Stage 4. When the patient initially presents, send deep ulcer swabs and tissue specimens for microbiology. Deep tissue taken at operative debridement must also go for culture.

Intravenous antibiotic therapy is similar to the treatment of severe deep infection: either piperacillin–tazobactam 4.5 g t.d.s. or quadruple therapy (amoxicillin 500 mg t.d.s., flucloxacillin 500 mg q.d.s., metronidazole 500 mg t.d.s. and ceftazidime 1 g t.d.s.) should be given. However, if the patient is allergic to penicillin, then vancomycin 1 g b.d. intravenously plus ciprofloxacin 400 mg b.d. intravenously and metronidazole

500 mg t.d.s. intravenously should be given. Antibiotic therapy should be adjusted when the results of cultures from tissues and operative specimens are available.

Intravenous antibiotics can be replaced with oral therapy after operative debridement and when infection is controlled. On discharge from hospital, oral antibiotics are continued and reviewed regularly in the foot clinic. When the wound is granulating well and swabs are negative then the antibiotics are stopped.

Dry necrosis

When dry necrosis develops secondary to severe ischaemia, antibiotics should be prescribed if discharge develops or the ulcer swab is positive and continued until there is no evidence of clinical or microbiological infection.

When toes have gone from wet to dry necrosis and are allowed to autoamputate, antibiotics should only be stopped if the necrosis is dry and mummified, the foot is entirely pain free, and there is no discharge exuding from the demarcation line.

Daily inspection is essential. Regular swabs should be sent for culture, and antibiotics should be restarted if the demarcation line becomes moist or swabs grow organisms.

Vascular control

All ischaemic feet that present with necrosis must have Doppler studies followed by Duplex angiography to show stenoses or occlusions of the arteries of the leg. The approach to the necrotic ischaemic diabetic foot is similar to that described in Chapter 5 for the infected ischaemic foot.

In wet necrosis, revascularization is necessary to heal the tissue deficit after operative debridement. In dry necrosis which occurs in the background of severe arterial disease, revascularization is necessary to maintain the viability of the limb.

When dry necrosis is secondary to emboli, a possible source should be investigated, and therefore the following should be performed:

- An ECG to detect atrial fibrillation or recent myocardial infarct
- Ultrasound of the abdomen to detect aortic aneurysm
- Angiography of the lower limbs to detect atherosclerotic plaque in iliac or femoral arteries.

Angioplasty

In some patients, increased perfusion following angioplasty may be useful. However, unless there is a very significant localized stenosis in iliac or femoral arteries, angioplasty rarely restores pulsatile blood flow to the foot, which is necessary to keep the limb viable in severe ischaemia or restore considerable tissue deficits secondary to necrosis. This is best achieved by arterial bypass.

Arterial bypass

Patients will have cardiovascular disease and need preoperative assessment to maximize cardiorespiratory status. Peripheral arterial disease is common in the tibial arteries, and distal bypass with autologous vein, isolated from leg or arm and identified by preoperative vein mapping, has become an established method of revascularization, in which a conduit is fashioned from either the femoral or popliteal artery down to a tibial artery in the lower leg, or the dorsalis pedis artery or plantar arteries of the foot. Patency rates and limb salvage rates after revascularization do not differ between diabetic patients and non-diabetic patients, and a more aggressive approach to such revascularization procedures should be promoted.

Hybrid procedures

Recently, combined hybrid procedures have been used to revascularize the foot. This commonly involves angioplasty of the superficial femoral artery followed by a distal bypass from the popliteal artery to arteries in the foot. Also, angioplasty is used to dilate anastomoses of distal bypasses when they become narrowed.

Postoperative care

Postoperatively, the leg has wounds both where the graft has been inserted and from where the vein has been harvested. Wounds overlying the arterial graft must be kept free from infection otherwise the graft will block. Such wounds need regular cleaning and covering with dry dressings, and any associated necrotic tissue which becomes bulky or moist should be gently debrided. Postoperative swelling is common and elevation of the leg is important. The patient should enter a graft surveillance programme.

Stem cell therapy

When there is no option for revascularization, intramuscular autologous bone marrow cell therapy is a feasible, relatively safe and potentially useful therapeutic approach.

Mechanical control

During the peri- and postoperative period, bed rest is essential with elevation of the limb to relieve swelling, but heels must be protected. These areas should be examined often and pressure-relieving measures taken to prevent pressure necrosis. Heels should be protected in bed. A pressure-relieving mattress should be used, and if there is any degree of drowsiness the patient should be turned regularly.

After operative debridement of the ischaemic foot, especially when revascularization has not been possible, non-weight-bearing is advised until the wound is healed. In the neuropathic foot, non-weight-bearing is advisable initially and then off-loading of the healing postoperative foot may be achieved by casting techniques.

If necrosis is to be treated conservatively by autoamputation, which can take several months, then the patient needs a wide-fitting shoe to accommodate the foot and dressings. Patients should walk as little as possible. The Scotchcast boot (see Chapter 4) is very useful for ischaemic patients with necrotic toes awaiting autoamputation.

Metabolic control

When patients present with necrosis, in the background of severe infection or ischaemia, they may be very ill, and will need close metabolic and haemodynamic monitoring. Considerable metabolic decompensation may occur, and full resuscitation is required with intravenous fluids and intravenous insulin sliding scale, which is often necessary to achieve good blood glucose control whilst the patient is infected or the leg severely ischaemic.

Patients who present with necrosis, especially ischaemic patients, usually have significant co-morbidities. They are often old and fragile and have cardiovascular disease and renal impairment. They will need careful monitoring to optimize the regulation of fluid balance, so as to avoid hypotension from underperfusion and hypertension and peripheral oedema from overperfusion. Many patients have autonomic neuropathy, which may contribute to impaired blood pressure control and cardiac arrhythmias.

Nutritional impairment may be denoted by a serum albumin of <3.5 g/L. A high-calorie diet should be instituted. A minimum of 1800 calories per day should be ingested to avoid the negative nitrogen balance that could accompany the depletion of protein stores. Dietary advice should be obtained and nasogastric feeding may be required. In patients with concomitant severe cerebrovascular disease and impaired swallowing, percutaneous endoscopic gastrostomy feeding may be necessary.

Educational control

Patient information

Patients who develop necrosis need careful education, including reassurance that much can be done to help them. We believe that practical and straightforward explanations are best, and advice should be given for when the patient is in hospital and at home.

In hospital
Your foot has developed a very serious problem.
- Please stay in bed to keep your feet up
- Your heels need to be protected
- Move your feet about in the bed and try not to lie in the same position for long periods
- Make sure your feet are not pressing against the end of the bed
- If you are allowed to sit out of bed on a chair, put your feet up on a stool covered by a pillow.

At home (for patients undergoing autoamputation)
- Rest your foot, keep it up and walk as little as possible
- You may want to obtain a wheelchair so that you can go out even before your foot has healed
- Your foot should be kept dry and covered with a dressing and bandage
- If you want to have a bath or shower you should cover your foot with a special wound-protecting plastic bag to keep it clean and dry
- It is important to take great care of the condition of the skin. The skin of your feet (not immediately next to the black areas) should be kept clean
- Moisturizing cream should be applied to prevent cracks
- Neglected skin is a common cause of foot problems
- A nurse should visit regularly to clean, dress and inspect your foot and check your other foot as well for cracks, splits, dry skin or new ulcers
- Ask for help with household chores. You should be resting, not working
- Return to the foot clinic immediately (the same day!) if your foot becomes swollen, painful, develops an unpleasant smell or part of your foot changes colour or discharges pus.

7

Managing Stage 6: the unsalvageable foot

PRESENTATION

Despite early intervention, some diabetic feet progress relentlessly to extensive necrosis, which compromises the viability and functional ability of the lower limb. There are two main reasons for the development of such an extensive necrosis:

- A massive acute reduction in arterial perfusion leading to necrosis that inexorably spreads up the foot (Fig. 7.1).
- Overwhelming infection that destroys the diabetic foot.

Also, there are other scenarios which need a major amputation:

- The severely ischaemic painful foot that cannot be revascularized and whose pain is very difficult to control.
- The unstable, inoperable Charcot hindfoot where external fixation or internal fixation is not possible.

Major amputation in a neuropathic foot should be a very rare event and is usually necessary only when infection has irretrievably destroyed the foot. This should be preventable in most cases. A non-healing ulcer should not necessarily be an indication for major amputation.

Patients needing major amputation have significant co-morbidity and are high risk for perioperative complications. They should be managed by a multidisciplinary team, consisting of surgeons, physiotherapists, prosthetists, occupational therapists, nurses, podiatrists and rehabilitation doctors.

Managing the Diabetic Foot, Third Edition. Michael E Edmonds and Alethea VM Foster.
© 2014 John Wiley & Sons, Ltd. Published 2014 by John Wiley & Sons, Ltd.

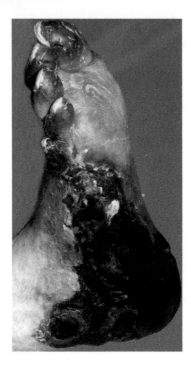

Fig. 7.1 Overwhelming necrosis secondary to popliteal artery thrombosis.

MAJOR AMPUTATION

Preoperative care

Cardiorespiratory status and metabolic control should be optimized. Patients should be encouraged to stop smoking. Malnutrition increases the risk of delayed wound healing. Weight loss and diminished appetite are common and patients should be seen by the dietician.

The level of amputation should be carefully considered to ensure that there is sufficient perfusion to achieve wound healing, and, when possible, a below-knee amputation should be carried out as this will conserve the knee joint and aid the fitting of a prosthesis. Antibiotic prophylaxis should be used. Once major amputation is planned, a lumbar epidural block with bupivacaine can be started 48 h beforehand to relieve postoperative pain.

Perioperative care
A major amputation puts the remaining foot at great risk. The heel should be protected on the operating table.

Postoperative care
Patients who undergo an amputation often suffer from shock, disbelief and sadness. Patient and family need attention, support, sympathy and reassurance. Amputation wounds are often slow to heal in ischaemic patients. Infection should be treated aggressively, but if there is poor arterial perfusion to the below-knee wound it may be necessary to convert it into an above-knee amputation.

Rehabilitation
Rehabilitation of the diabetic amputee is extremely difficult and is characterized by long stays in hospital. Only 25% of diabetic amputees will ever walk again. Morbidity and mortality associated with major amputation are very high. Major amputation, therefore, must not be taken lightly. It does not guarantee a future ulcer-free existence.

Before the definitive prosthesis is issued, some patients may be suitable for mobility aids. The amputee mobility aid is suitable for below- and through-knee amputees only. The stump is supported and stabilized by an inflatable bag, which also assists in reducing swelling. The pneumatic postamputation mobility aid has a pneumatic sleeve extending from the groin to below amputation residuum enclosed by a frame cage and is suitable for above-knee, through-knee and below-knee amputees.

The definitive prosthesis contains a stump sheath worn inside a customized thermoplastic socket fitted onto a modular prosthesis. Donning and doffing may be difficult for patients with neuropathic hands and poor eyesight.

Stump oedema may be a problem. Compression stump shrinkers provide good oedema control, both short and long term.

Once healed, the stump should be inspected daily for skin breakdown. Neuropathic stumps are prone to ulceration. This is preceded by callus, which should be debrided with a scalpel. After amputation, the value of the remaining limb should not be underestimated: even if the patient never walks again they will need their leg to transfer from chair to bed and toilet and thus maintain a little independence.

A major amputation will put the remaining foot at great risk of ulceration. The heel of the surviving foot should be protected. Amputees undergoing rehabilitation should be provided with suitable footwear. The key for success is careful follow-up. Regular foot checks and preventive foot care are essential. There should be close links between the diabetic foot team, the rehabilitation team and ward staff. Everyone must understand the need to avoid trauma to the remaining foot at all costs. Major amputees are among the most high risk of all diabetic foot patients.

Palliative care

In some rare cases when patients have multiple co-morbidities and will not be fit enough to withstand major surgery, then palliative care may be a suitable alternative with the emphasis on symptom relief, particularly pain control. This particularly applies to patients who have a terminal illness and a very limited life expectancy.

Appendix: Problems of differential diagnosis

Managing the Diabetic Foot, Third Edition. Michael E Edmonds and Alethea VM Foster.
© 2014 John Wiley & Sons, Ltd. Published 2014 by John Wiley & Sons, Ltd.

Further reading

Ashley, C. and Currie, A. (2009) *The Renal Drug Handbook*, 3rd edition, Radcliffe Publishing, Oxford.

Boulton, A.J.M., Cavanagh, P.R. and Rayman, G. (2006) *The Foot in Diabetes*, 4th edition, John Wiley & Sons, Ltd, Chichester.

Bus, S.A.,Valk, G.D., van Deursen, R.W. *et al.* (2008) Specific guidelines on footwear and offloading 2007. *Diabetes/Metabolism Research and Reviews*, **24** (Suppl. 1), S192–S193.

Edmonds, M.E., Foster, A.V.M. and Sanders, L. (2008) *A Practical Manual of Diabetic Foot Care*, 2nd edition, Blackwell Publishing.

Foster, A.V.M. and Edmonds, M.E. (2011) *Diabetic Foot Care: Case Studies in Clinical Management*, Wiley–Blackwell.

Rogers, L.C., Frykberg, R.G., Armstrong, D.G. *et al.* (2011) The Charcot foot in diabetes. *Diabetes Care*, **34**, 2123–2129.

Schaper, N., van Houtum, W. and Boulton, A. (eds) (2012) Proceedings of the 6th International Symposium on the Diabetic Foot. *Diabetes/Metabolism Research and Reviews*, **28** (Suppl. S1).

The Schaper *et al.* (2012) supplement includes the following guidelines:

Bakker K., Apelqvist, J. and Schaper, N.C. (2012) Practical guidelines on the management and prevention of the diabetic foot 2011. *Diabetes/Metabolism Research and Reviews*, **28** (Suppl. S1), 225–231.

Game, F.L., Hinchliffe, R.J., Apelqvist, J. *et al.* (2012) Specific guidelines on wound and wound-bed management 2011. *Diabetes/Metabolism Research and Reviews*, **28** (Suppl. S1), 232–233.

Lipsky BA., Peters, E.J.G., Berendt, A.R. *et al.* (2012) Specific guidelines for the treatment of diabetic foot infections 2011. *Diabetes/Metabolism Research and Reviews*, **28** (Suppl. S1), 234–235.

Schaper, N.C., Andros, G., Apelqvist, J. *et al.* (2012) Specific guidelines for diagnosis and treatment of peripheral arterial disease in patients with diabetes and ulceration of the foot 2011. *Diabetes/Metabolism Research and Reviews*, **28** (Suppl. S1), 236–237.

Index

Page numbers in *italics* denote figures and those in **bold** denote tables

---

Managing the Diabetic Foot, Third Edition. Michael E Edmonds and Alethea VM Foster.
© 2014 John Wiley & Sons, Ltd. Published 2014 by John Wiley & Sons, Ltd.

Index

Index

Printed and bound by CPI Group (UK) Ltd, Croydon, CR0 4YY

09/10/2024

14571429-0001